S0-BOD-345

DECISION MAKING IN
Pain Management

Clinical Decision Making™ Series

Berman:
  Pediatric Decision Making
Bready, Smith:
  Decision Making in Anesthesiology
Bucholz, Lippert, Wenger, Ezaki:
  Orthopaedic Decision Making
Callaham, Barton, Schumaker:
  Decision Making in Emergency Medicine
Cibis, Tongue, Stass-Isern:
  Decision Making in Pediatric Ophthalmology
Cohn, Doty, McElvein:
  Decision Making in Cardiothoracic Surgery
DeCherney, Polan, Lee, Boyers:
  Decision Making in Infertility
Greene:
  Decision Making in Medicine
Karlinsky, Lau, Goldstein:
  Decision Making in Pulmonary Medicine
Korones, Bada-Ellzey:
  Neonatal Decision Making
Levine:
  Decision Making in Gastroenterology
Marsh:
  Decision Making in Plastic Surgery
Nichols, Hyslop, Bartlett:
  Decision Making in Surgical Sepsis
Ramamurthy, Rogers:
  Decision Making in Pain Management
Resnick, Caldamone, Spirnak:
  Decision Making in Urology
Schein:
  Decision Making in Oncology
van Heuven, Zwaan:
  Decision Making in Ophthalmology
Weisberg, Strub, Garcia:
  Decision Making in Adult Neurology

DECISION MAKING IN

Pain Management

Somayaji Ramamurthy, M.D.
Professor
Department of Anesthesiology
Director, Pain Management Clinic
The University of Texas Health Science Center
at San Antonio
San Antonio, Texas

James N. Rogers, M.D.
Assistant Professor
Department of Anesthesiology
The University of Texas Health Science Center
at San Antonio
San Antonio, Texas

B.C. Decker
An Imprint of Mosby–Year Book, Inc.

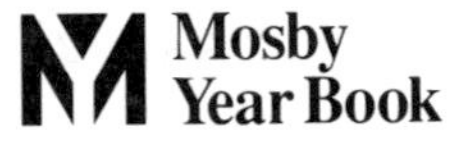

Dedicated to Publishing Excellence

BC Decker

Executive Editor: Susan M. Gay
Senior Managing Editor: Lynne Gery
Project Supervisor: Linda J. Daly

NOTICE: The authors and publisher have made every effort to ensure that the patient care recommended herein, including choice of drugs and drug dosages, is in accord with the accepted standard and practice at the time of publication. However, since research and regulation constantly change clinical standards, the reader is urged to check the product information sheet included in the package of each drug, which includes recommended doses, warnings, and contraindications. This is particularly important with new or infrequently used drugs.

Printed in the United States of America

Mosby–Year Book, Inc.
11830 Westline Industrial Drive
St. Louis, Missouri 63146

Library of Congress Cataloging in Publication Data

Decision making in pain management / [edited by] Somayaji Ramamurthy, James N. Rogers.
p. cm. — (Clinical decision making series)
Includes bibliographical references and index.
1. Pain—Treatment—Decision making. 2. Analgesia—Decision making. 3. Anesthesia—Decision making. I. Ramamurthy, Somayaji. II. Rogers, James N. (James Norman) III. Series.
[DNLM: 1. Pain—diagnosis. 2. Pain—therapy. 3. Palliative Treatment. WL 704 D294]
RB127.D43 1992
616'.0472—dc20
DNLM/DLC 92-23026
for Library of Congress CIP

ISBN 1-55664-370-5

96 CL/MY 9 8 7 6 5 4 3

CONTRIBUTORS

JEFFERY J. BAEUERLE, M.D.
Clinical Assistant Professor, Department of Anesthesiology, University of Texas Health Science Center, San Antonio, Texas

DOUGLAS BARBER, M.D.
Attending Physician, St. Rose Rehabilitation Hospital, San Antonio, Texas

RICHARD BAROHN, M.D.
Assistant Professor of Medicine (Neurology), University of Texas Health Science Center, San Antonio, Texas

BARI BENNETT, M.D.
Assistant Professor, Department of Anesthesiology, University of Texas Health Science Center, San Antonio, Texas

TIMOTHY CASTRO, Jr., M.D.
Clinical Assistant Professor, University of Texas Health Science Center and Northwest Medical Center, Houston, Texas

DOUGLAS E. CHAPMAN, M.D.
Staff Anesthesiologist, Fitzsimons Army Medical Center, Aurora, Colorado

TARA L. CHRONISTER, M.D.
Resident Anesthesiologist, Brooke Army Medical Center, San Antonio, Texas

RAYMOND M. COSTELLO, Ph.D.
Professor, Department of Psychiatry, and Director, Psychodiagnostic and Neuropsychology Laboratory, University of Texas Health Science Center, San Antonio, Texas

ROBERT D. CULLING, D.O.
Director, Lovelace Center for Pain Management, Albuquerque, New Mexico

SUSAN J. DREYER, M.D.
Associate, Georgia Spine and Sports Physicians, Atlanta, Georgia

PAUL DREYFUSS, M.D.
Private Practice, The Neuro-Skeletal Center, Tyler, Texas

J. P. DUCEY, M.D.
Clinical Assistant Professor of Medicine and Surgery, Uniformed Services University of the Health Sciences, Bethesda, Maryland

JAY S. ELLIS, Jr., M.D.
Chairman, Department of Anesthesiology, Wilford Hall Medical Center, and Clinical Associate Professor, University of Texas Health Science Center, San Antonio, Texas

NORMAN G. GALL, M.D.
Associate Professor, Department of Rehabilitation Medicine, University of Texas Health Science Center; Chief of Rehabilitation Medicine, Veterans' Administration Hospital, San Antonio, Texas

DIANE GILBERT, M.D.
Assistant Professor, Department of Rehabilitation Medicine, University of Texas Health Science Center, San Antonio, Texas

JAMES GRIFFIN, P.T., A.T.C.
Department of Anesthesiology, University of Texas Health Science Center, San Antonio, Texas

MARY ANN GURKOWSKI, M.D.
Assistant Professor, Department of Anesthesiology, University of Texas Health Science Center, San Antonio, Texas

MARC B. HAHN, D.O.
Department of Army, Walter Reed Army Medical Hospital, Washington, D.C.

NANCY E. HAMBLETON, R.N., B.S.N.
Senior Research Nurse, Department of Anesthesiology, University of Texas Health Science Center, San Antonio, Texas

ROSEMARY HICKEY, M.D.
Associate Professor, Department of Anesthesiology, University of Texas Health Science Center, San Antonio, Texas

JOAN HOFFMAN, R.N., M.S.N.
Instructor, Department of Anesthesiology, University of Texas Health Science Center, San Antonio, Texas

W. CORBETT HOLMGREEN, D.D.S., M.D.
Associate Professor, Department of Anesthesiology, University of Texas Health Science Center, San Antonio, Texas

PAUL T. INGMUNDSON, Ph.D.
Clinical Assistant Professor of Psychiatry and Medicine (Neurology), University of Texas Health Science Center, and Audie L. Murphy Memorial Veterans Hospital, San Antonio, Texas

KEVIN L. KENWORTHY, M.D., C.P.T., M.C.
Staff Anesthesiologist, Tripler Army Medical Center, Honolulu, Hawaii

LAURIE G. KILBOURN, M.D.
Staff Anesthesiologist, Brazos Port Memorial Hospital, Lake Jackson, Texas

JOHN KING, M.D.
Medical Director, Chronic Pain Management Program, Rehabilitation Institute of San Antonio, San Antonio, Texas

KELLY GORDON KNAPE, M.D.
Assistant Professor, Director of Analgesia Management Service, and Director of Obstetric Anesthesia, Department of Anesthesiology, University of Texas Health Science Center, San Antonio, Texas

ERIC B. LEFEVER, M.D.
Staff Anesthesiologist, Naval Hospital, Oakland, California

ELLEN LEONARD, M.D.
Assistant Professor, Department of Rehabilitation Medicine, University of Texas Health Science Center, San Antonio, Texas

JONATHAN P. LESTER, M.D.
Associate, Georgia Spine and Sports Physicians, Atlanta, Georgia

ALFONSO MAYTORENA, M.D.
Clinical Assistant Professor, Department of Anesthesiology, University of Texas Health Science Center, San Antonio, Texas

JOHN S. McDONALD, D.D.S., M.S., F.A.C.D.
Professor of Clinical Otolaryngology and Maxillofacial Surgery, and Associate Professor of Clinical Anesthesia and Pain Control, University of Cincinnati College of Medicine, Cincinnati, Ohio

EMIL J. MENK, M.D.
Chief of Anesthesiology, Brooke Army Medical Center, San Antonio, Texas

GREGORY J. MEREDITH, M.D., M.P.H.
Resident Anesthesiologist, University of Texas Health Science Center, San Antonio, Texas

JOHN D. MERWIN, M.D.
Assistant Professor, Louisiana State University School of Medicine, Shreveport, Louisiana

ROBERT E. MIDDAUGH, M.D.
Staff Anesthesiologist and Director of Pain Management Service, St. Vincent's Infirmary Medical Center, Little Rock, Arkansas

SCOTT D. MURTHA, M.D.
Staff Anesthesiologist, Walter Reed Army Medical Center, Washington, D.C.

ANTHONY PELLEGRINO, M.D.
Staff Anesthesiologist, David Grant United States Air Force Medical Center, Travis Air Force Base, California

JAMES C. PHERO, D.M.D., F.A.C.D.
Chief, Section of Head and Neck Pain, University Pain Control Center, University of Cincinnati College of Medicine, Cincinnati, Ohio

JEFFREY PRIEST, M.D.
Staff Anesthesiologist, Tripler Army Medical Center, Honolulu, Hawaii

SOMAYAJI RAMAMURTHY, M.D.
Director of Pain Management Clinic, and Professor, Department of Anesthesiology, University of Texas Health Science Center, San Antonio, Texas

ROLAND REINHART, M.D.
Staff Anesthesiologist, Eisenhower Memorial Hospital, Rancho Mirage, California

JAMES N. ROGERS, M.D.
Assistant Professor, Department of Anesthesiology, University of Texas Health Science Center, San Antonio, Texas

MARK E. ROMANOFF, M.D.
Clinical Assistant Professor, Department of Anesthesiology, University of Texas Health Science Center; Director, Pain Clinic, Wilford Hall Medical Center, San Antonio, Texas

RICHARD ROSENTHAL, M.D.
Resident Anesthesiologist, Department of Anesthesiology, University of Texas Health Science Center, San Antonio, Texas

DOMINIQUE SCHIFFER, M.D.
Resident Anesthesiologist, Brooke Army Medical Center, San Antonio, Texas

LAWRENCE S. SCHOENFELD, Ph.D.
Professor, Departments of Psychiatry, Anesthesiology, and Rehabilitation Medicine, University of Texas Health Science Center, San Antonio, Texas

DALE SOLOMON, M.D.
Assistant Professor, Department of Anesthesiology, University of Texas Health Science Center, San Antonio, Texas

ROBERT SPRAGUE, M.D.
Chief of Anesthesia, Blanchfield Army Community Hospital, Fort Campbell, Kentucky

JEFFERY E. STEDWILL, M.D.
Resident, Department of Rehabilitation Medicine, University of Texas Health Science Center, San Antonio, Texas

WILLIAM E. STRONG, M.D.
Staff Anesthesiologist, Brooke Army Medical Center, San Antonio, Texas

JEFFERY T. SUMMERS, M.D.
Director of Pain Management, University of Mississippi Medical Center, Jackson, Mississippi

DONALD B. TALLACKSON, M.D.
Resident Anesthesiologist, Brooke Army Medical Center, San Antonio, Texas

LINDA TINGLE, M.D.
Assistant Professor, Department of Anesthesiology, University of Texas Health Science Center, San Antonio, Texas

DAVID VANOS, M.D.
Staff Anesthesiologist, Fairchild Air Force Base, Washington

DAWN E. WEBSTER, M.D.
Assistant Professor, Department of Anesthesiology, University of Texas Health Science Center, San Antonio, Texas

ROGER L. WESLEY, M.D.
Staff Anesthesiologist, and Director, Pain Clinic, Brooke Army Medical Center, San Antonio, Texas

To Alon P. Winnie, M.D.,
a great teacher and friend,
in appreciation of his achievements and
his continuing, tireless efforts to reduce human suffering

To our families,
Rajam, Sendhil, and Sujatha Ramamurthy
and
Diana, Jennifer, Jim, and Jaime Rogers,
for their unconditional love and support

PREFACE

Decision Making in Pain Management provides an algorithmic approach to the evaluation, testing, and treatment of pain for all physicians engaged in the management of pain. It is not meant to replace in-depth, highly referenced textbooks on pain, but to act as a supplement, providing the physician with a logical, concise, stepwise approach to the identification, diagnosis, and management of various acute or chronic painful conditions or syndromes. It is a convenient source for the physician to review familiar concepts quickly in preparation for board examinations and patient care.

A multidisciplinary approach is provided, with input from specialists in anesthesiology, physical medicine and rehabilitation, neurology, psychology, dentistry, physical therapy, and nursing. The book is divided into sections on the evaluation of pain, acute and chronic pain syndromes, pain occurring in specific regions of the body, therapeutic modalities, and specific nerve blocks used in the diagnosis and treatment of pain. Each chapter consists of a decision tree and related textual comments. The comments provide information on designated decision points within the trees and are supported by references. In areas of controversy, the chapters may reflect the preferences of the individual contributor.

We would like to thank our many contributors for their enthusiastic response to our requests for chapters. We would also like to thank Lynne Gery and Linda Daly at Mosby–Year Book for their help, support, and most of all patience in seeing this endeavor to its conclusion. Special thanks to Diana Rogers for her invaluable help in preparing and retyping this manuscript. Truly, without her selfless devotion, this book would never have been completed.

Somayaji Ramamurthy
James N. Rogers

CONTENTS

SPECIFIC BLOCKS

APPENDICES

EVALUATION

Initial Management of Acute Pain
Evaluation of the Chronic Pain Patient
Psychological Evaluation
Post-traumatic Stress Disorder
Sleep Disturbances and Chronic Pain
Pain Measurement
Thermography
Pentothal Testing
Testing and Treatment with Intravenous Local Anesthetics
Differential Epidural/Spinal Blockade
Diagnostic Neural Blockade

INITIAL MANAGEMENT OF ACUTE PAIN

Kelly Gordon Knape, M.D.

It is very important to patients with new or recent onset of pain to have it treated promptly. They must first be thoroughly evaluated so that the correct diagnosis is made. Both the cause and the symptom can then be treated to ensure the effectiveness of the therapy. There are many common causes of acute pain: trauma, infection, inflammation, and exacerbations of chronic medical problems, as well as postoperative pain. Psychological causes are rare. Historically, acute pain has been undertreated for many reasons, with no realization that this can lead to secondary morbidity. It is therefore in the patient's best interest to be precise and expeditious in diagnosis and treatment.

A. History taking should be complete, to including possible systemic and local causes. Examples include single joint pain as a manifestation of ankylosing spondylitis, or acute abdominal pain. Documentation of onset, duration, intensity, and quality of pain should be specific. Any previous use of analgesics should be noted. Previous self-treatment often occurs and provides early information about the effectiveness of treatment; however, it also may mask the intensity of pain and other symptoms such as fever. Stoicism or anxiety in patients may decrease or increase complaints, respectively.

B. Further evaluation includes a complete physical examination and close scrutiny of the site of the pain. Observation should focus on any associated induration, erythema, and edema. Palpation identifies areas of firmness and crepitance as well as eliciting or accentuating the pain. Auscultation is important in the evaluation of chest and abdominal pain. Passive and active range of motion is also assessed with joint-related complaints. Any neurologic disorders, including areas of hypo- or hyperalgesia and associated weakness, must be noted, especially when there is extremity pain. Radiographic evaluation is often helpful. Routine blood tests (cell counts, electrolytes) may help focus on a systemic-related diagnosis. Additional serologic tests may be necessary to pinpoint a cause.

C. Quantification of pain is necessary to direct the degree of intervention needed. The location of pain is a preliminary guide and should match the patient's own report of severity. At least 60% of surgical patients have moderate to severe pain. Scoring systems have been developed to better quantify and follow the trends in intensity. These include the Visual Analogue Scale (VAS) and 10-point Verbal Scale. A visual scale using various facial expressions (smile to frown) has been useful in children and other patients who have difficulty using the other scales. In noncommunicative patients such as infants, it is necessary to use other methods, including observation of grimacing or inability to sleep. Signs of increased sympathetic outflow (tachycardia, hypertension, sweating), restlessness, and agitation may indicate significant discomfort.

D. Therapeutic goals include not only pain relief but alleviation of anxiety, preservation of function, and avoidance of complications. If associated disease or injury is severe, preservation of life and limb takes priority but not to the complete exclusion of other goals. Once the cause is identified, pain control is often initiated simultaneously with treatment of the primary process. Whenever possible, analgesic agents should be started during the initial evaluation, provided that they do not interfere with priority care or delay the diagnosis. Knowledge of the pathophysiology of the specific cause of the pain will direct the choice of the most effective therapy. For example, inflammatory pain responds better to NSAIDs, and visceral pain responds well to narcotics. In choosing a specific analgesic regimen with known efficacy, the goals should be "the 3 L's": the *lowest* effective dose that provides the *longest* duration with the *least* side effects.

E. Safe and effective analgesia can result if dosing is titrated initially. This is usually labor-intensive but can minimize problems later. Oral regimens are more time consuming, but titration can be accomplished even at home if there is thorough patient education and close and frequent initial follow-up. IV and continuous regional block techniques are usually reserved for inpatient management and are more quickly titrated to effect. Patient-controlled techniques, including intravenous patient-controlled analgesia (PCA) and PCEA (epidural), allow patients to titrate the analgesia to what they consider is a tolerable level with an acceptable amount of any side effects that may occur (p 26). It is important to involve patients to minimize their loss of control.

F. Side effects may develop despite careful titration. Often these are related to a relative overdose and commonly include sedation and nausea, especially when narcotic regimens are used. If the dose cannot be decreased without increasing pain, the side effects should be treated. Promethazine is used to treat nausea and acts to potentiate analgesia. Other adjuncts such as NSAIDs can be added to help reduce the dosage of the primary analgesic. The offending analgesic agent or regimen may need to be changed entirely if the side effects persist. Continuous regional techniques can optimize analgesia and reduce side effects by means of low concentrations of local anesthetics with lipid-soluble narcotics such as fentanyl, but their use is limited by their invasiveness and the inherent risks.

G. Communication must be maintained with patients, families, and primary referring physicians so that care does not become complicated or confused. Involvement of an Acute Pain Service can help coordinate

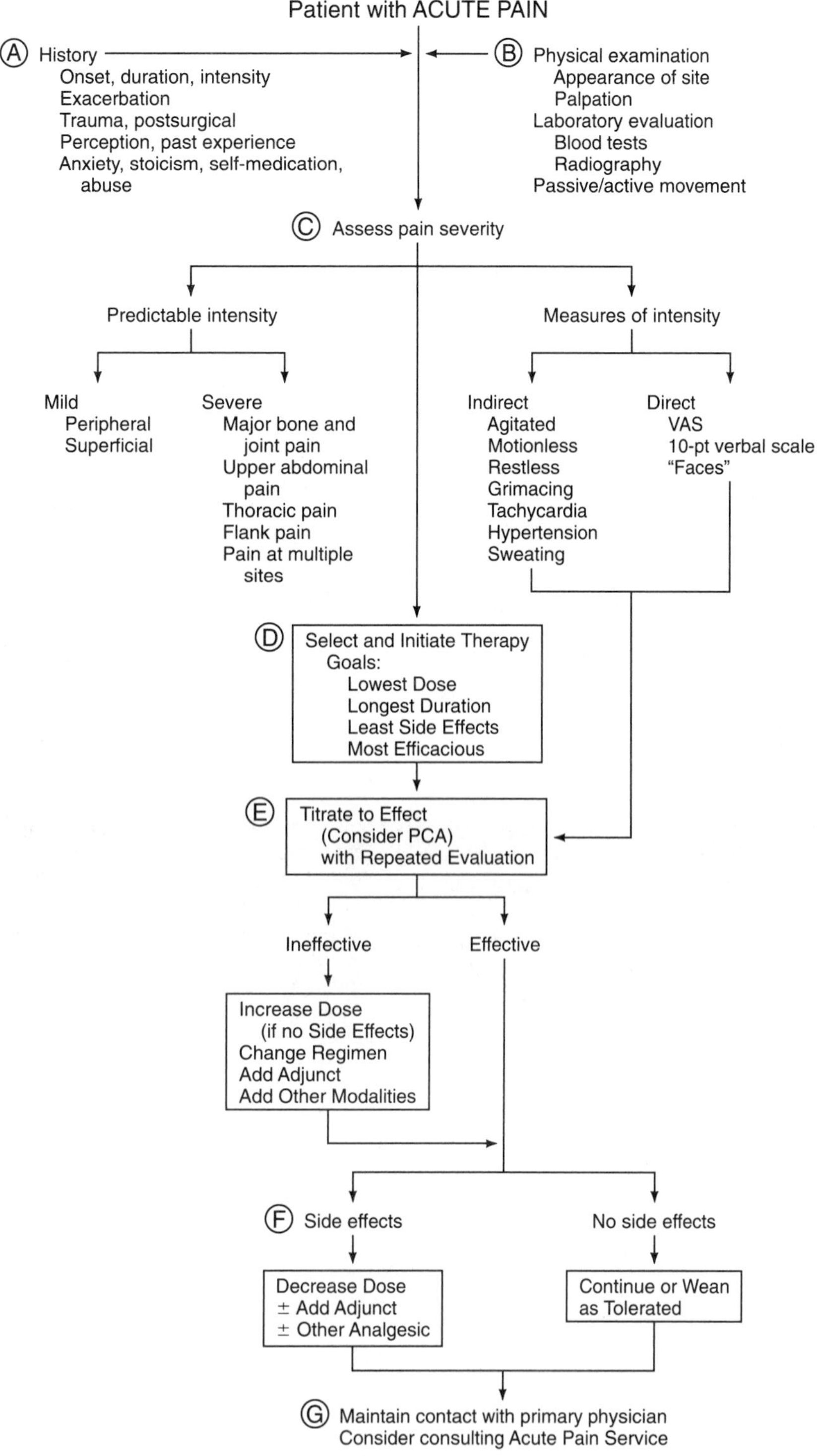

care and education as well as offer a broad spectrum of analgesic tools.

References

Bonica JJ. General considerations of acute pain. In: Bonica JJ, Loeser JD, Chapman CR, Fordyce WE, eds. The management of pain. 2nd ed. Philadelphia: Lea & Febiger, 1990, p. 159.

Egan KJ. What does it mean to a patient to be "in control"? In: Ferrante FM, Ostheimer GW, Covino BG, eds. Patient-controlled analgesia. Boston: Blackwell Scientific Publications, 1990:17.

Mackersie RC, Karagianes TG. Pain management following trauma and burns. In: Oden RV, Benumof JL, eds. Management of postoperative pain. Anesthesiol Clin North Am 1989; 7:211.

Ready LB. Acute pain services: An academic asset. Clin J Pain 1989; 5(Suppl 1):S28.

EVALUATION OF THE CHRONIC PAIN PATIENT

James N. Rogers, M.D.

Chronic pain is defined as pain that persists past the time of healing or has been present for more than 3 months. The evaluation of chronic pain can be difficult, as evidenced by the fact that many patients will have had extensive diagnostic work-ups and still carry the diagnosis of simple back pain. A multidisciplinary approach, involving anesthesiologists, psychologists, and other appropriate medical specialists, works best in evaluating these patients.

A. Pain is a subjective experience for the patient and is difficult for the physician to quantify objectively. The physician must rely on the history obtained, which should focus on the duration, intensity, and character of the pain as well as any aggravating or mitigating factors. Location and precise description of any radiation of the pain is important. The physical examination should focus on neurologic functioning as well as identifying the existence of provocative maneuvers that reproduce the painful symptoms. The presence or absence of temperature, or sweating differences should be recorded.

B. Psychological testing can help determine the existence of psychological factors that may influence future management. Personal, social, employment, and family histories should be obtained. Lawsuits and other forms of compensation may have a significant influence on the success of treatment. In selected patients, psychological intervention or behavior modification may be all that is needed to manage the pain.

C. If provocative tests such as supine straight leg raising reproduce pain, a Pentothal test (p 16) can be used to distinguish somatic pain from central pain syndromes, psychogenic pain, or malingering by repeating the provocative maneuver during the period of sedation.

D. If the provocative maneuver during the Pentothal examination fails to reproduce the pain, a differential spinal or epidural block should be used to further identify the cause. If there is no pain relief despite complete motor and sensory blockade, central pain, psychogenic pain, or malingering is indicated. Further psychological evaluation is then necessary to distinguish between these three entities.

E. If there is evidence suggestive of sympathetically mediated pain, a diagnostic sympathetic block of the affected area should be performed. Pain relief with documented sympathetic blockade and the absence of motor or sensory blockade confirm the diagnosis of reflex sympathetic dystrophy (RSD) as well as providing initial therapy.

F. If the presence of somatic pain has been confirmed in this initial evaluation, further diagnosis and treatment is described in subsequent chapters.

References

Bonica DJ. Treatment of cancer pain: Current status and future needs. In: Fields HL, et al, eds. Advances in pain research and therapy. Vol 9. New York: Raven Press, 1985:589.

Fordyce WE. The validity of pain behavior measurement. In: Melzack R, ed. Pain measurement and assessment. New York: Raven Press, 1983.

Mendelsson G. Compensation, pain complaints and psychological disturbances. Pain 1984; 20:169.

Merskey H, ed. Classification of chronic pain. Description of chronic pain syndromes and definitions of pain terms. Pain 1986; 3[Suppl]:1.

Savitz D. Medical evaluation of the chronic pain patients. In: Aronoff GM, ed. Evaluation and treatment of chronic pain. Baltimore: Urban & Schwarzenberg, 1985:39.

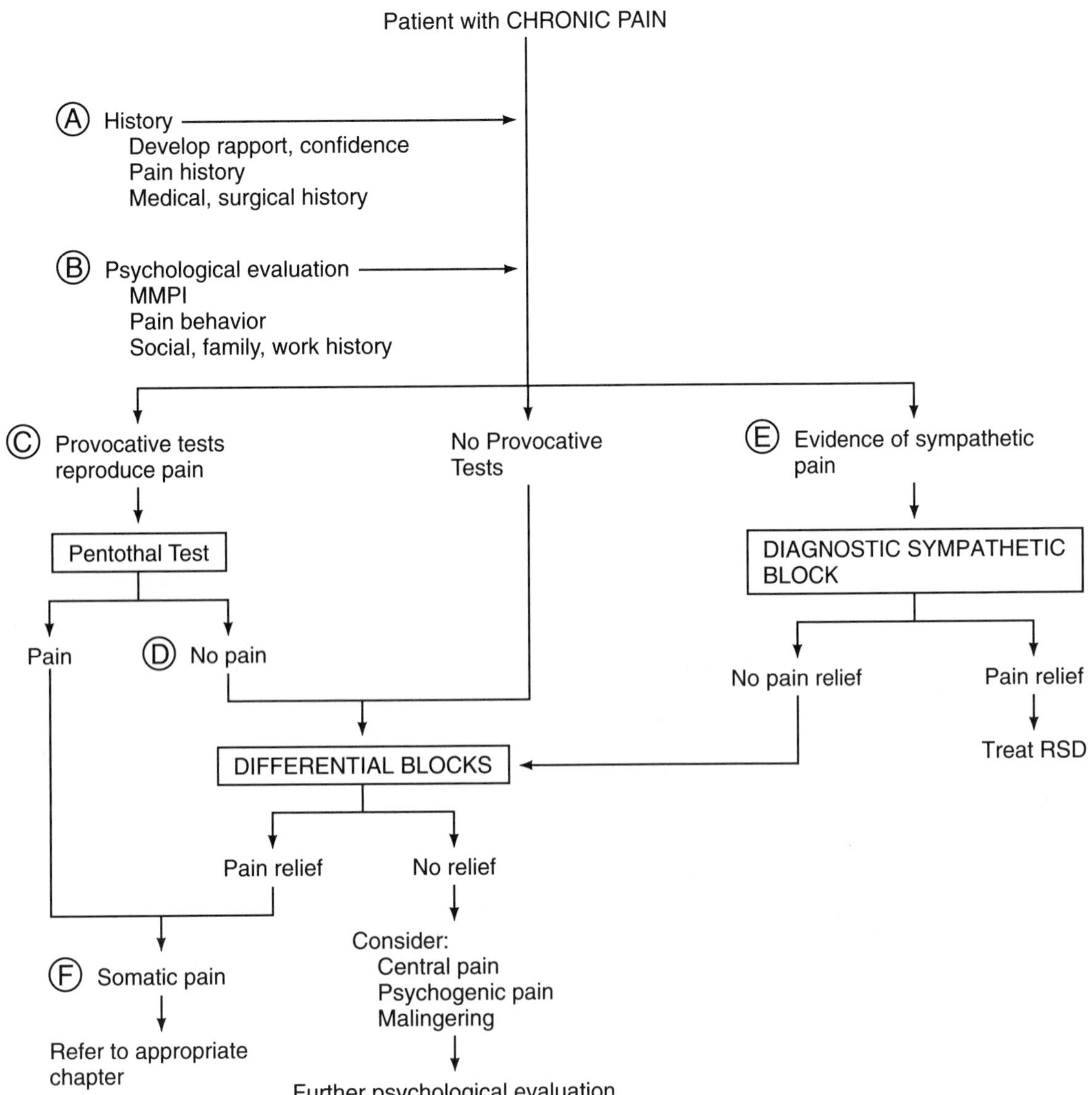

Patient with CHRONIC PAIN
(A) History
Develop rapport, confidence
Pain history
Medical, surgical history
(B) Psychological evaluation
MMPI
Pain behavior
Social, family, work history
(C) Provocative tests reproduce pain
No Provocative Tests
(E) Evidence of sympathetic pain
Pentothal Test
DIAGNOSTIC SYMPATHETIC BLOCK
Pain
(D) No pain
No pain relief
Pain relief
Treat RSD
DIFFERENTIAL BLOCKS
Pain relief
No relief
(F) Somatic pain
Refer to appropriate chapter
Consider:
Central pain
Psychogenic pain
Malingering
Further psychological evaluation

PSYCHOLOGICAL EVALUATION

Lawrence S. Schoenfeld, Ph.D.
Raymond M. Costello, Ph.D.

Chronic pain is a psychobiologic process with affective, cognitive, motivational, and somatic components. A psychological evaluation therefore is an essential part of the comprehensive evaluation of patients with chronic pain. The evaluation often includes both an interview and selective psychometric instruments. Psychophysical measures of the pain experience are sometimes employed. Successful management of the chronic pain patient is facilitated by the clarification of psychosocial factors contributing to the pain experience. Psychological interventions can then be offered and invasive somatic procedures avoided.

A. A comprehensive psychodiagnostic interview of the patient with chronic pain requires a mental health professional skilled both in interview techniques and in the field of chronic pain. A thorough knowledge of the professional chronic pain literature helps the clinician to gather appropriate data important to the integration of relevant psychological, sociologic, and economic factors. A detailed pain and developmental history often provides a context for understanding the chronicity of the pain syndrome.

B. Various psychophysical techniques assess the intensity of pain experienced and maximum pain tolerance. Cold pressor testing has shown that at any given age Anglo-Saxon males have the highest pain tolerance, followed by non–Anglo-Saxon males, Anglo-Saxon females, and finally non–Anglo-Saxon females.

C. Psychometric assessment provides standardized methods for evaluating mood, cognition, motivation, personality style, extent of disability, and illness behavior. The educational level of the patient must be sufficient for the instruments chosen. Chronic pain patients often are reluctant to complete personality tests. Testing should occur in the context of more comprehensive interdisciplinary evaluations.

D. The visual analog scale is usually a 10 cm line with end points defined as "no pain" and "severe pain." The patient is asked to mark the severity of pain. End points may also define improvement ("no improvement" versus "total improvement") and degree of disability ("no disability" versus "total disability") as well as other important dimensions. This is a simple, widely used instrument that enables the patient to communicate in a standard fashion.

E. The MMPI has been used more than any other psychological instrument in the assessment of personality factors contributing to the experience of chronic pain. A number of MMPI typologies are based on research involving empirical clustering of MMPI pain profiles into prototypes. The MMPI typology labeled P-A-I-N appears to have important clinical and demographic correlates. Classification rules have been proposed to allow patient-typing without a computer.

References

Costello RM, Hulsey TL, Schoenfeld LS, Ramamurthy S. P-A-I-N: A four cluster MMPI typology for chronic pain. Pain 1987; 30:199.

Costello RM, Schoenfeld LS, Ramamurthy S, Hobbs-Hardee B. Sociodemographic and clinical correlates of P-A-I-N. J Psychosom Res 1989; 33:315.

Melzack R, ed. Pain measurement and assessment. New York: Raven Press, 1983.

Walsh NE, Schoenfeld LS, Ramamurthy S. Normative model for cold pressor test. Am J Phys Med Rehabil 1989; 68:6.

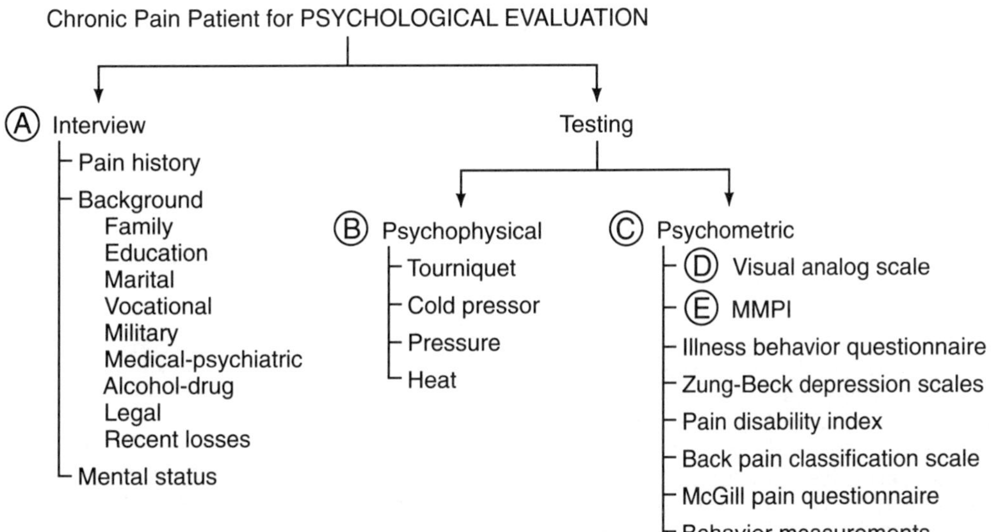
Chronic Pain Patient for PSYCHOLOGICAL EVALUATION
(A) Interview
Pain history
Background
Family
Education
Marital
Vocational
Military
Medical-psychiatric
Alcohol-drug
Legal
Recent losses
Mental status
Testing
(B) Psychophysical
Tourniquet
Cold pressor
Pressure
Heat
(C) Psychometric
(D) Visual analog scale
(E) MMPI
Illness behavior questionnaire
Zung-Beck depression scales
Pain disability index
Back pain classification scale
McGill pain questionnaire
Behavior measurements

POST-TRAUMATIC STRESS DISORDER

Paul T. Ingmundson, Ph.D.

Post-traumatic stress disorder (PTSD) refers to a constellation of psychiatric symptoms sometimes observed after a psychologically distressing event. The syndrome is officially classified as an anxiety disorder, although patients in whom the diagnosis is made may manifest features of other mental disorders, including major depressive and dissociative disorders. The syndrome has been observed among war veterans, trauma victims, and residents of communities exposed to disaster. The lifetime prevalence has been estimated at 1% in the general population, 3.5% in victims of physical assault, and 20% among veterans wounded during the Vietnam war. Recognition of the syndrome is of particular importance for the clinician evaluating a pain complaint because of the frequent co-occurrence of anxiety symptoms and pain symptoms after traumatic injury, and the tendency of some of these patients to present psychologic disturbances in the form of physical complaints.

A. The essential feature of the syndrome is exposure to a traumatic event outside the range of normal human experience, such as a natural disaster, a physical assault or rape, or combat. The experience may be associated with intense feelings of terror, rage, or helplessness. Simple bereavement, financial reversals, or marital discord are generally considered within the range of common experience and do not qualify for the diagnosis. The precipitating event is frequently, although not necessarily, life threatening.

B. The traumatic event is persistently re-experienced in the form of intrusive recollections, disturbing dreams, episodes of acting or feeling as though one were reliving the event ("flashbacks"), or intense distress when one is exposed to symbolic reminders of the event.

C. Stimuli associated with the event are persistently avoided. The pattern of avoidance may be associated with an inability to recall aspects of the event (psychogenic amnesia) and may generalize into social withdrawal, alienation, feelings of detachment or estrangement, restriction of range of affect (e.g., not being able to have caring feelings toward a spouse or child), and a fatalistic sense of helplessness about the future.

D. Increased levels of autonomic arousal may be manifested by symptoms such as difficulty falling or staying asleep, irritability and anger, concentration difficulties, hypervigilance, exaggerated startle responses, and physiologic reactivity to stimuli that may symbolize or resemble the traumatic event.

E. The symptoms must persist for at least 1 month. Syndromes of brief duration may be considered acute situational reactions or adjustment disorders and may benefit from supportive, prophylactic measures.

F. A delayed form of the syndrome, in which symptoms develop at least 6 months after the traumatic stressor, has also been described, although this is probably less frequent.

G. Individual psychotherapy, in which the patient works through the memories of the event along with associated feelings of guilt or helplessness, has often been found helpful, but may be prolonged and expensive.

H. Success has been reported with behavior therapies, which may involve graduated re-exposure to the traumatic stimulus (systematic desensitization), exaggerated re-exposure (flooding), or imaginal re-exposure coupled with simultaneous relaxation and a restructuring of associated negative thoughts and feelings (eye movement desensitization). These approaches are generally of shorter duration (one to ten sessions) than insight-oriented psychotherapy.

I. Group treatment has been a popular and often effective psychotherapeutic tool, particularly with patients (e.g., combat veterans, holocaust survivors) whose group identification was linked with exposure to the traumatic events.

J. Pharmacotherapy has frequently been reported to be helpful but is rarely considered sufficient and is generally focused on target symptoms. Tricyclic antidepressants have been particularly popular, and successes have also been reported with other antidepressant therapies (e.g., monoamine oxidase inhibitors, fluoxetine). Benzodiazepines are often used and may benefit some patients, although problems with tolerance and dependence make their use with chronic forms of the disorder particularly difficult. Cyproheptadine is generally well tolerated and has been reported to have specific efficacy in the treatment of sleep disturbances associated with combat nightmares.

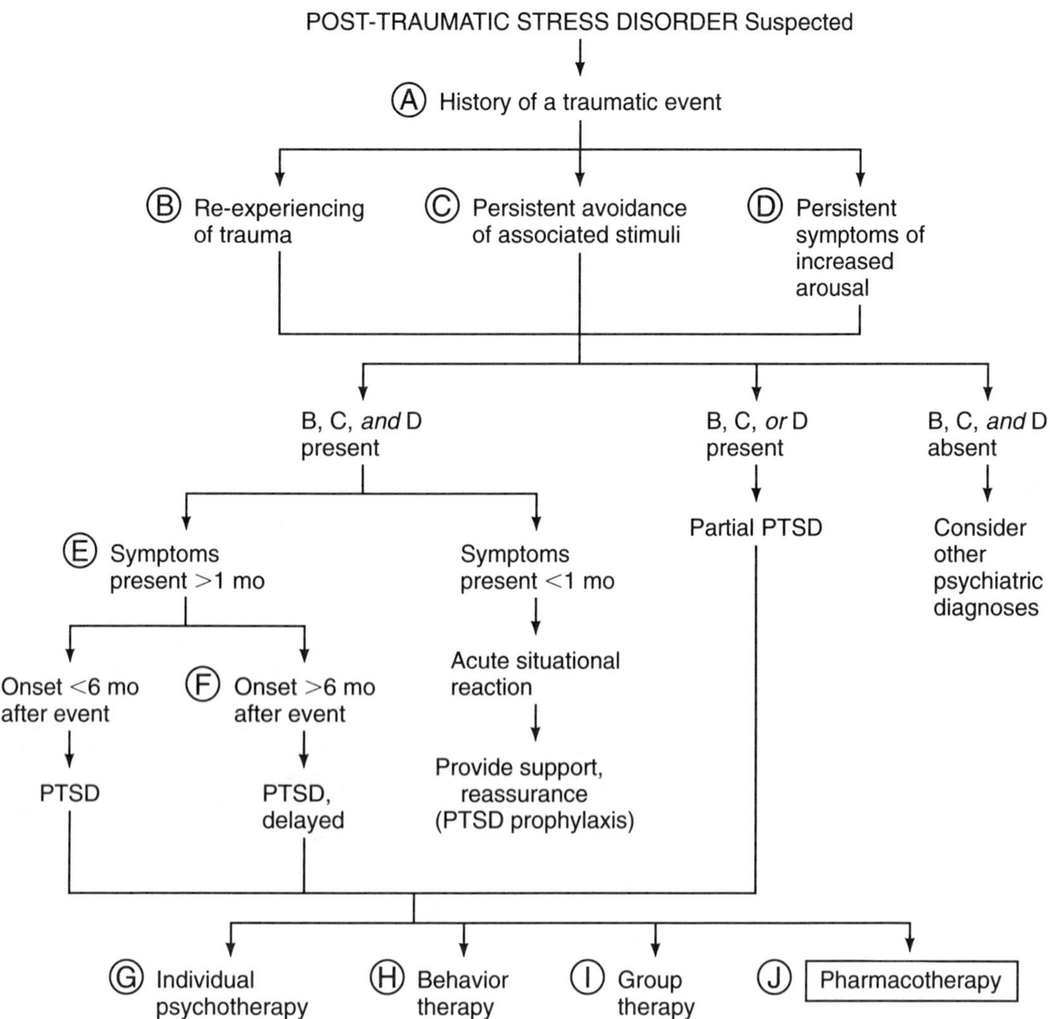

References

American Psychiatric Association. Diagnostic and statistical manual of mental disorders. 3rd ed, revised. Washington, DC: American Psychiatric Association, 1987.

Brophy MH. Cyproheptadine for combat nightmares in post-traumatic stress disorder and dream anxiety disorder. Milit Med 1991; 156:100.

Fairbank JA, Brown T. Current behavioral approaches to the treatment of post-traumatic stress disorder. Behav Ther 1987; 3:57.

Friedman M. Toward rational pharmacotherapy for post-traumatic stress disorder: An interim report. Am J Psychiatry 1988; 145:281.

Helzer JE, Robins LN, McEvoy L. Post-traumatic stress disorder in the general population. N Engl J Med 1987; 317:1630.

Shapiro F. Eye movement desensitization: A new treatment for post-traumatic stress disorder. J Behav Ther Exp Psychiatry 1989; 20:211.

Wolpe J, Abrams J. Post-traumatic stress disorder overcome by eye-movement desensitization: A case report. J Behav Ther Exp Psychiatry 1991; 22:39.

SLEEP DISTURBANCES AND CHRONIC PAIN

Paul T. Ingmundson, Ph.D.

Sleep disturbances are common among chronic pain patients; complaints of poor sleep occur in up to 70% in some reported series. A variety of sleep disorders are associated with complaints of pain.

A. The basis for the diagnosis of any sleep disorder is a history of the sleep complaint, including a review of the medical and psychiatric history and use of medications. A collateral history from the bed partner, including information about the frequency and types of movements, arousals, and any respiratory abnormalities, is often critical in arriving at a tentative diagnosis. A sleep log, documenting hours spent in bed, time asleep, and daytime naps, also may yield useful data for the initial assessment.

B. A variety of extrinsic factors need to be assessed in evaluating a sleep complaint. Noisy sleep environment; inappropriate use of alcohol, stimulants, or sedative hypnotic medications; poor sleep hygiene; jet lag; and shift work are all examples of extrinsic factors that may contribute to a complaint of poor sleep.

C. Disorders of excessive daytime sleepiness are sometimes termed hypersomnias. A complaint of hypersomnia accompanied by loud, irregular snoring raises the suspicion of obstructive sleep apnea, which must be confirmed in an overnight laboratory study (nocturnal polysomnography). Associated features may include hypertension, obesity, and morning headaches.

D. Disorders associated with repetitive movement during sleep may be associated with complaints of pain and fatigue on awakening. Restless legs syndrome (RLS) consists of creeping, painful sensations in the lower extremities that can only be relieved by movement and may be associated with difficulties in initiating sleep. Periodic limb movements during sleep (PLMS) are stereotyped, repetitive movements of the extremities that occur during sleep. Virtually all patients with RLS have PLMS, although the converse is not true. The incidence of PLMS increases with age and may occur without an associated complaint of disturbed sleep. Clonazepam, 0.5 mg to 2.0 mg, or temazepam, 30 mg, has been reported to be effective. Reports of successful treatment with bromocriptine and L-dopa may implicate dopaminergic mechanisms in the etiology of the disorder.

E. Nocturnal bruxism, or tooth grinding, is frequently associated with complaints of facial pain and may involve destruction of dental and joint tissue. The cause is unknown, although psychosocial stressors are frequently implicated as trigger factors. Treatment generally consists of an occlusive splint, or nightguard. Biofeedback or relaxation training may be helpful in some cases, although the clinical efficacy of these for bruxism remains to be established.

F. Psychiatric conditions, particularly anxiety and depression, are often associated with disturbed sleep, although the presence of psychiatric symptoms should not preclude investigation of other possible etiologies.

G. Chronic musculoskeletal pain, in the absence of specific laboratory findings or evidence of connective tissue or metabolic disease, has been labeled fibrositis, fibromyalgia, or myofascial pain. The disorder is frequently associated with complaints of nonrestorative sleep. Nocturnal polysomnography in such patients often demonstrates alpha-frequency (8 to 11.5 Hz) intrusions in the EEG, or nonrapid eye movement sleep. The alpha EEG finding is also observed during febrile illness and postviral syndromes, but is generally absent in insomnia or depressive disorders. Treatment generally consists of a sedating tricyclic (e.g., amitriptyline) in conjunction with nonsteroidal anti-inflammatory analgesics. The use of short half-life benzodiazepines such as triazolam is generally discouraged, although benzodiazepines with intermediate range half-lives (e.g., nitrazepam) have proved useful in some cases. Behavioral approaches to treatment may often be helpful.

H. Idiopathic insomnia is a childhood-onset disorder of initiating or maintaining sleep that cannot be attributed to other psychiatric or medical factors. Psychophysiologic, or "learned," insomnia usually has an adult onset and is associated with agitation and somatized tension. Patients in both groups are frequently prescribed benzodiazepines, although the chronic nature of the complaint may lead to problems with tolerance or dependence. Ultimate resolution of the disturbance often requires some form of behavioral intervention.

I. Chronic pain patients typically report spending much time in bed or at rest, although they also describe their sleep as disturbed and frequently unrestorative. Behavioral approaches to sleep disturbances focus on modifying maladaptive sleep behaviors. The stimulus control method focuses on altering cues in the sleep environment that may be associated with arousal rather than sleep. The sleep restriction method titrates the amount of time spent in bed to the patient's sleep efficiency, a ratio of sleep time to the amount of time spent in bed. Both approaches, or combinations thereof, may help consolidate the sleep phase and improve the subjective quality of sleep.

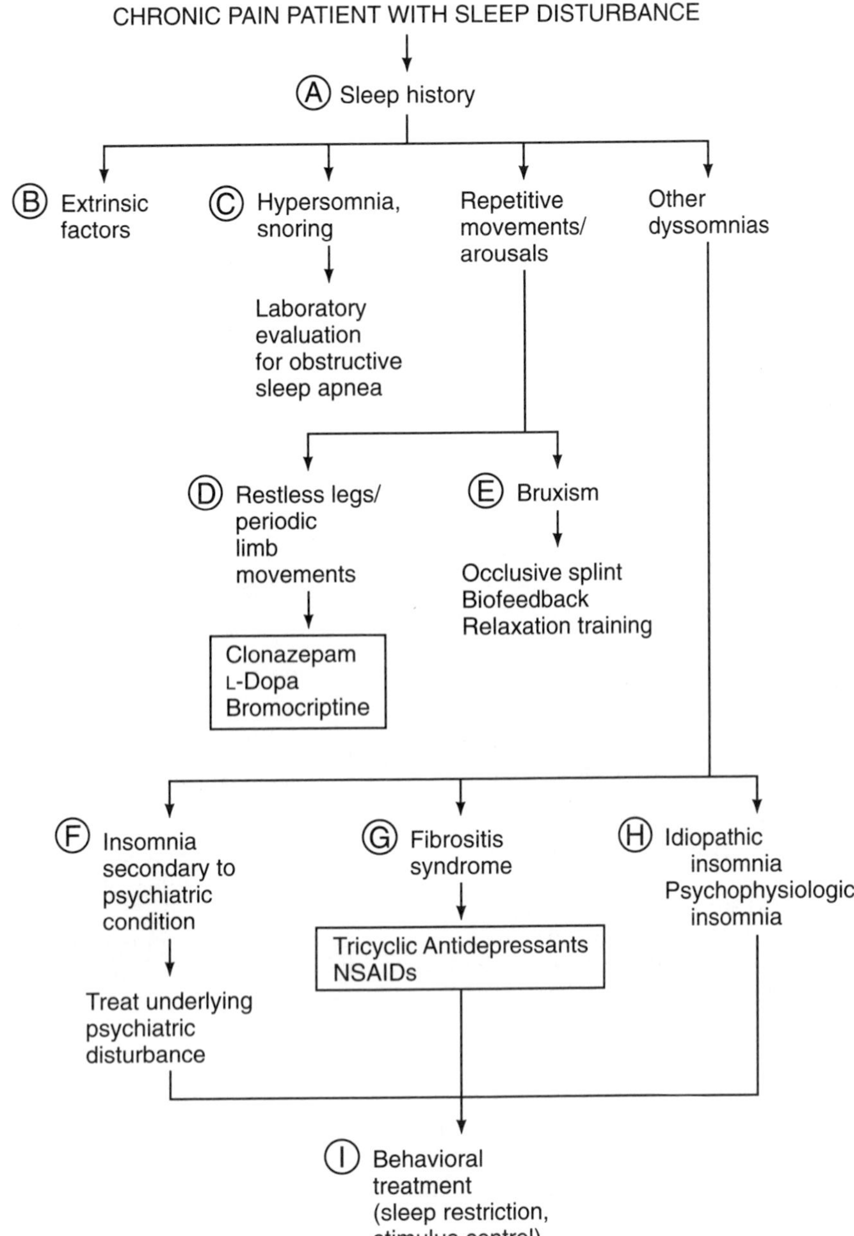

References

American Sleep Disorders Association. The international classification of sleep disorders. Lawrence, KS: Allen Press, 1990.

Moldofsky H. Sleep and fibrositis syndrome. Rheum Dis Clin North Am 15:91.

Montplaisir J, Godbout R. Restless legs syndrome and periodic movements during sleep. In: Kryger MH, Roth T, Dement WC, eds. Principles and practice of sleep medicine. Philadelphia: WB Saunders, 1989.

Morin CM, Kowatch RA, Wade JB. Behavioral management of sleep disturbances secondary to chronic pain. J Behav Ther Exp Psychiatry 1989; 20:295.

Pilowksky I, Crettendon I, Townley M. Sleep disturbance in pain clinic patients. Pain 1985; 23:27.

PAIN MEASUREMENT

Joan Hoffman, R.N., M.S.N.

The measurement of pain is difficult because of the variation in individual responses to painful stimuli and the subjective nature of pain. Nevertheless, numerous methods have been developed for the measurement of pain. The most commonly used methods are described here. When choosing a method, one must consider the type of setting, the ease of administration and scoring, and patient population characteristics such as educational level. One must also consider the reliability and validity of the specific device, especially when conducting research.

A. Verbal descriptor scales measure pain intensity using three to five numerically ranked words (Fig. 1). Degree of pain relief can also be measured in this manner, using categories ranging from "no relief" to "complete relief." Verbal descriptor scales are easy to administer and score.

B. The visual analog scale (VAS), which can be used to measure a variety of subjective symptoms, is commonly used to measure pain intensity. The VAS consists of a 10 cm line with verbal anchors at either end (Fig. 2). A variation of the VAS places descriptive words (anchors) along the scale. Like the verbal descriptor scales, the VAS is easy to administer and score. A small percentage of patients have difficulty conceptualizing their pain and marking its intensity on a straight line. Although the anchor words may make the scale easier to understand, the fact that answers tend to be grouped near anchor words is a disadvantage.

C. A numerical rating scale of 0 to 100 or 0 to 10 can be used to measure pain intensity. This scale is probably the easiest to administer verbally, making it the most practical for clinical use. Usually 0 represents no pain and 10 represents the worst pain imaginable, although 10 also can be defined as the worst pain the patient has experienced or the baseline pain prior to treatment. It is important that the end points be consistent so that patients and clinicians are clear about what the number represents.

D. The McGill pain questionnaire utilizes twenty lists of words that describe sensory, affective, and evaluative dimensions of pain. The words in each group are ranked from least pain to most pain. The patient is asked to choose the one word in each list that describes his or her pain. This scale takes more time than the other scales to complete as well as to score. The word descriptors are difficult for some patients to understand, especially those with limited formal education, thus limiting the population in which this questionnaire may be used.

E. In chronic pain patients, the measurement of pain behaviors, along with pain measurement, can be useful in determining the success of treatment. Home recording of physical activity, medications use, and pain intensity on an hour-to-hour basis in diary form has been described by Fordyce. Methods of direct observation of pain behaviors also have been developed. The University of Alabama Birmingham (UAB)

_______ 1. NONE

_______ 2. MILD

_______ 3. MODERATE

_______ 4. SEVERE

_______ 5. UNBEARABLE

Figure 1 Verbal Descriptor Scale for Measurement of Pain Intensity.

No pain ____ Pain as bad as it could possibly be

No pain ____ Pain as bad as it could possibly be

Mild Moderate Severe

Figure 2 Visual Analog Scales for Measurement of Pain Intensity.

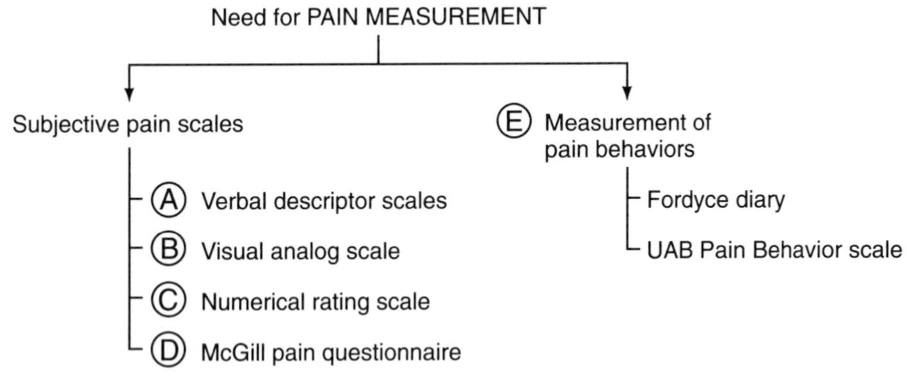

Pain Behavior scale is an objective assessment of the following pain behaviors: verbal vocal complaints, nonverbal vocal complaints, time spent lying down, facial grimaces, standing posture, mobility, body language, use of visible supportive equipment, stationary movement, and medication. Both the Fordyce diary and the UAB scale are fairly simple to use and can provide important information to the clinician treating patients with chronic pain.

References

Fordyce WE, Lansky, S, Calsyn DA, et al. Pain measurement and pain behavior. Pain 1984; 18:53.

Melzack R. The McGill Pain Questionnaire: Major properties and scoring methods. Pain 1975; 1:275.

Richards JS, Nepomuceno C, Riles M, et al. Assessing pain behavior: The UAB pain behavior scale. Pain 1982; 14:393.

THERMOGRAPHY

Nancy E. Hambleton, R.N., B.S.N.
James N. Rogers, M.D.

Thermography is a process for measuring regional skin temperatures by either conduction or detection of infrared radiation produced by the body surface. It is primarily used as a diagnostic tool and a physiologic test to correlate pathologic changes with physical findings. Thermography does not show pain because pain is a perception. It does not take the place of other diagnostic tests, but does provide early information not previously available with other assessment tools. The imaging technique is claimed to supply objective documentation of the patient's complaint of pain that can be correlated with the history, physical findings, and/or laboratory results. In practice, it is useful only as a tool to measure skin temperature over a wide area of the body.

A. Two types of thermographic techniques are currently used: (1) liquid crystal, or contact, thermography; and (2) infrared, or tele-electronic, thermography. Liquid crystal thermography uses cholesteric crystals that change color with variations in surface temperature. The lowest temperature range is displayed as a dark brown color and changes with progressive temperature elevation to tan, reddish brown, yellow, green, blue, and dark blue. Eleven "air pillow" Thermoflex Detectors progressively numbered 24 through 35, corresponding to the median Celsius temperature ranges of their incorporated liquid crystal Flexitherm sheets, are available. Each air pillow has an approximate temperature range of 4° to 5° C, making the total possible range obtainable approximately 19° to 40° C. The temperature reproducibility is typically ± 0.2° C. A fixed distance frame attached to an instant Polaroid camera provides support for the air pillow and facilitates photography. Infrared thermography consists of a television-like camera that detects the infrared radiation produced at the body surface. The high-speed infrared scanning camera is focused on the patient, and the heat emission from the body surface is projected to an infrared radiation detector, converted to electric signals, and displayed on a color monitor. A Polaroid or 35-mm picture of the monitor screen is taken. Some scanning cameras can be connected directly to a computer and the data stored for future use on a disk system.

B. The advantages of contact thermography over infrared thermography include lower overall price, equipment portability and simplicity, and higher color contrast. The major advantages of infrared thermography are that larger body areas can be evaluated on each view, and contact with the patient's skin is not required. Other general advantages of thermography are that it is noninvasive and painless and no potentially harmful radiation is produced. It is safe to use in pregnant women and children. Chronic pain patients who may have previously undergone many invasive and painful procedures tolerate either technique well. Thermography can be adapted to any region of the body.

C. Thermography is an extremely sensitive test that must be performed under carefully controlled conditions. Two types of interference exist: environment related and patient related. The environment must be a draft-free room at a temperature of 68° to 72° F with no sunlight or reflecting surfaces (Table 1).

D. Thermography permits more decisive diagnosis and treatment plans for the clinician when used in conjunction with other tests.

E. The primary indication for use of thermography is as a diagnostic tool. Claims have been made that it can be used by the clinician to detect neuropathic, myofascial, circulatory, and skeletal pain syndromes. Temperature changes secondary to changes in circulation as a result of injury to nerves, ligaments, muscles, or joints are shown by thermography. In reflex sympathetic dystrophy, a diffuse pattern of decreased temperature is usually seen over the entire limb, more pronounced distally. Thermography can help identify carpal tunnel syndrome, chronic low back pain, and spinal root irritation, in which temperature changes in the corresponding dermatomes may be seen. Because thermography records infrared heat emission from joints, it has been used to study inflammatory joint disease.

F. Qualitative and quantitative evaluation of sympathetic function after a sympathetic block or sympathectomy is another value of thermography. Information as to whether the appropriate fibers have been blocked or surgically denervated can be obtained. The efficacy of

TABLE 1 Patient Preparation for Thermography

No smoking for *4 hr* before test
No powder, cosmetics, or lotions to skin surface to be imaged
No physical therapy *24 hr* previously
No TENS, acupuncture, or EMG *24 hr* previously
No brace or splint to affected area *6 hr* previously
No sunburn *10 days* previously
Note previous fractures, surgeries, superficial scars, gout, diabetes, arthritis, and any medications, especially topical
Note any changes since last thermography (e.g., injections, bumps, bruises, insect bites, injuries)

TENS, Transcutaneous electrical nerve stimulation.

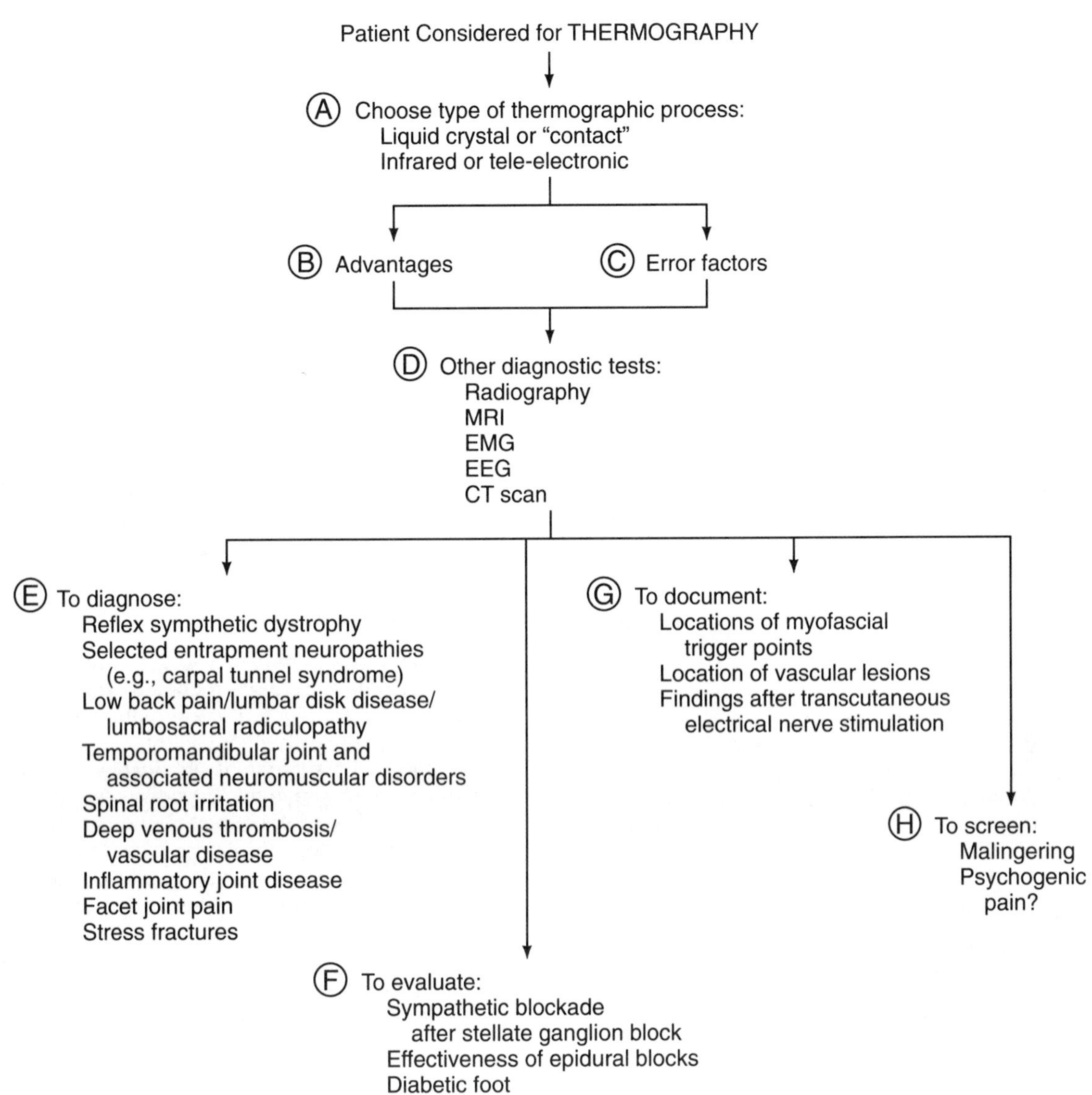

mography pictures by a dramatic increase in temperature in the affected extremity, indicating increased blood flow.

G. Documentation of thermographic objectivity in pain syndromes is also obtainable. Myofascial pain syndrome usually shows trigger areas with a 1° to 2° F temperature elevation. The appearance of trigger points on the thermograms is typically a disk 5 to 10 cm in diameter, or irregularly shaped spots compared with the corresponding opposite side.

H. It is claimed that thermography provides the clinician with a useful tool for screening of malingering and psychogenic pain syndromes. These claims have not been confirmed by convincing studies.

References

Edwards BE, Hobbins WB. Pain management and thermography. In: Raj PP, ed. Practical management of pain. 2nd ed. St. Louis: Mosby-Year Book, 1992:168.

Flexitherm. A subsidiary of E-Z-EM, Inc. New York: The Flexitherm System.

LeRoy PL, Filasky R. Thermography. In: Bonica JJ, ed. The management of pain. 2nd ed. Vol I. Philadelphia: Lea & Febiger, 1990:610.

Mahoney L, McCulloch J, Csima A: Thermography in back pain. Thermology 1:43, 1985.

Newman R, Seres J, Miller E: Liquid crystal thermography in the evaluation of chronic back pain. Pain 20:298, 1984.

Pochaczevsky R. Assessment of back pain by contact thermography of extremity dermatomes. Orthop Rev 1983; 12:45.

PENTOTHAL TESTING

Roger L. Wesley, M.D.

Frequently we encounter "complex pain" patients who present diagnostic or therapeutic dilemmas. These patients may have pain of multifactorial, uncertain, or unknown etiology with a confusing or inconsistent course; the pain may not respond to conventional therapy; and there may be more pronounced symptoms than the organic etiology would predict. This may be related to psychosocial overlay, since pain is a subjective experience, sometimes influenced heavily by cultural learning, psychological and social variables, and secondary gain. Before subjecting these patients to expensive or invasive diagnostic tests, intensive or risky treatment regimens, or surgical intervention, it is desirable to identify those in whom a psychological etiology prevails, so as to minimize risk to the patient, conserve medical resources, and provide more appropriate therapy. Pentothal testing is a useful diagnostic aid for these patients.

A. Traditionally, psychological testing such as the MMPI or Eysenck personality inventory has been used to identify those patients who may be predisposed to a nonorganic etiology for their pain. Similarly, diagnostic neural blockade (p 22) has been used to assess the relative influence of organic and psychosocial factors in chronic pain patients.

B. Pentothal testing is a modification of the sodium amytal interview, initially developed in 1961 and subsequently described in detail by Soichet, in which a detailed psychological and physical examination is performed during increasing levels of sedation. It is believed that barbiturate sedation may eliminate the influence of malingering or psychosocial overlay on the examination. Pentothal testing involves assessment of a previously painful physical maneuver under sodium pentothal sedation. The basis of the test is the fact that while a patient is under light sedation, he is capable of demonstrating a primitive reaction to pain and is unable to demonstrate a supratentorial response.

C. The patient fasts overnight, and informed consent is obtained. After IV cannulation, monitors are applied, including continuous ECG, pulse oximetry (SpO_2), and BP cuff. Equipment for airway resuscition, including positive pressure ventilation, and resuscitative drugs are kept close at hand.

D. The response to a previously painful maneuver is assessed. For example, a grimace or withdrawal in response to a straight leg raise test is documented.

E. Sodium pentothal is administered in 50 mg increments until loss of voice response and lash reflex is attained.

F. A stimulus known to be painful (Achilles heel pinch or 50 Hz Ministim tetanus) is applied, and a grimace or withdrawal response is documented.

G. The previously painful maneuver is repeated, and a response or lack of one is recorded. The presence of a response is considered confirmation of peripheral pathology, and further conventional treatment, neurolytic block, or surgery, if applicable, may be instituted. Lack of a painful response suggests a nonperipheral etiology, indicating that the patient may have central or psychogenic pain or may be malingering, and that invasive, neurolytic block, or surgical treatment is unlikely to benefit the patient. Psychological therapy may be helpful.

References

Krempen JF, Silver RA, Hadley J. An analysis of differential epidural spinal anesthesia and pentothal pain study in the differential diagnosis of back pain. Spine 1979; 4:452.

Soichet RP. Sodium amytal in the diagnosis of chronic pain. Can Psychiatr Assoc J 1978; 23:219.

Walters A. Psychogenic regional pain alias hysterical pain. Brain 1961; 84:1.

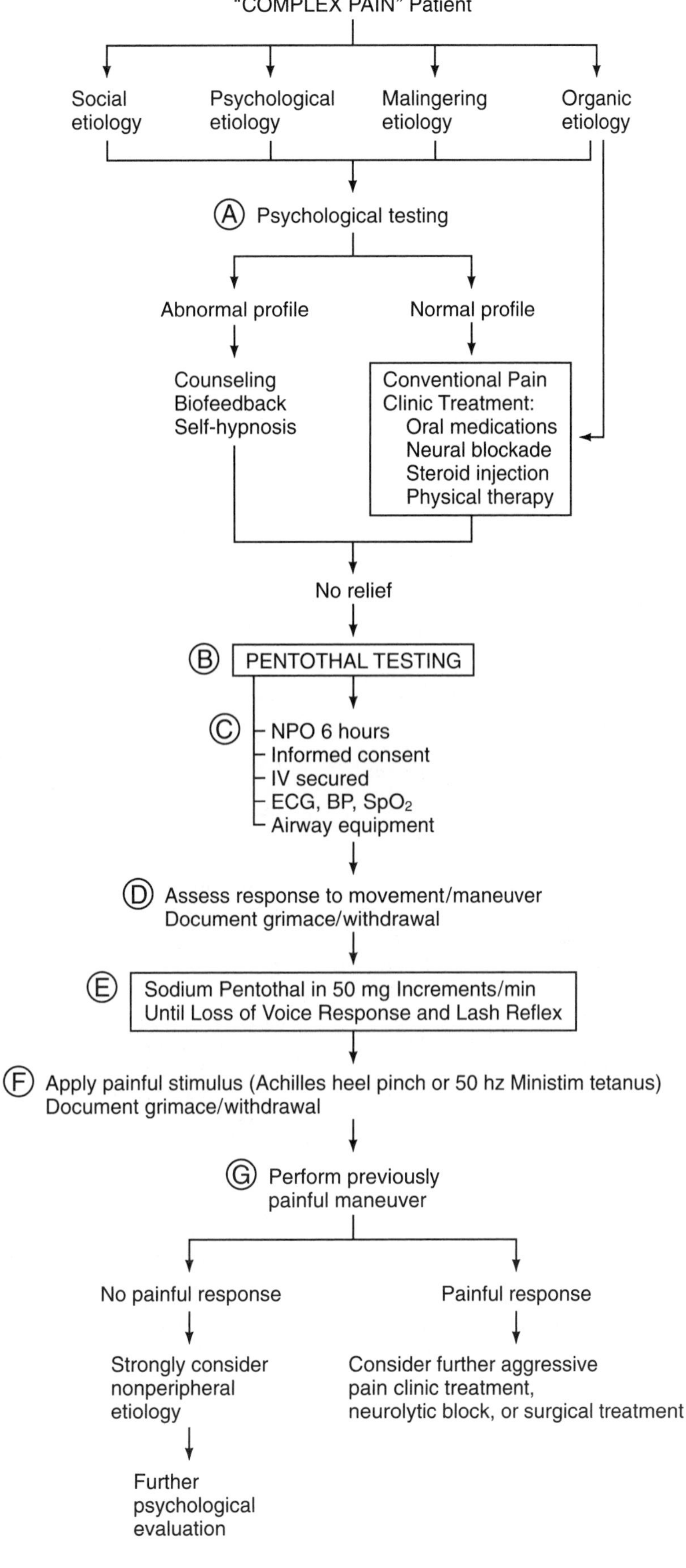

"COMPLEX PAIN" Patient
Social etiology
Psychological etiology
Malingering etiology
Organic etiology
(A) Psychological testing
Abnormal profile
Normal profile
Counseling
Biofeedback
Self-hypnosis
Conventional Pain Clinic Treatment:
Oral medications
Neural blockade
Steroid injection
Physical therapy
No relief
(B) PENTOTHAL TESTING
(C) NPO 6 hours
Informed consent
IV secured
ECG, BP, SpO2
Airway equipment
(D) Assess response to movement/maneuver
Document grimace/withdrawal
(E) Sodium Pentothal in 50 mg Increments/min
Until Loss of Voice Response and Lash Reflex
(F) Apply painful stimulus (Achilles heel pinch or 50 hz Ministim tetanus)
Document grimace/withdrawal
(G) Perform previously painful maneuver
No painful response
Painful response
Strongly consider nonperipheral etiology
Further psychological evaluation
Consider further aggressive pain clinic treatment, neurolytic block, or surgical treatment

TESTING AND TREATMENT WITH INTRAVENOUS LOCAL ANESTHETICS

J. P. Ducey, M.D.

In 1938 Leriche and Fonotaine reported the intravascular administration of local anesthetics for the relief of chronic pain. Numerous reports since then have supported the use of intravascular procaine, lidocaine, chloroprocaine, and even tetracaine for the treatment of central pain, deafferentation syndromes, sympathetic pain, neuropathies, myofascial pain, and other chronic pain syndromes. The mechanism of their action has been debated, but probably involves both anesthesia of small nerve endings in regions of tissue injury, and interruption of C-fiber synaptic transmission in the spinal cord with deafferentation syndromes.

A. Pain syndromes for which intravenous local anesthetics may be beneficial include central pain, deafferentation syndrome, phantom limb pain, neuritis/neuropathy, sympathetically mediated pain, postherpetic neuralgia, and myofascial pain.

B. IV lidocaine testing should be used to determine the efficacy of the treatment. Inform the patient that several injections will be given to see if any alleviation of the pain can be achieved. Obtain a baseline visual analog pain scale (VAS) from the patient before beginning the injections. After ECG, pulse oximetry, and noninvasive BP monitors are placed, slowly administer the first injection of normal saline over 5 minutes. Determine the VAS again 5 minutes after the injection has been completed. If there has been <50% improvement in the VAS score, perform a second injection of normal saline. If there is >50% improvement in the VAS, the patient is a placebo responder and no further injections are made. If the response is <50%, slowly administer the third injection, consisting of 1.5 to 2.0 mg/kg of lidocaine, 40 mg at a time. Observe the patient for 90 minutes after treatment. Alternatively, 2-chloroprocaine can be used.

C. If there is an adverse response to the anesthetic, stop the infusion and take the appropriate steps to address the complication. If CNS toxicity is manifested by seizure, administration of oxygen after drug discontinuation may be adequate. Administer a benzodiazepine if seizures persist, and consider airway control. If the adverse response is an allergic reaction to an ester anesthetic, undertake repeat testing with lidocaine at a later date. In a case of CNS toxicity, retesting at a later date with a smaller dose may be considered.

D. If pain relief is achieved with the first infusion, repeat the procedure weekly for 3 to 4 weeks. Lidocaine may be infused at 4 mg/min for 60 minutes or 5 mg/kg over 30 to 60 minutes. Each infusion should provide better, longer-lasting relief. If the benefits are only transient such that each infusion fails to provide more substantial relief of longer duration, the technique should probably be abandoned.

E. If IV anesthetics prove successful, consider chronic oral therapy with tocainide or mexiletine, agents with actions very similar to lidocaine. Monitor the serum levels of these agents carefully to avoid toxicity. At least one study suggests that the response to oral antiepileptic agents is accurately predicted by the initial response to IV anesthetics. Therefore, phenytoin and carbamazepine may also be considered after successful initial testing.

F. If IV anesthetics fail to provide adequate pain relief, consider anxiolytics such as alprazolam or the use of narcotics. The effectiveness of these agents may also be predicted with IV testing. Conventional methods of pain management, including nonsteroidal analgesics, physical therapy, and local anesthetic injections, may be continued as indicated.

References

Ackerman WE, Phero JC, McDonald JS. Analgesia with intravenous local anesthetics. In: Raj PP, ed. Practical management of pain. 2nd ed. St. Louis: Mosby–Year Book, 1992:851.

Boas RA, Covino BG, Shahnarian A. Analgesic responses to IV lignocaine. Br J Anaesth 1982; 54:501.

Edwards WT, Farajallah H, Burney RG, et al. Intravenous lidocaine in the management of various chronic pain states. Reg Anesth 1985; 10:1.

Phero JC, McDonald JS, Raj PP, et al. Controlled intravenous administration of chloroprocaine for intractable pain management. Reg Anesth 1984; 9:50.

Woolf CJ, Wiesenfeld-Hallin Z. The systemic administration of local anaesthetics produces a selective depression of C-afferent fibre evoked activity in the spinal cord. Pain 1985; 23:361.

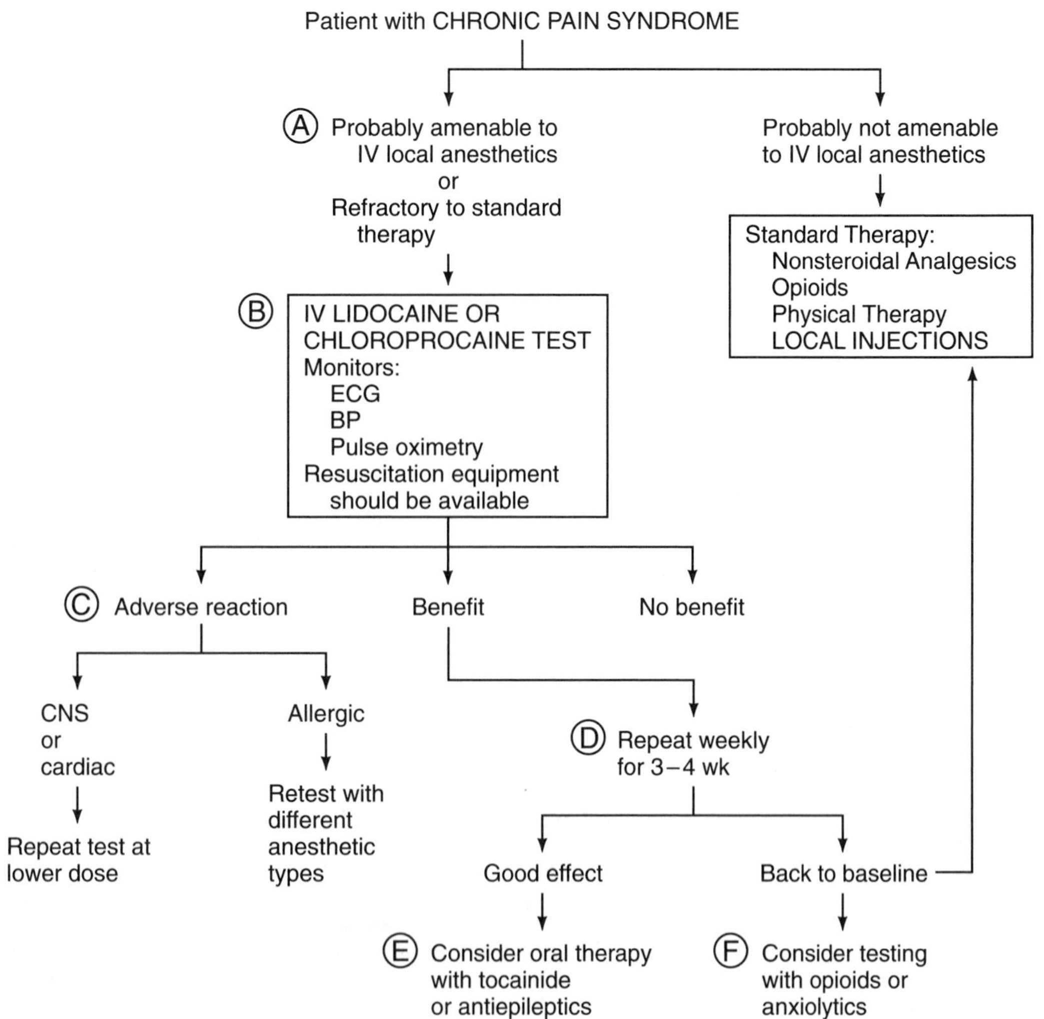

Patient with CHRONIC PAIN SYNDROME
(A) Probably amenable to IV local anesthetics or Refractory to standard therapy
Probably not amenable to IV local anesthetics
Standard Therapy: Nonsteroidal Analgesics Opioids Physical Therapy LOCAL INJECTIONS
(B) IV LIDOCAINE OR CHLOROPROCAINE TEST Monitors: ECG BP Pulse oximetry Resuscitation equipment should be available
(C) Adverse reaction
Benefit
No benefit
CNS or cardiac
Allergic
Repeat test at lower dose
Retest with different anesthetic types
(D) Repeat weekly for 3–4 wk
Good effect
Back to baseline
(E) Consider oral therapy with tocainide or antiepileptics
(F) Consider testing with opioids or anxiolytics

DIFFERENTIAL EPIDURAL/SPINAL BLOCKADE

William E. Strong, M.D.

Many patients are referred to the pain clinic with a chronic pain problem of unknown etiology despite extensive evaluation. A differential epidural/spinal block can help identify the mechanism of pain. Its usefulness is based on the differential sensitivity of nerve fibers to local anesthetic agents (Table 1). This procedure is most useful for patients with pain in the lower extremities, lower abdomen, pelvis, or low back. The epidural form can be used for thoracic pain. The purpose of the block is to define the mechanism of pain, whether sympathetic, somatic, or central in origin. The procedure is useful in diagnosis and prognosis and can be therapeutic. Differential spinal block was first described by Sarnoff and Arrowood, and recently was modified by Raj and Ramamurthy to include the differential epidural blocks.

A. A thorough history and physical examination are required in the initial evaluation of all patients at the pain clinic. Additional studies such as x-ray and EMG are made as indicated, although in most cases these studies have already been completed. A psychological profile including MMPI completes the initial evaluation. At this point the diagnosis can usually be ascertained and treatment begun. If the etiology is still unclear, a differential nerve block is an appropriate next step.

B. The differential block can be performed as a spinal, continuous spinal, or continuous epidural block. An advantage of the continuous techniques is that the patient does not have to lie on his or her side for the entire procedure with a needle in the back. Disadvantages of the epidural technique are slower onset and less clear-cut end points. It should be emphasized that these patients are receiving a central neuraxial block, and the usual monitoring, IV access, and airway resuscitation equipment should be immediately available.

C. Perform the spinal or epidural block in the usual manner. For the spinal technique (noncontinuous), the patient must remain on his or her side with the needle in the subarachnoid space during the entire procedure. All injections should be made with syringes that have the same volume and appearance so that the patient will be unaware of which solution is being used. Test sensation with pinprick, and test sympathetic function with a cutaneous temperature probe or sympathogalvanic response before and 5 minutes after each injection. Whether an epidural or spinal technique is chosen, the initial injection should be with 0.9% saline as a placebo. If the patient gets pain relief with this injection, he or she is considered a placebo responder. This does not rule out an organic etiology, because 30 to 35% of patients whose pain has an organic cause obtain relief with a placebo (p 204). However, the relief is generally temporary. Those who obtain long-lasting pain relief most likely have psychogenic pain.

D. If the patient receives no pain relief with the placebo, inject a low concentration of local anesthetic (0.25% procaine for spinal, 0.5% lidocaine for epidural) to produce a sympathetic block to the painful region. If pain relief occurs after documenting sympathetic block, but with intact sensation, the pain is most likely sympathetic-mediated. This patient may respond to a series of sympathetic blocks.

E. If the patient still has pain after a sympathetic block, inject a higher concentration of local anesthetic (0.5% procaine for spinal, 1% lidocaine for epidural). If pain

TABLE 1 Classification of Nerve Fibers on the Basis of Fiber Size (Relating Fiber Size to Fiber Function and Sensitivity to Local Anesthetics)

Group	*Fiber Diameter*	*Conduction Velocity*	*Modality Subserved*	*Sensitivity to Local Anesthetics (Subarachnoid Procaine)*
A (myelinated)				
Alpha	20 μ	100 mps	Large motor, priopriception (reflex activity)	1%
Beta	20 μ	100 mps	Small motor, touch and pressure	1%
Gamma	20 μ	100 mps	Muscle spindle fibers (muscle tone)	1%
Delta	4 μ	5 mps	Temperature and sharp pain, possibly touch	0.5%
B (myelinated)	3 μ	3–14 mps	Preganglionic autonomic fibers	0.25%
C (unmyelinated)	0.5–1 μ	1.2 mps	Dull pain, temperature, touch (like delta, but slower)	0.5%

mps = meters per second
From Ramamurthy S, Winnie AP. Regional anesthetic techniques for pain relief. Semin Anesth 1985; 4:237; with permission.

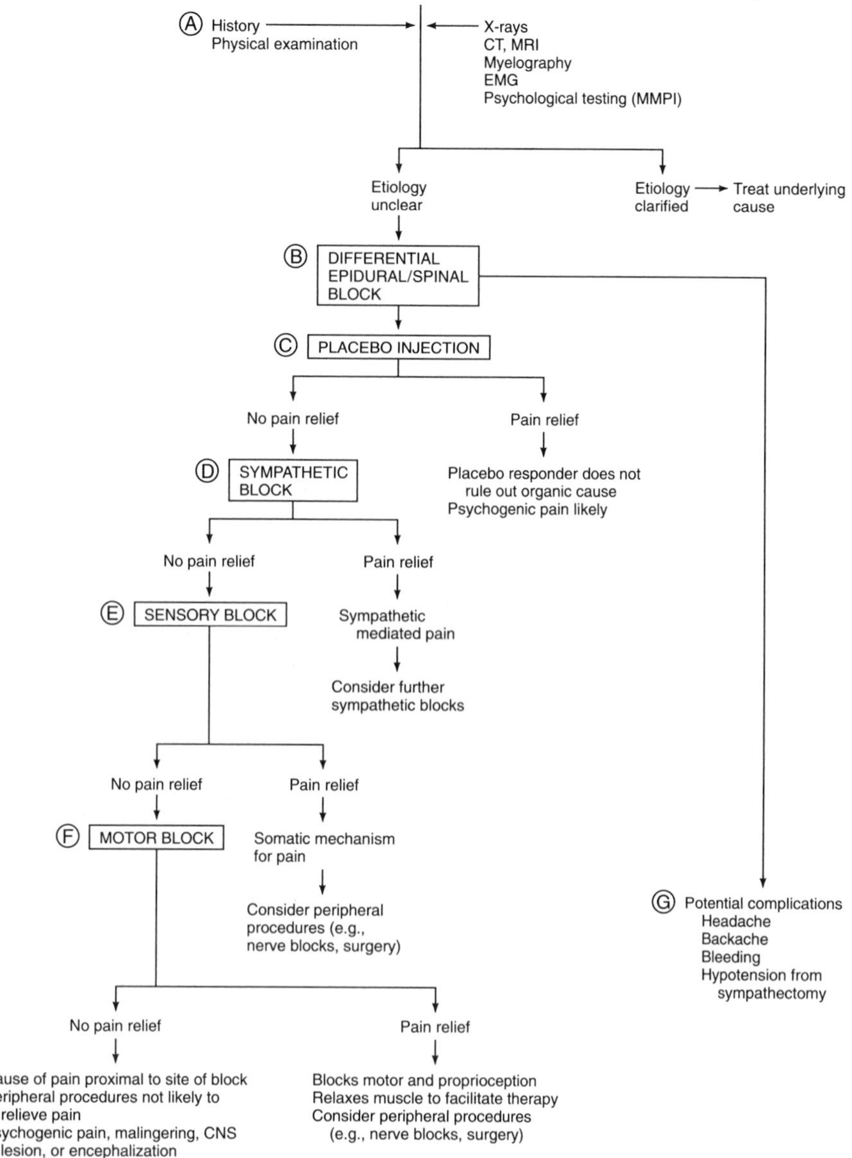

is relieved after loss of sensation to pinprick is documented, a somatic etiology is likely, and the patient may be a candidate for further peripheral nerve blocks or surgery.

F. If pain is not relieved with a sensory block, inject a higher concentration of local anesthetic (1% or higher concentration of procaine for spinal, 2% lidocaine for epidural) to completely block sensory and motor fibers. If pain is relieved, a somatic etiology is likely, and peripheral nerve blocks or surgery may be helpful. If the patient obtains no pain relief with complete somatic nerve block, the etiology of the pain is proximal to the site of the block, and neither peripheral blocks nor surgery will be of benefit. No pain relief with this procedure can occur with a CNS lesion, encephalization, malingering, or psychogenic pain.

G. Complications of the differential epidural/spinal block procedure are the same as for other epidural or spinal procedures. These include headache (most likely from dural puncture), backache, bleeding (including epidural hematoma), and hypotension from sympathectomy. The patient should be informed of these potential complications prior to any block.

References

Gasser HS, Erlanger J. Role of fiber size in establishment of nerve block by pressure or cocaine. Am J Physiol 1929; 88:581.

Raj PP, Ramamurthy S. Differential nerve block studies. In Raj PP, ed. Practical management of pain. Chicago: Year Book, 1988; 173.

Sarnoff SJ, Arrowood JG: Differential spinal block. Surgery 1946; 20:150.

DIAGNOSTIC NEURAL BLOCKADE

William E. Strong, M.D.

Nerve blocks frequently are employed for treatment of painful disorders. However, in many instances, nerve blocks can be useful in making accurate diagnosis and predicting prognosis in various painful disorders. This becomes extremely useful when dealing with a patient whose painful disorder remains undiagnosed after the usual diagnostic work-up. The approach described here has been outlined in detail by Ramamurthy and Winnie.

A. Evaluation of all patients for possible nerve block should include a complete history, physical examination, and indicated laboratory and radiographic studies. A psychological evaluation and MMPI can provide additional insight (p 6). If no obvious etiology for the pain can be ascertained, after the evaluation is completed, consider a diagnostic neural block.

B. A differential epidural/spinal block may help diagnose certain painful disorders, (p 20) but it is limited to pain localized in the lower extremities, lower abdomen, pelvis, and low back. A diagnostic neural block can be applied to pain in any region; in addition, the sympathetic fibers can be blocked separately from the somatic nerve fibers. The results of the diagnostic nerve block can predict whether more permanent interruption of that nerve pathway may result in long-term pain relief.

C. The choice of the site to block is based on the most likely origin of the pain (Table 1). For example, facial pain mediated through the sympathetic nervous system can be blocked by performing a stellate ganglion block; somatic pain associated with trigeminal neuralgia can be blocked at the trigeminal ganglion or at individual branches of the nerve.

D. The initial injection should be a placebo such as 0.9% saline. Pain relief obtained with a placebo does not rule out an organic etiology, because 30 to 35% of patients with an organic source of pain will receive some relief with a placebo injection (p 204). However, most patients who have pain with an organic etiology will receive short-term relief with a placebo, whereas those that obtain long-term relief with a placebo most likely have psychogenic pain.

E. If the patient receives no relief from the placebo injection, the next step is to attempt a sympathetic block. For example, a block of the stellate ganglion will selectively block the sympathetic nerve supply to the head, neck, and upper extremity. This block usually does not result in a somatic nerve block (p 242). Before making any diagnostic decision, it is important to demonstrate successful sympathetic block of the painful region (e.g., increased skin temperature, loss of sympathogalvanic response), while demonstrating an intact sensory nerve supply. If the patient does obtain pain relief with a sympathetic block, additional sympathetic blocks may provide more sustained pain relief.

F. If the patient obtains no pain relief with a sympathetic block, attempt a somatic block of the nerves that supply the painful region. For example, hand pain not relieved with a stellate ganglion block may be relieved with a brachial plexus block or block of an individual peripheral nerve. If the pain is relieved with a somatic nerve block, additional nerve blocks or surgery may be of benefit. Remember that peripheral nerves carry sympathetic and somatic fibers; this emphasizes the need to perform a selective sympathetic block initially to help identify the precise pain mechanism. In addition, in some instances the mechanism is complex and may involve both sympathetic and somatic nerve fibers. If the patient receives no relief with complete sympathetic and somatic block, the pain originates at a site proximal to the level of the block. No pain relief with this procedure can occur with a CNS lesion,

TABLE 1 Procedural Sequence: Differential Diagnostic Nerve Blocks

	Solutions To Be Injected		
Site of Pain	*Saline*	*Sympathetic Local Anesthetic*	*Somatic Local Anesthetic*
Head	Placebo block	Stellate ganglion block	Block C-2, block of trigeminal I, II, III (or branches)
Neck	Placebo block	Stellate ganglion block	Cervical plexus block (or individual nerve)
Arm	Placebo block	Stellate ganglion block	Brachial plexus block (or individual nerve)
Thorax	Placebo block	Dilute thoracic epidural, paravertebral block, intercostal block	Concentrated thoracic epidural, paravertebral block, intercostal block
Abdomen	Placebo block	Celiac plexus block	Paravertebral block, intercostal block
Leg	Placebo block	Lumbar paravertebral sympathetic block	Lumbar paravertebral somatic block (or individual nerve)

From Ramamurthy S, Winnie AP. Regional anesthetic techniques for pain relief. Semin Anesth 1985; 4:237; with permission.

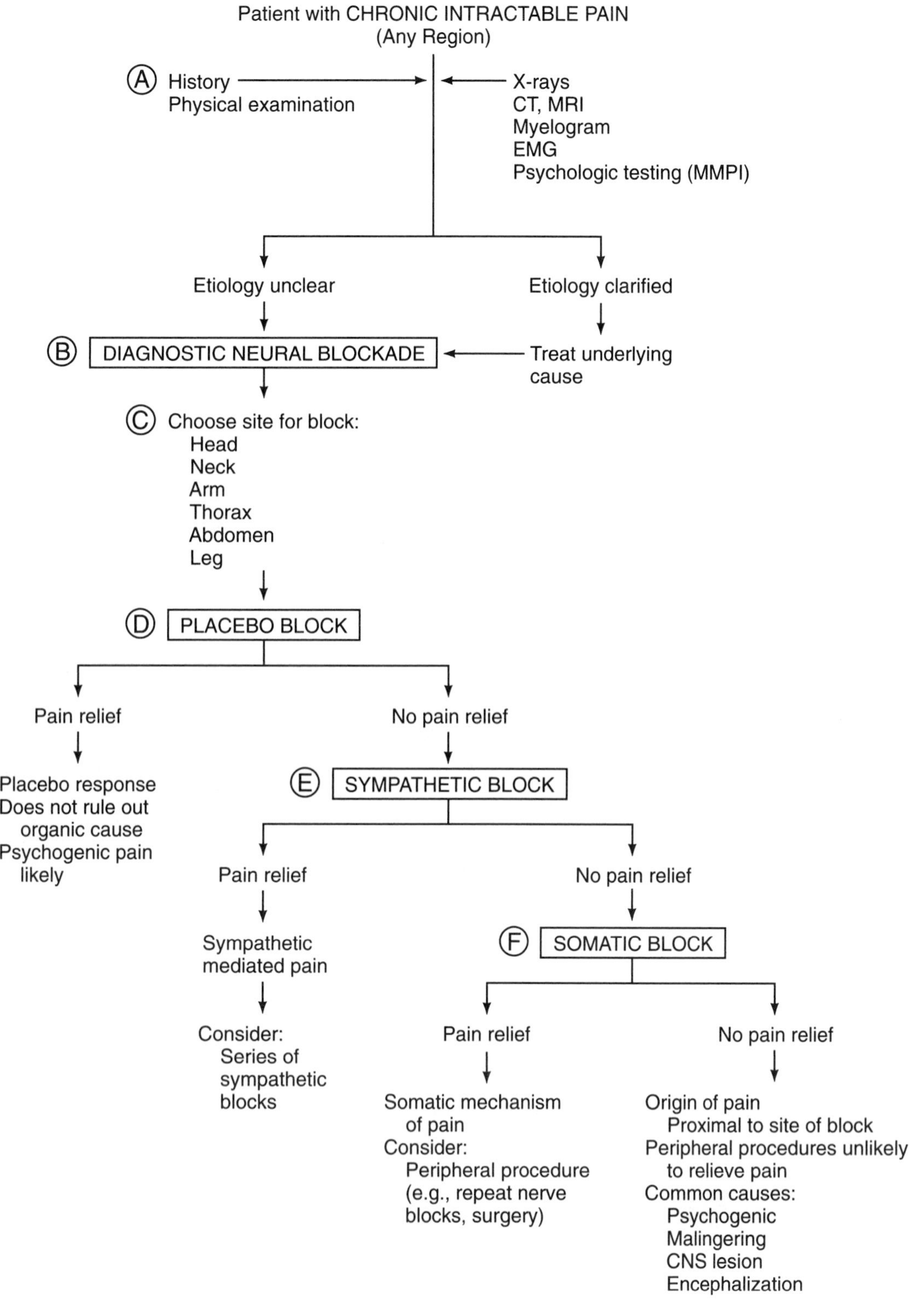

encephalization,* malingering, or psychogenic pain. Further nerve blocks or surgical treatment are unlikely to relieve pain.

*Encephalization is a severe pain, originally noted peripherally, which moves centrally after a prolonged time.

Reference

Ramamurthy S, Winnie AP. Regional anesthetic techniques for pain relief. Semin Anesth 1985; 4:237.

ACUTE PAIN

PATIENT CONTROLLED ANALGESIA

Nancy E. Hambleton, R.N., B.S.N.
James N. Rogers, M.D.

Patient controlled analgesia (PCA) was first reported in the early 1970s and has since become popular across the globe. PCA can bypass the complexities of individual pharmacodynamics and pharmacokinetics that are responsible for interpatient variation in drugs required for pain management. It provides a clear profile of drug dosages needed in each patient to achieve comfort. In addition, PCA allows patients to take an active role in the management of their pain. The goal is a comfortable, nonsedated patient.

A. PCA can be used in IV, subcutaneous (SQ), epidural, or intrathecal drug delivery systems. It has proved successful in managing acute postoperative pain, labor pain, cancer pain, and burn pain. It has been used safely in intensive care and general inpatient and outpatient settings. Even children can be instructed to use the pump to provide pain relief; in the case of very young children, the parents can be instructed to use the PCA pump, which allows them to be part of the pain management team.

B. The advantages of PCA are many. It provides rapid control of severe pain and establishes the hourly dose needed for continuous IV infusion. Plasma concentration is maintained. PCA also eliminates the need for painful intramuscular (IM) injections and requires less nursing time. Individual analgesic consumption remains almost constant, and less drug is required than with IM injections.

C. A disadvantage can be the initial cost in acquiring the PCA pumps. Narcotics given regularly cause side effects regardless of the route of administration. Constipation, nausea, vomiting, sedation, and respiratory depression are most common. Most patients reach a balance between comfort and side effects. When side effects are a major difficulty, they should be aggressively treated.

D. The PCA pump is an infusion device interfaced with a microprocessor connected to a push-button held by the patient that will deliver a predetermined dose of narcotic when pressed. The pump should have the ability to deliver a bolus injection on demand over a baseline continuous infusion. After delivery of a bolus, the device becomes refractory to any further demands for a preset time (lock-out time). All PCA systems have data storage capabilities. A display panel shows how long the system has been in use, the number of doses received, the number of times the button was pushed, and how much medication is left. Security features such as a key and set of code numbers prevent tampering.

E. Patient instruction is crucial for appropriate and optimal use of the PCA pump. Instructions should include information about narcotics (e.g., misconceptions, side effects) and an explanation of realistic expectations for pain relief. When patients have direct control, they should be told how often they can administer the bolus, whether they will receive a dose each time they make an attempt, what the drug is, and what the dosage is. Patients should be told to administer additional medication as soon as the pain returns or increases, or before a painful event such as ambulation. Well-informed patients manage their pain more effectively.

F. An effective protocol, especially useful in managing postoperative pain, begins with an initial IV bolus of morphine titrated to patient comfort over 20 to 30 minutes. At that point the PCA is made available for the patient and connected to an IV access site. In adults, 1 to 2 mg of morphine is made available at each request with a lock-out time of 10 to 15 minutes. After the first 8 hours, the narcotic use is accessed and an hourly narcotic requirement determined. A continuous infusion can then be started with the PCA pump, and bolus IV dosing used for break-through pain.

G. PCA neuraxial analgesia can be provided by either the epidural or subarachnoid route. These routes can be helpful in controlling postoperative pain after thoracic, orthopedic, and abdominal surgery and in managing cancer pain poorly controlled by other methods. Contraindications include spinal abnormalities, infection, bleeding or clotting abnormalities, or lack of patient or family willingness or resources to provide this level of care at home or in a hospice.

References

Forrest WH, Smethurst PWR, Kienetz ME. Self-administration of intravenous analgesics. Anesthesiology 1970; 33:363.

Lehamann KA. Practical experience with demand analgesia for postoperative pain. In: Harmer M, Rosen M, Vickers MD, eds. Patient-controlled analgesia. Oxford: Blackwell, 1985.

Sechzer PH. Studies in pain with the analgesic demand system. Anesth Analg 1971; 50:1.

Tamsen A, Sjoestroem S, Hartvig P. The Uppsala experience of patient-controlled analgesia. In: Foley KM, Inturrisi CE, eds. Advances in pain research and therapy. Vol 8. New York: Raven Press, 1986.

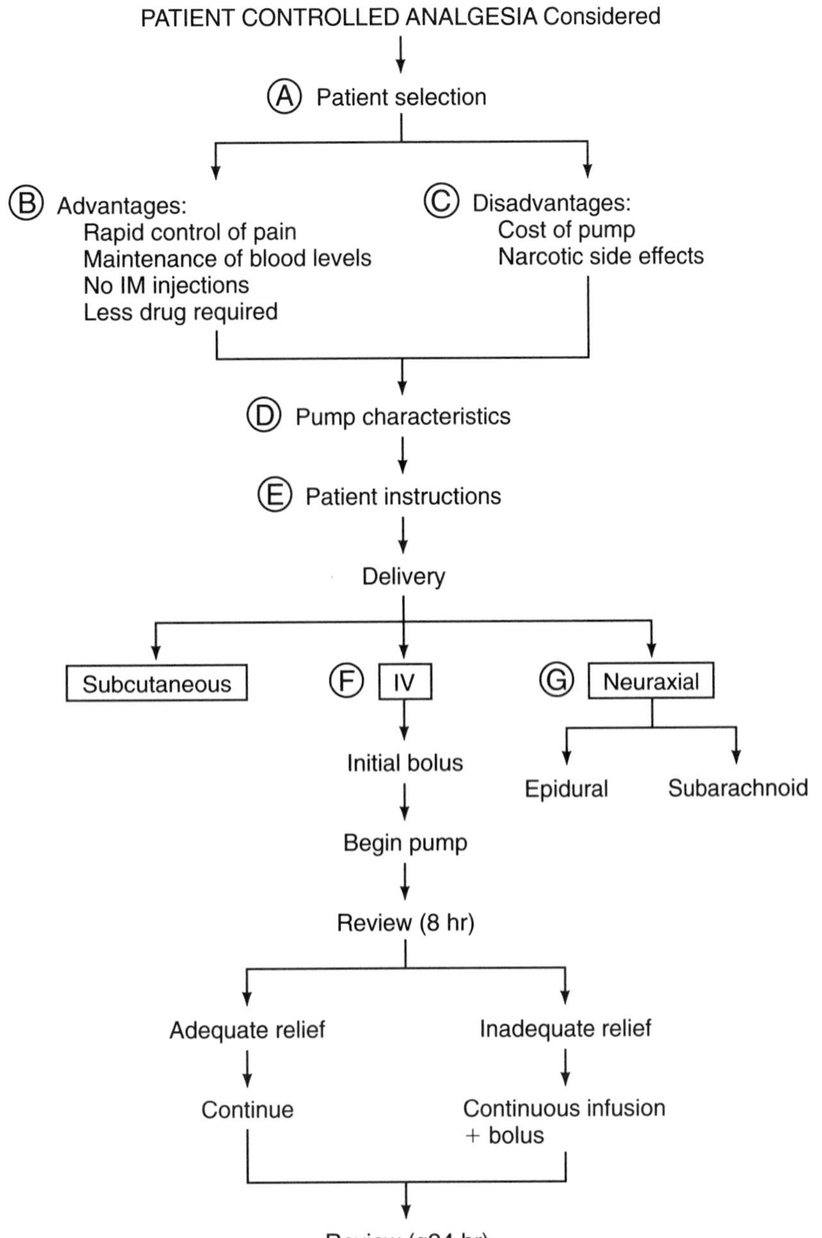
PATIENT CONTROLLED ANALGESIA Considered
(A) Patient selection
(B) Advantages:
Rapid control of pain
Maintenance of blood levels
No IM injections
Less drug required
(C) Disadvantages:
Cost of pump
Narcotic side effects
(D) Pump characteristics
(E) Patient instructions
Delivery
Subcutaneous
(F) IV
(G) Neuraxial
Initial bolus
Begin pump
Review (8 hr)
Epidural
Subarachnoid
Adequate relief
Inadequate relief
Continue
Continuous infusion
+ bolus
Review (q24 hr)

ACUTE HERPES ZOSTER

Robert Sprague, M.D.

Herpes zoster (HZ) is a common problem seen in the pain management clinic. It is a debilitating pain syndrome that may be difficult to diagnose and may lead to the chronic problem of postherpetic neuralgia (PHN). HZ is a reactivation of the varicella virus, causing intense hemorrhagic inflammation in the dorsal root ganglion extending to the peripheral nerve. Basically the disease afflicts the immunocompromised (i.e., the young and the elderly). Children <2 years of age make up 5 to 8% of cases, whereas patients 50 to 70 years old make up 40% of cases. PHN is primarily a disease of patients over 50 years of age.

A. A thorough history and physical examination are important in delineating the dermatomal levels involved (Table 1); they also may uncover the underlying cause of the immunodeficiency, such as an undiagnosed malignancy.

B. Ocular HZ may lead to blindness and should be treated by an ophthalmologist. A stellate ganglion block may be helpful (p 242).

C. Although somewhat arbitrary, 2 months postvesicular eruption is used to differentiate PHN and HZ. This is extremely important in devising treatment modalities.

D. Therapeutic interventions are aimed at pain relief and prevention of PHN.

E. Analgesia is of the utmost concern to the patient, as this syndrome is extremely painful. Oral narcotics combined with NSAIDs may provide relief. This modality, however, will not prevent the onset of PHN. In clinical trials, oral or intralesional steroids have been shown to decrease pain and possibly prevent PHN.

F. Antiviral agents such as acyclovir decrease the pain of HZ and speed lesion healing but have no effect on the prevention of PHN.

G. Sympathetic block definitely provides pain relief and speeds healing in the treatment of HZ, but its role in the prevention of PHN is open to debate. The preponderance of positive clinical experience and relatively low risk in this procedure sways one toward employing this therapy if the patient is seen early in the course of the disease.

H. Adjuvant therapy such as transcutaneous electrical nerve stimulation (TENS) and topical agents such as lidocaine or aspirin/chloroform mixtures have had limited success.

TABLE 1 Dermatomal Distribution of Herpes Zoster

Cranial (includes trigeminal nerve)	25%
Cervical	12%
Thoracic	55%
Lumbar	14%
Sacral	3%
Generalized	1%

References

Eaglestein WH, et al. The effects of early corticosteroid therapy on the skin eruption and pain of herpes zoster. JAMA 1970; 211:168.

Epstein E. Corticosteroid therapy of zoster: Oral vs sublesional injection. Hawaii Med J 1982; 41:420.

Portenoy RK, et al. Acute herpes zoster and postherpetic neuralgia: Clinical review and current management. Ann Neurol 1986; 20:1.

Portenoy RK, et al. Postherpetic neuralgia: A workable treatment plan. Geriatrics 1986; 41:34.

Watson CP. Postherpetic neuralgia: Postmortem analysis of a case. Pain 1988; 34:129.

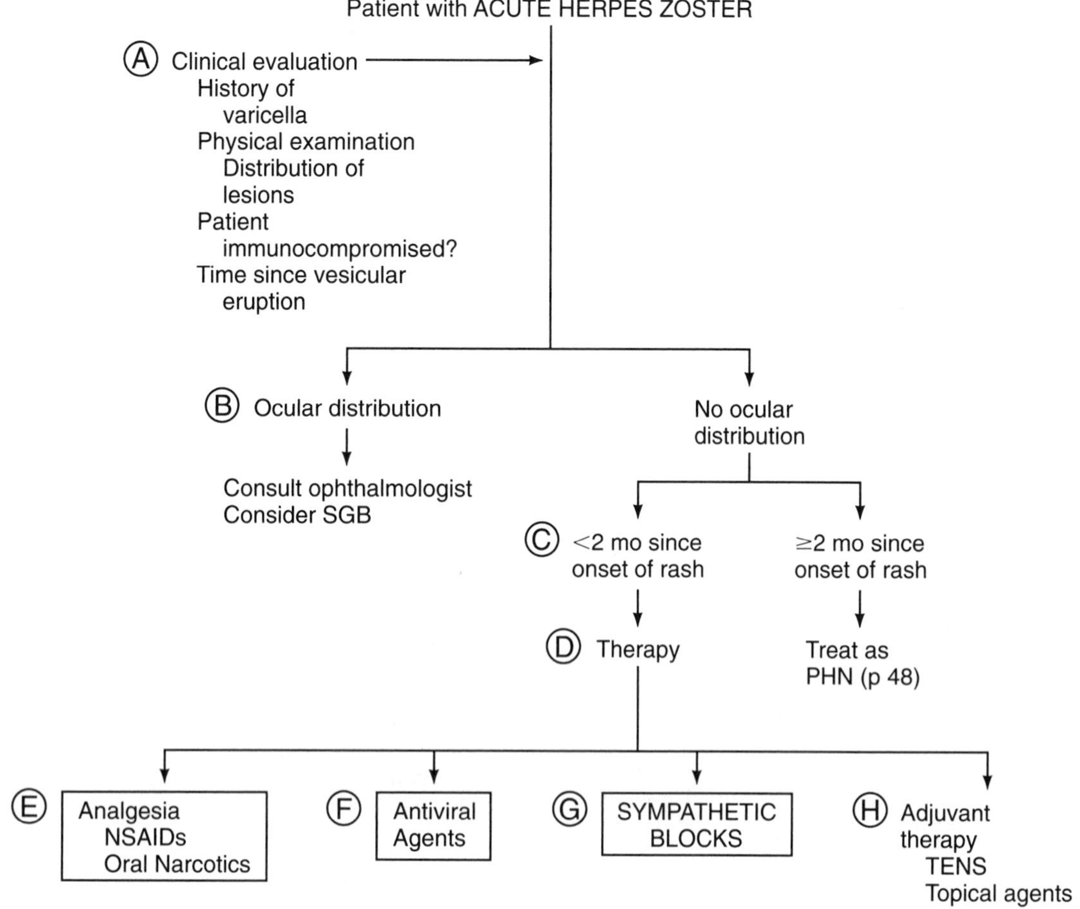

Patient with ACUTE HERPES ZOSTER
Ⓐ Clinical evaluation
History of varicella
Physical examination
Distribution of lesions
Patient immunocompromised?
Time since vesicular eruption
Ⓑ Ocular distribution
Consult ophthalmologist
Consider SGB
No ocular distribution
Ⓒ <2 mo since onset of rash
≥2 mo since onset of rash
Ⓓ Therapy
Treat as PHN (p 48)
Ⓔ Analgesia
NSAIDs
Oral Narcotics
Ⓕ Antiviral Agents
Ⓖ SYMPATHETIC BLOCKS
Ⓗ Adjuvant therapy
TENS
Topical agents

ACUTE UPPER EXTREMITY PAIN

Mary Ann Gurkowski, M.D.

Most acute upper extremity pain is secondary to trauma or limb ischemia, including bone fractures, lacerations, abrasions, puncture wounds, and embolism. Regional anesthetic techniques and analgesic medications are the mainstays of treatment of acute upper extremity pain.

A. The choice of upper extremity blocks should depend on the innervation to the injured area and the location of the injury. The choice of blocks includes brachial plexus block, musculocutaneous nerve block, suprascapular nerve block, radial nerve block, ulnar nerve block, median nerve block, and digital nerve block. The brachial plexus can be blocked by one of four approaches: interscalene, supraclavicular, infraclavicular, and axillary (p 260).

B. The primary indication for performing these blocks is to relieve pain. This makes the patient much more comfortable and cooperative for manipulation, cleansing, and splinting or casting of the arm. Other indications include the desire for sympathectomy or motor blockade. Sympathectomy enhances blood flow to the injured area. The advantage of nerve blocks is that pain relief is applied only to the affected area. Unless systemic medications are given, the patient is usually much more alert and cooperative.

C. Contraindications (relative and absolute) to regional blocks include patient refusal, infection at the site of needle insertion, coagulopathy, nerve injury, and compartment syndrome. The disadvantage is that it requires patient cooperation and can be painful to administer. The risk of compartment syndrome may also be a disadvantage.

D. The primary complications of regional blocks include intravascular injection, seizures, failed block, local anesthetic toxicity, nerve injury, infection, and bleeding. The risk of intravascular injection can be reduced if epinephrine (1:200,000) is used in the local anesthetic, a test dose is given, the total dose is injected incrementally, and aspiration is performed before injection.

E. The other methods of pain relief that can be used include patient controlled analgesia (p 26), timed IV, or as needed oral, intramuscular (IM), or IV pain medications. These medications may include sedatives, narcotics, NSAIDs, and mixed agonist/antagonist drugs. Contraindications to pain medications include a history of allergic reaction, and patient refusal. Disadvantages include the risk of oversedation, respiratory depression, and incomplete pain relief. IM injections take approximately 20 to 30 minutes to become effective and are painful when administered. The complications of pain medications include overdosage, administration of the wrong drug, anaphylactic reaction, respiratory depression, and nausea/vomiting.

References

Blumberg H, Griessen HJ, Hornyak ME: Mechanisms and role of peripheral blood flow dysregulation in pain sensation and edema. In Stanton-Hicks M, Jänig W, Boas RN eds: Reflex sympathetic dystrophy, Boston, 1989, Kluwer Academic.

Dolene VV: Contemporary treatment of peripheral nerve and brachial plexus lesions, Neuro Surg Rev 9:149, 1986.

Wall PD: The prevention of postoperative pain (editorial) PAIN, 33:289, 1988.

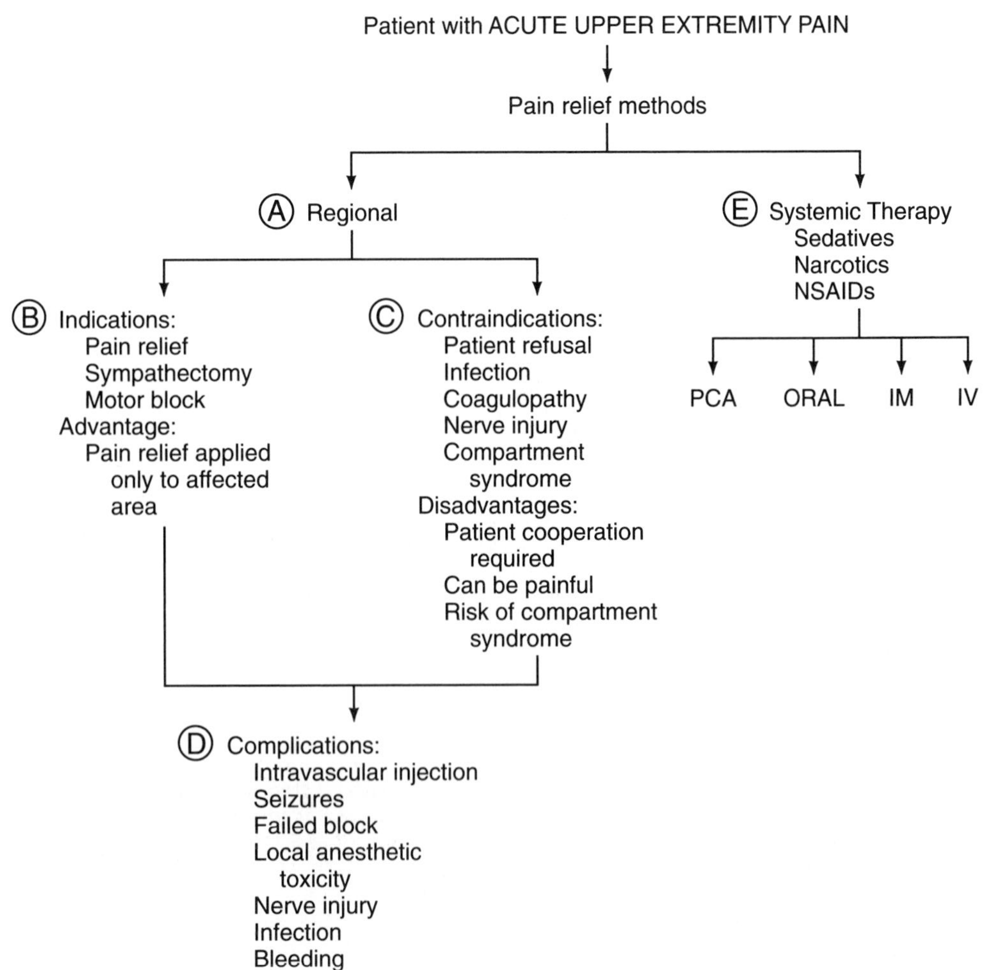
Patient with ACUTE UPPER EXTREMITY PAIN
Pain relief methods
Ⓐ Regional
Ⓑ Indications:
Pain relief
Sympathectomy
Motor block
Advantage:
Pain relief applied only to affected area
Ⓒ Contraindications:
Patient refusal
Infection
Coagulopathy
Nerve injury
Compartment syndrome
Disadvantages:
Patient cooperation required
Can be painful
Risk of compartment syndrome
Ⓓ Complications:
Intravascular injection
Seizures
Failed block
Local anesthetic toxicity
Nerve injury
Infection
Bleeding
Ⓔ Systemic Therapy
Sedatives
Narcotics
NSAIDs
PCA
ORAL
IM
IV

ACUTE LOWER EXTREMITY PAIN

Kelly Gordon Knape, M.D.

The management of acute lower extremity pain is similar to that of other forms of acute pain. It is important to determine the cause or source of the discomfort and treat that as well as the symptom. Lower extremity pain, especially musculoskeletal pain, is one of the most common complaints. Fractures are among the most common acute causes of moderate to severe pain; tibia-fibula fractures are common in young, active patients and femoral neck fractures more common in those >50 years. New complaints are not always acute, so chronic or systemic disease must also be considered.

A. The history should be complete in order to rule out systemic as well as local causes. Destructive arthritides should be considered if the joint pain has lasted >1 month. Vascular insufficiency manifests as crescendo muscle pain during exercise. Onset, duration, intensity, and quality of pain should be very specific. Difficulty in localizing pain can mean involvement of deep structures but may also suggest something chronic. Earlier use of analgesics should be noted. Previous self-treatment is often a factor and gives preliminary information about treatment efficacy, but it also may mask the intensity of pain as well as other symptoms such as fever. Referred pain may actually be the presenting symptom, as in ipsilateral knee pain with primary hip pathology. Consult specialists (rheumatologist, orthopedist, vascular surgeon) to confirm or assist in diagnosis, treatment, and follow-up.

B. Further evaluation involves a complete physical examination, including close scrutiny of the site of the pain. Always compare with the unaffected extremity. Note induration, erythema, swelling, and edema. Palpation evaluates firmness and crepitance as well as eliciting or accentuating the pain. Especially with underlying fractures, consider hidden blood loss and compartment syndrome, especially if regional anesthetic block is to be used. The neurologic status, including areas of hypo- or hyperalgesia and associated weakness, must also be determined. Assess passive and active range of motion (ROM) as well as weightbearing and effect on ambulation.

C. Clinical testing includes radiographic evaluation and blood studies. Radiographic views assess such factors as extension, rotation, abduction, and adduction. Use views of the unaffected side for comparison. Elevated WBC counts, especially with fever, suggest infection. Additional serologic tests (rheumatoid factor, sedimentation rate) may be necessary. Aspirate synovial joint fluid for analysis in patients with isolated joint complaints for evidence of infection, arthritis, or gout.

D. Once pain is no longer useful as a means of evaluation, initiate analgesia immediately; this facilitates additional evaluation. For example, evaluation of a joint with passive ROM becomes easier when a regional anesthetic block is in place because of both pain relief and muscle relaxation. Immobilization using a form of traction, splinting, or casting is then initiated as therapy, or as a temporizing measure until surgery.

E. Regional anesthesia for manipulation or surgery can provide postoperative analgesia and other potential benefits, although compartment syndrome must always be anticipated. If a long-acting agent such as bupivacaine is used for major nerve block, analgesia can persist for approximately 12 hours. Continuous epidural infusions can be maintained for several days using a narcotic, a local anesthetic, or both. Local anesthetics provide sympathectomy to optimize perfusion and minimize embolic complications, although orthostasis can occur and high concentrations may affect ambulation. A patient controlled analgesia (PCA) device can also be connected to an epidural catheter. Epidural or intrathecal administration of preservative-free morphine provides approximately 24 hours of superior relief; the common side effects of pruritus and urinary retention are easily managed. Postoperative epidural analgesia can reduce perioperative pulmonary complications in high-risk patients.

F. Joint infiltration is an effective alternative for analgesia, especially for outpatients undergoing knee arthroscopy. Infiltration of 30 ml 0.5% bupivacaine can reduce the additional need for analgesics and promotes mobilization; injection of 0.5 to 1.0 mg of morphine may also be effective.

G. Administration of parenteral narcotics is most efficacious when a PCA device is used. PCA pumps afford the patient some control and independence. A "background" infusion can be added. Transdermal fentanyl is another sustained narcotic alternative. Balanced analgesia can be provided by adding IM or oral NSAIDs to act peripherally and potentially reduce narcotic requirements. The partial opioid agonists (buprenorphine and dezocine) can be used with efficacy similar to that of morphine, with a ceiling for side effects. Adjunctive agents such as promethazine can potentiate analgesia and reduce nausea, but sedation may result. Tricyclic antidepressants (TCAs) or clonidine given at bedtime can facilitate sleep as well as analgesia.

H. Conservative therapies are generally the simplest but usually less effective. Immobilization and positioning can alleviate some pain, and with elevation may reduce swelling. Additional analgesia is often necessary to initiate ambulation early to prevent problems such as stiff or "frozen" joint, reflex sympathetic dystrophy, weakness, or deep venous thrombosis and potential emboli. Cryotherapy using fluoromethane or ethylchloride spray or the application of ice packs is also helpful. Transcutaneous electrical nerve stimulation (TENS) and acupuncture have also been used.

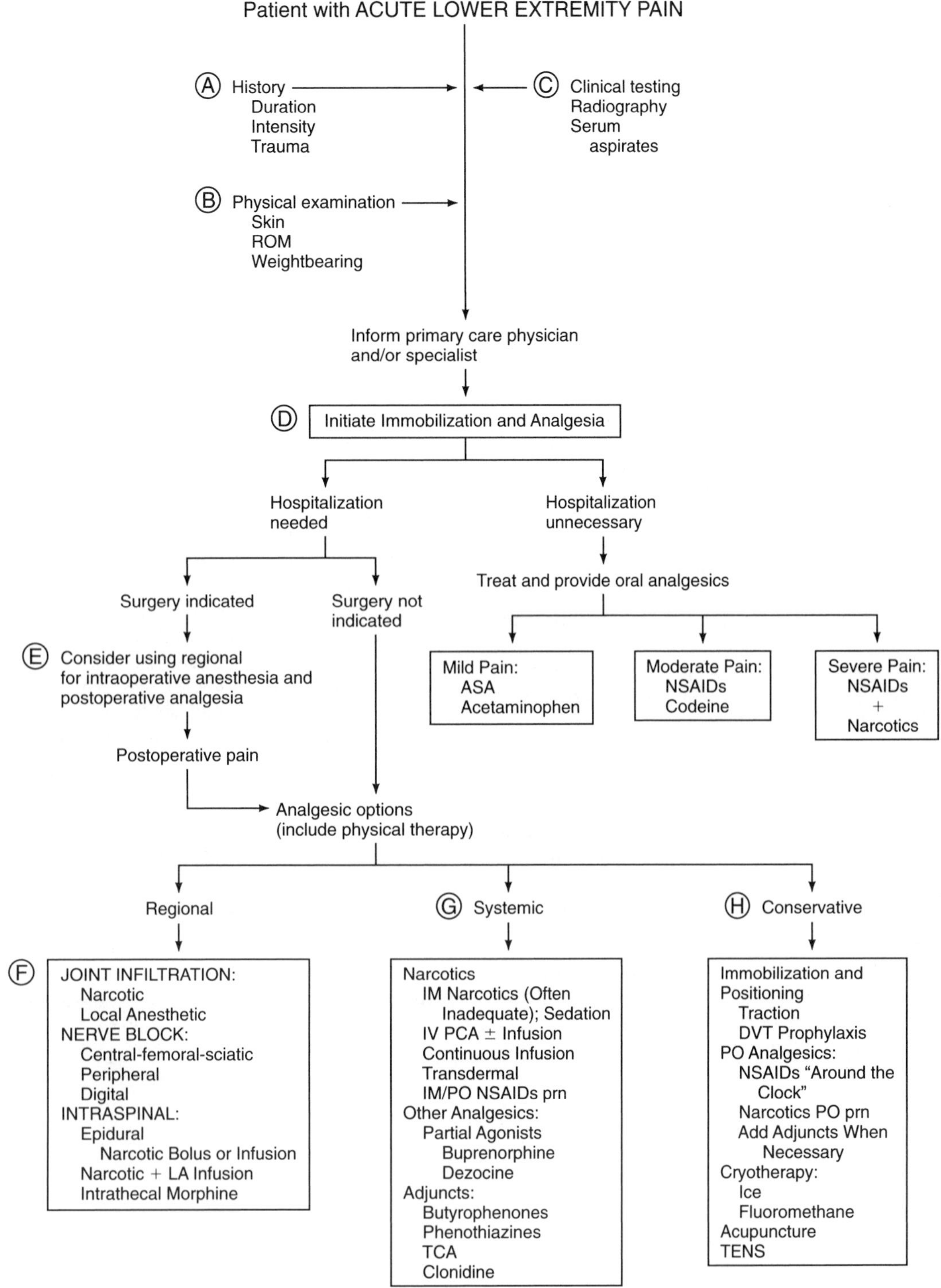

References

Bonica JJ. General considerations of acute pain. In: Bonica JJ, ed. The management of pain. 2nd ed. Philadelphia: Lea & Febiger, 1990:163.

Ferrante FM, Ostheimer GW, Covino BG, eds. Patient-controlled analgesia. Boston: Blackwell Scientific Publications, 1990.

Modig J, Borg T, Karistrom G, et al. Thromboembolism after total hip replacement: Role of epidural and general anesthesia. Anesth Analg 1983; 62:174.

Smith I, Van Hemeirijck J, White PF, Shively R. Effects of local anesthesia on recovery after outpatient arthroscopy. Anesth Analg 1991; 73:536–539.

Stein C, Comisel K, Haimerl E, et al. Analgesic effect of intra-articular morphine after arthroscopic knee surgery. N Engl J Med 1991; 325:1123.

Yeager M. Outcome of pain management. In: Benumof JL, ed. Management of postoperative pain. Philadelphia: WB Saunders, 1989:246.

ACUTE THORACIC PAIN

John D. Merwin, M.D.

There are many causes of acute thoracic pain and most are easily diagnosed. Occasionally the cause is difficult to identify, especially since the afferent nerves of the heart, aorta, esophagus, lungs, and chest wall share a common pathway in the spinal cord, and lesions may cause similar pain. Acute thoracic pain should be treated only after a diagnosis has been made, so that the resultant analgesia does not affect the clinical assessment of the disease.

A. A thorough history and physical examination are crucial for identifying the source of the pain. The history should focus on speed of onset, site, radiation, quality, and intensity of pain. It is important to identify factors that aggravate or alleviate the pain, such as breathing, feeding, positioning, or exercising. A history of sharp aggravation of pain with deep breathing or coughing usually indicates pleura, pericardium, or chest wall disorders. Associated symptoms such as palpitations, dyspnea, coughing, expectoration, hemoptysis, nausea, vomiting, and gaseous distention of abdominal organs help to indicate the correct diagnosis. Laboratory tests, electrocardiography, and imaging studies may prove helpful.

B. Life-threatening conditions such as acute myocardial infarction should be managed in an intensive care unit with either medical or surgical intervention. Pain secondary to an infectious process is best treated by antimicrobial agents, surgical drainage, or both.

C. Visceral chest pain may occur from the esophagus, myocardium, trachea, bronchi, pericardium, pulmonary arteries, and aorta, in descending order of frequency. Visceral pain is usually poorly localized, vague, colicky, cramping, aching, and squeezing and often referred and associated with internal factors. This intensity and quality of the stimulus are important. Systemic narcotics or cervicothoracic sympathetic blockade of the visceral afferent neurons may provide pain relief.

D. Acute lateral chest wall pain suggests muscle injury or rib fracture, although pulmonary embolism or pneumothorax must be ruled out. Segmental pain with vesicles suggests acute herpes zoster (p 28). Postoperative pain from mastectomy or thoracotomy may be severe. Systemic or epidural narcotics can provide analgesia. Intercostal (p 252), paravertebral (p 254), or interpleural nerve blocks (p 250) should be considered. Inflammatory reactions such as costochondritis respond well to NSAIDs.

E. Sudden acute chest pain may cause significant anxiety, apprehension, and fear, especially in patients who believe they are having a heart attack. Emotional reactions should be carefully assessed and treated aggressively. Acute anxiety attacks, depression, conversion reactions, and hypochondriasis can be primary causes of thoracic pain. The exclusion of any systemic organic pathology and the presence of psychological factors help confirm that there is a psychological cause of thoracic pain.

References

Conacher ID. Pain relief after thoracotomy. Br J Anaesth 1990; 65:806.

Cousins MJ. Acute pain and the injury response: Immediate and prolonged effects. Reg Anesth 1989; 14:162.

Ramamurthy S. Thoracic and low back pain. In: Raj PP, ed. Practical management of pain. Chicago, Year Book, 1986:470.

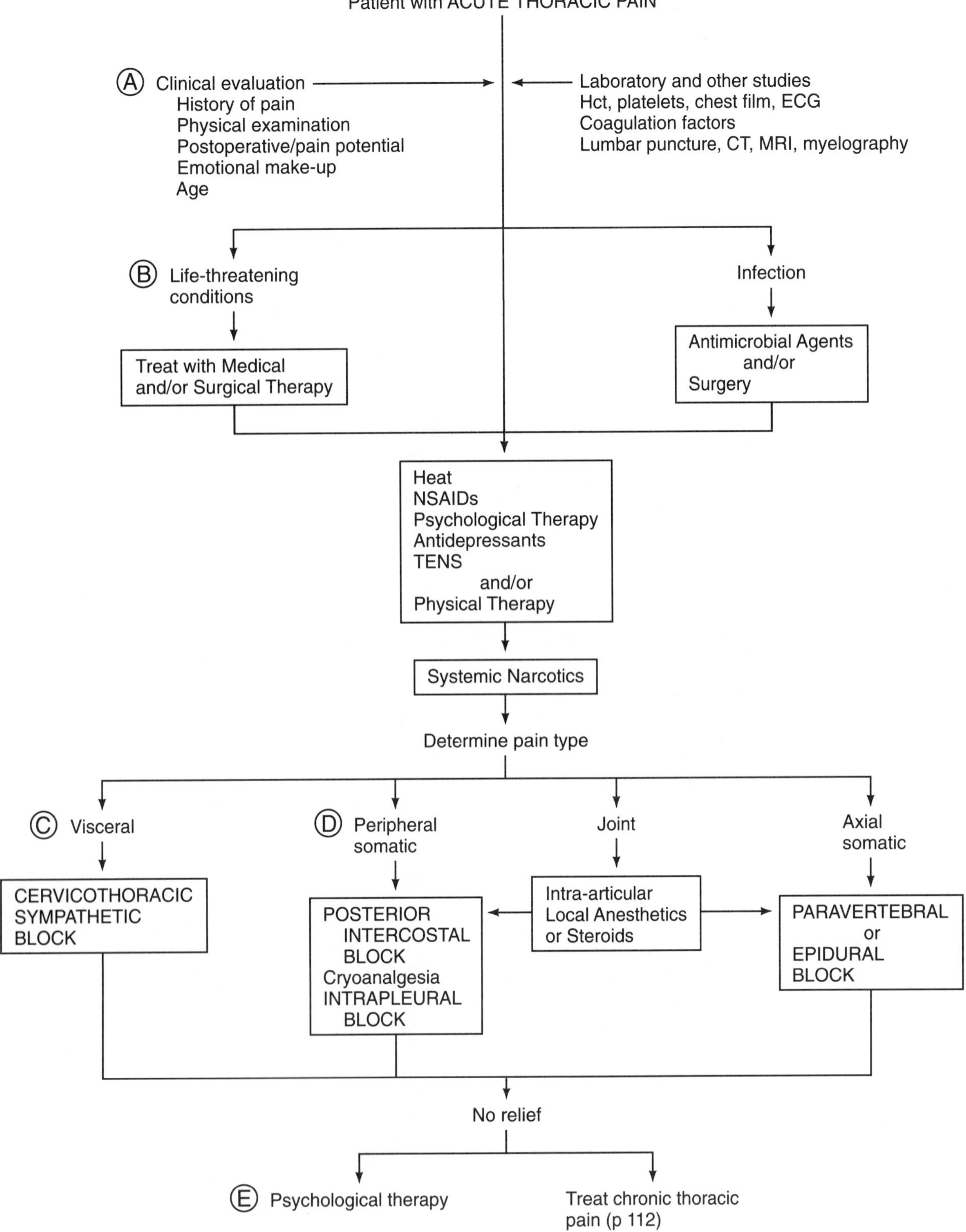
Patient with ACUTE THORACIC PAIN
(A) Clinical evaluation
History of pain
Physical examination
Postoperative/pain potential
Emotional make-up
Age
Laboratory and other studies
Hct, platelets, chest film, ECG
Coagulation factors
Lumbar puncture, CT, MRI, myelography
(B) Life-threatening conditions
Treat with Medical and/or Surgical Therapy
Infection
Antimicrobial Agents and/or Surgery
Heat
NSAIDs
Psychological Therapy
Antidepressants
TENS
and/or
Physical Therapy
Systemic Narcotics
Determine pain type
(C) Visceral
CERVICOTHORACIC SYMPATHETIC BLOCK
(D) Peripheral somatic
POSTERIOR INTERCOSTAL BLOCK
Cryoanalgesia
INTRAPLEURAL BLOCK
Joint
Intra-articular Local Anesthetics or Steroids
Axial somatic
PARAVERTEBRAL or EPIDURAL BLOCK
No relief
(E) Psychological therapy
Treat chronic thoracic pain (p 112)

ACUTE ABDOMINAL PAIN

Kelly Gordon Knape, M.D.

Discomfort in the abdomen is common. It usually arises from the viscera or the parietal peritoneum, yet referred pain from intrathoracic disease is also common, making differential diagnosis difficult. Referred pain may be experienced in the skin and body wall, as in inguinal and testicular pain from ureteral stones. True visceral pain is early, dull and aching, vague, diffuse, and difficult to pinpoint, although usually described as being in the midline and deep despite the location of the involved organ. Visceral pain is due to spasm of the smooth muscles of hollow organs; contraction against an obstruction; sudden or extensive stretch of the organ or its capsule; inflammation or ischemia; chemical or mechanical irritation of inflamed membranes; stretch, traction, or twisting of the mesentery and/or ligaments or vessels; and necrosis.

Parietal pain is sharp and sometimes stabbing, and may be localized or referred. Both sources are accompanied by reflex guarding, tenderness, hyperalgesia, and (when severe) nausea and/or vomiting. Sympathetic stimulation including sweating, or vagal stimulation with bradycardia, is also possible.

A. The history should be complete in order to rule out systemic as well as extra-abdominal disease, such as diabetes, uremia, porphyria, sickle crisis, black widow spider bite, lead poisoning, lower rib fractures or dislocation of costochondral cartilages, acute myocardial infarction, pulmonary embolism, pneumothorax, tabes, spinal cord compression, herpetic problems, and psychological disorders. Duration is important: severe pain lasting longer than 6 hours in a previously healthy patient is an "acute abdomen" and needs immediate diagnosis and possible surgical intervention. Onset should be classified as sudden (rupture, perforation, embolism), rapid (acute inflammation, colic, torsion, obstruction, toxic or metabolic disease), or gradual (chronic inflammation, ectopic pregnancy, tumor, infarct). Quality is described as sharp (cutaneous or somatic, including nerve root compression), burning (neuralgia, upper GI inflammation of mucous membranes), tearing (dissecting aortic aneurysm, anal fissure), and vague (visceral disease). Temporal features (continuous: peritonitis, colicky stones, or hernia; constant: cancer, migratory, emotional), factors that aggravate or relieve, relation to other body functions (menstruation, defecation), and associated signs and symptoms (nausea, diarrhea, segmental distribution, spasm of rectus, abdominal distention) are also noted and must be specific. Menstrual history is taken in all women. Any previous use of analgesics and other medications for associated symptoms is also documented. Earlier therapies may mask the intensity of pain and other symptoms such as fever. Consult appropriate specialties (internal medicine, ob/gyn, general surgery) to confirm or assist in diagnosis, treatment, and follow-up.

B. A complete physical examination is essential. Vital signs can suggest sepsis (fever, tachycardia, hypotension). Any distention or hernia, stillness (peritonitis) or restlessness (ureteral stones), and concomitant sweating and/or pallor should be noted. Gently palpate, noting guarding (voluntary or involuntary) and the presence of rebound pain. Percussion detects organomegaly, ascites (fluid wave), or masses. Careful auscultation notes silence or hyperperistalsis. Perform a rectal and/or pelvic examination unless a specialist is available.

C. Clinical testing requires blood and urine sampling as well as radiography. Serum electrolyte as well as urine ketone and specific gravity tests suggest the degree of dehydration. Elevated WBC counts, especially with fever, suggest infection, and low hematocrit suggests nonacute blood loss. Sample stool for occult blood. X-rays films should include not only the chest but also abdominal views. ECG is also helpful. Additional tests include peritoneal lavage (trauma) and CT scan.

D. If pain is not useful for evaluation, initiate analgesia immediately. This may facilitate additional evaluation, especially that requiring patient cooperation. Nausea may be caused by pain, and adequate relief may treat it. Analgesics, especially narcotics, do not mask pertinent findings, and a "constipating" effect may relieve pain secondary to peristalsis. Immobilization may offer temporary relief. Hydration must also be initiated early and vital signs monitored. Respiratory therapy should be started early and is used to estimate the effectiveness of analgesia.

E. Infiltration of a local anesthetic (LA) by the surgeon or anesthetist at the end of the procedure is an effective alternative to analgesia, especially in outpatients (e.g., wound infiltration for inguinal herniorrhaphy). A long-acting agent such as bupivacaine can reduce the need for analgesics and promote mobilization.

F. Regional anesthesia can provide postoperative analgesia and other potential benefits. Continuous epidural infusions can be maintained for several days with a narcotic, LA, or both. An LA provides sympathectomy to optimize perfusion, although orthostasis can occur and high concentrations may affect ambulation. Intraspinal narcotics by epidural or intrathecal routes are effective, especially for visceral pain. Adding narcotic to LA can improve the quality of analgesia, especially for mobilization and cough, and reduces the dosage of each required. Recommended dosages include 0.03125 to 0.0625% bupivacaine with 2 to 5 μg/ml fentanyl, to run at 0.5 to 1.5 μg/kg/hr. A patient controlled analgesia (PCA) device can be connected to an epidural catheter. Epidural or intrathecal administration of preservative-free morphine provides approximately 24 hours of superior relief; the common side effects of pruritus and urinary retention are easily

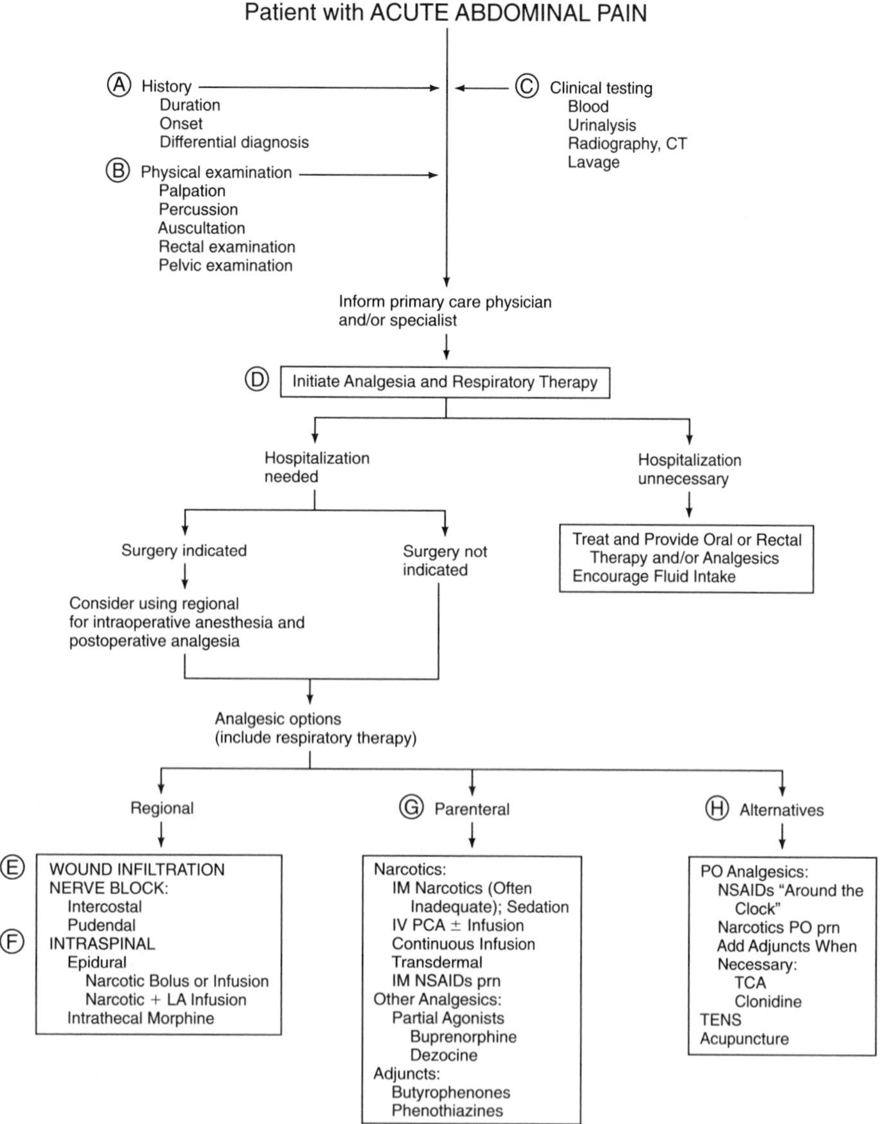

managed. Doses are 0.05 mg/kg and 0.002 to 0.005 mg/kg, respectively. Addition of fentanyl (100 μg) or sufentanil (10–30 μg) can speed the slow onset of epidural morphine. Postoperative epidural analgesia can reduce perioperative pulmonary complications in high-risk patients.

G. Administration of parenteral narcotics is most efficacious when a PCA device is used. PCA pumps provide the patient with some control and independence. A "background" infusion can be added. Transdermal fentanyl is another sustained narcotic alternative. "Balanced analgesia" can be provided by adding NSAIDs to reduce narcotic requirements. The partial opioid agonists can be used with efficacy similar to that of morphine, with a ceiling for side effects. Adjunctive agents such as promethazine can potentiate analgesia and reduce nausea, but sedation may result.

H. Oral adjuncts can be added (tricyclic antidepressants [TCAs] or clonidine), which when given at bedtime can improve sleep and provide analgesia. TENS and acupuncture have also been used.

References

Bonica JJ. General considerations of acute pain. In: Bonica JJ, Loeser JD, Chapman CR, Fordyce WE, eds. The management of pain. 2nd ed. Philadelphia: Lea & Febiger, 1990: 1146.

Dahl JB, Kehlet H. Non-steroidal anti-inflammatory drugs: Rationale for use in severe postoperative pain. Br J Anaesth 1991; 66:703.

Dahl JB, Rosenberg J, Hanssen BL, et al. Differential analgesic effects of low-dose epidural morphine and morphine-bupivacaine at rest and during mobilization after major abdominal surgery. Anesth Analg 1992; 74:362.

Gwirtz KH. Intraspinal narcotics in the management of postoperative pain. Anesthesiol Rev 1990; 17:17.

Sinatra RS, Sevarine FB, Chung JH, et al. Comparisons of epidurally administered sufentanil, morphine, and sufentanil-morphine combination for postoperative analgesia. Anesth Analg 1991: 72:522.

Yamaguchi H, Watanabe S, Motokawa K, et al. Intrathecal morphine dose-response data for pain relief after cholecystectomy. Anesth Analg 1990; 70:168.

ACUTE PANCREATITIS

Robert Sprague, M.D.

Acute pancreatitis (AP) is a relatively common disease, and anesthesiologists may be consulted for pain management of this malady. In the United States, AP is usually related to excessive alcohol ingestion, but it also may be secondary to gallstones, trauma, or metabolic disorders or may be induced iatrogenically via drugs. The abdominal pain occurring in this disease is often incapacitating and may be severe enough to lead to respiratory failure.

A. Medical intervention, in which the anesthesiologist is usually not directly involved, is directed at pancreatic rest via nasogastric suctioning, intravenous hydration, and correction of metabolic and physiologic disruptions. Narcotic analgesics are often part of the treatment regimen.

B. Celiac plexus block (CPB) may be performed to alleviate the severe pain of this malady (p 246). Not only is pain relief obtained, but also the course of the disease may be altered. Spasm of the ducts and sphincters of the pancreas is believed to be the source of the pain in AP. A CPB with local anesthetic solutions combined with methylprednisolone has been shown to decrease the severity of the attack, presumably by releasing ductal pressures. The block should be performed with 20 to 25 cc of 0.25% bupivacaine per side, mixed with 80 to 160 mg of methylprednisolone in depot form. Before CPB is performed, it is extremely important to evaluate fully the physical status of the patient and his or her ability to withstand the physical stress of the block. These patients are often hypovolemic secondary to the disease process, and the hypotension caused by the sympatholysis of CPB may be hazardous. Therefore, full monitoring of the patient, including blood pressures, should be done during the block. These patients also may manifest a low-grade disseminated intravascular coagulopathy, along with respiratory embarrassment secondary to splinting of the chest wall and pleural effusions. Pancreatic ascites may also be present, making the prone position necessary for CPB difficult.

C. Continuous epidural blockade relieves the pain of AP in a fashion similar to CPB, with the relief of ductal spasm. The hazards of placing an epidural catheter in a patient with low-grade DIC must be appreciated. The risk of epidural abscess must also be realized, as these patients are often bacteremic. If performed, the regimen should consist of 7 to 10 days of daily injections with 10 cc of 0.25% bupivacaine through a catheter placed near the twelfth thoracic vertebra, as the sympathetic input to the celiac plexus arises near this level.

D. Psychological evaluation and management of substance abuse must be part of the treatment program. Obviously, alcohol abuse must be treated, or the entire cycle will be repeated. The patient must also be evaluated for chronic oral narcotic addiction.

References

Bridenbaugh PO, Cousins MJ. Neural blockade in clinical anesthesia and management of pain. 2nd ed. Philadelphia: JB Lippincott, 1988.

Greenberger NJ, Toskes PP. Approach to the patient with pancreatic disease. In Wilson JD, et al (eds): Principles of internal medicine. 12th ed. New York: McGraw Hill, 1991.

Leung JWC, et al. Celiac plexus block for pain in pancreatic cancer and pancreatitis. Br J Surg 1983; 70:730.

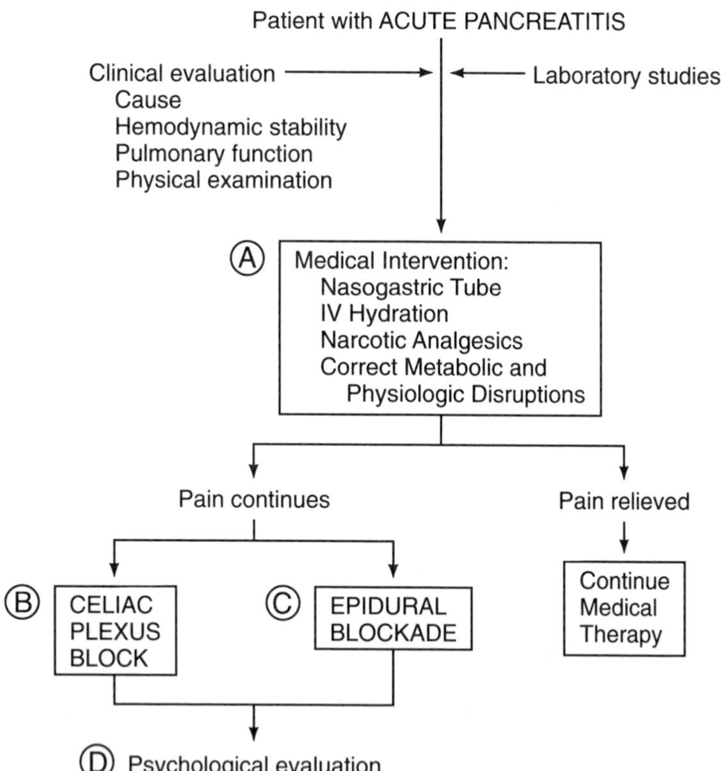
Patient with ACUTE PANCREATITIS
Clinical evaluation
Cause
Hemodynamic stability
Pulmonary function
Physical examination
Laboratory studies
A
Medical Intervention:
Nasogastric Tube
IV Hydration
Narcotic Analgesics
Correct Metabolic and Physiologic Disruptions
Pain continues
Pain relieved
B
CELIAC PLEXUS BLOCK
C
EPIDURAL BLOCKADE
Continue Medical Therapy
D
Psychological evaluation

OBSTETRIC PAIN

Bari Bennett, M.D.

The obstetric patient poses a significant challenge to the anesthesiologist, since both maternal and fetal welfare must be considered. Physiologic changes of pregnancy render the obstetric patient at high risk for anesthesia (aspiration, failed intubation), yet more than 50% of patients request or require anesthesia during labor and delivery. A thorough understanding of fetal physiology and of obstetrics must be attained to provide maternal comfort without fetal or neonatal depression.

A. Evaluate maternal status, including other risk factors (e.g., preeclampsia) and fetal status. Determine whether there are contraindications to regional anesthesia (coagulopathy, infection, hypovolemia, patient refusal). Coagulation studies should be made if risk factors are present (preeclampsia, abruptio).

B. Pain in the first stage of labor primarily results from dilatation of the cervix and lower uterine segment, as well as distention of the body of the uterus. Noxious impulses from the cervix and uterus are transmitted by afferent nerves that accompany sympathetic pathways, pass into the lumbar and lower thoracic sympathetic ganglia, and travel via the white rami and posterior roots of T10-L1 into the spinal cord. In early labor, only roots T11-T12 are involved, but as labor progresses T10 and L1 are recruited. The first stage of labor is further subdivided into latent and active phases. A cervical dilatation of 4 to 5 cm in primigravidas or 3 to 4 cm in multigravidas usually coincides with the change from latent to active phase. IV sedation or epidural/intrathecal opiates can be used in the first stage, with varying degrees of pain relief and a high incidence of side effects (Table 1). Epidural anesthesia with a local anesthetic is the safest technique that can provide complete pain relief during labor and delivery. The addition of small doses of opiates augments the analgesia produced by more dilute concentrations of local anesthetics and thus decreases the incidence of motor blockade. Paracervical blocks are effective but have an 8% to 40% incidence of fetal bradycardia. Lumbar sympathetic blocks require bilateral injections, are more difficult technically, and do not provide analgesia for the second stage of labor.

C. The second stage of labor is heralded by complete cervical dilatation and descent of the fetus. Pain is produced by stretching of the perineum and is transmitted by the pudendal nerve derived from S2-S4. Pudendal nerve blocks or major conduction anesthesia are most commonly employed for this stage. Inhalational anesthetic agents may be used, but the loss of maternal protective airway reflexes and neonatal depression are major concerns. Ketamine (<1 mg/kg) can provide good analgesia without significant neonatal depression.

D. Most side effects associated with anesthesia are minor and easily treated. The sympathetic block and associated hypotension seen with regional techniques are particularly worrisome and should be treated aggressively, since the placental blood flow is not autoregulated. In general, obstetric patients should be hydrated with approximately 1 L of crystalloid before a regional block and be positioned with left uterine displacement. Although rare, more serious complications of anesthesia include IV injection of local anesthetics and high epidural/spinal blocks. For epidural and caudal techniques, a test dose of local anesthesia is mandatory to avoid unintentional IV or subarachnoid injections. The addition of epinephrine as a marker in the obstetric patient has been questioned, since tachycardia secondary to labor is common and epinephrine may have deleterious effects on the fetus by decreasing uterine blood flow. Dural puncture is generally easily recognized, but unintentional total spinal blocks may occur. To avoid disastrous complications, it is best to aspirate before each injection, give small incremental doses of 3 to 5 ml, and allow sufficient time to detect a subarachnoid or IV injection. Resuscitation equipment should always be immediately available, and frequent communication is paramount, since the patient is the best monitor.

TABLE 1 Epidural Doses for First-Stage Labor (T10-L1)

Agent	*Load*	*Infusion*	*Rate (ml/hr)*
Bupivacaine	8–10 ml of 0.25%	0.25%	7
	8–10 ml of 0.25%	0.125%	12–14
	8–10 ml of 0.25% with 50 μg of fentanyl	0.0625–0.125% with 2 μg/ml of fentanyl	10–12
Lidocaine	8–10 ml of 1% with 50 μg of fentanyl	0.75% with 2 μg/ml of fentanyl	10
Chloroprocaine	8–10 ml of 2%	0.5%	<30

(Continued on page 42)

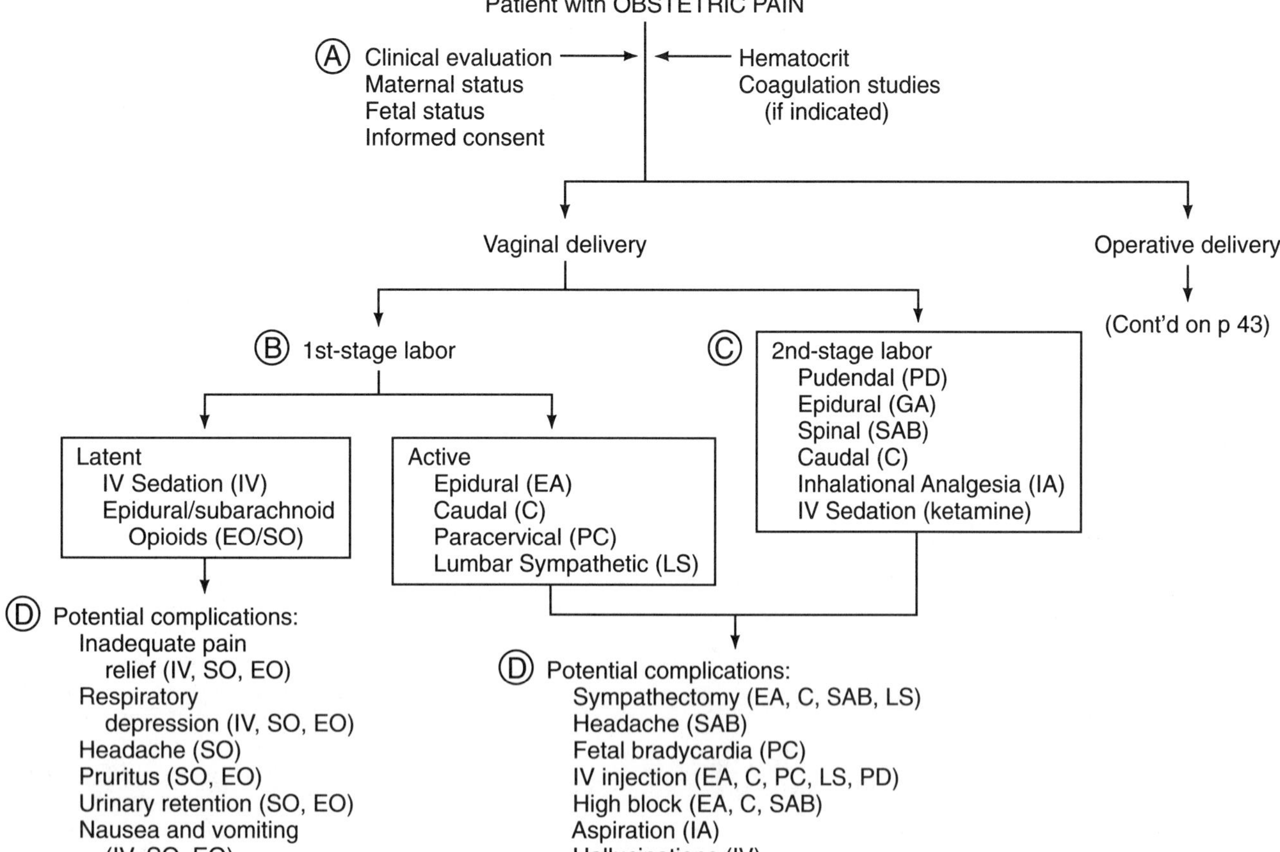

Patient with OBSTETRIC PAIN
(A) Clinical evaluation
Maternal status
Fetal status
Informed consent
Hematocrit
Coagulation studies
(if indicated)
Vaginal delivery
Operative delivery
(Cont'd on p 43)
(B) 1st-stage labor
(C) 2nd-stage labor
Pudendal (PD)
Epidural (GA)
Spinal (SAB)
Caudal (C)
Inhalational Analgesia (IA)
IV Sedation (ketamine)
Latent
IV Sedation (IV)
Epidural/subarachnoid
Opioids (EO/SO)
Active
Epidural (EA)
Caudal (C)
Paracervical (PC)
Lumbar Sympathetic (LS)
(D) Potential complications:
Inadequate pain relief (IV, SO, EO)
Respiratory depression (IV, SO, EO)
Headache (SO)
Pruritus (SO, EO)
Urinary retention (SO, EO)
Nausea and vomiting (IV, SO, EO)
(D) Potential complications:
Sympathectomy (EA, C, SAB, LS)
Headache (SAB)
Fetal bradycardia (PC)
IV injection (EA, C, PC, LS, PD)
High block (EA, C, SAB)
Aspiration (IA)
Hallucinations (IV)

TABLE 2 Anesthetic Doses for Cesarean Section (T4-S5)

Agent	*Epidural*	*Spinal*
Bupivacaine	20–30 ml of 0.5% ± 50–100 μg fentanyl ± 1:200,000 epinephrine	10–12.5 mg hyperbaric
Lidocaine	20–30 ml of 2% ± 50–100 μg fentanyl ± 1:200,000 epinephrine	60–75 mg hyperbaric
Chloroprocaine	20–30 ml of 2% ± 50–100 μg fentanyl ± 1:200,000 epinephrine	–
Tetracaine	–	8–10 mg hyperbaric

E. If operative delivery is needed, all obstetric patients should receive 15 to 30 ml of a clear, nonparticulate antacid approximately 30 minutes before surgery. Given adequate time, an H_2-receptor antagonist may also be given to increase intragastric pH. Metoclopramide has been used to accelerate gastric emptying time and increase lower esophageal sphincter tone, but its efficacy in cesarean section patients has not been proved and its routine use has not been recommended. Sedatives and narcotics should be avoided because of potential fetal and neonatal depression.

F. Choose the anesthetic technique based on surgical urgency and maternal and fetal conditions. Regional anesthesia reduces the risks of maternal aspiration and neonatal depression and should be used when immediate delivery is not crucial. Subarachnoid block (SAB) is rapid, easily administered, and reliable but is more difficult to control. A T4-T6 to S5 block is necessary for patient comfort (Table 2). General endotracheal anesthesia (GETA) is required when either the mother or fetus is in immediate danger (hemorrhage, fetal distress).

G. If general anesthesia is required, the patient should be prepped and draped and surgeons should be ready to begin before the induction in order to avoid prolonged anesthetic exposure before delivery. A rapid-sequence induction should be used with thiopental (3 to 4 mg/kg), ketamine (1 mg/kg), or a combination of both followed by succinylcholine. If difficult intubation is suspected, an awake look or intubation should be used. Anesthesia should be maintained with 50% N_2O. After delivery, narcotics and muscle relaxants may be used as needed. Low concentrations of inhalational agents may also be used to decrease intraoperative awareness without affecting the neonate or uterine response to oxytocic agents. Patients should be fully awake before extubation.

H. Postoperative analgesia after cesarean section may be provided by epidural opiates, intrathecal opiates, or patient controlled analgesia (PCA). Epidural morphine (preservative free) in doses of 3 to 5 mg provides 16 to 24 hours of satisfactory analgesia in most patients. Intrathecal morphine in doses of 0.1 to 0.25 mg provides excellent analgesia for 18 to 27 hours. Side effects are usually minimal but include pruritus, urinary retention, and nausea. Respiratory depression may be immediate or delayed and remains the most serious side effect. All patients should be monitored for 24 hours after receiving epidural or intrathecal opiates. For patients undergoing general anesthesia, PCA provides pain control superior to intramuscular morphine with a high patient acceptance.

References

Eisenach JC, Grice SC, Dewan DM. Patient-controlled analgesia following cesarean section: A comparison with epidural and intramuscular narcotics. Anesthesiology 1988; 68:444.

Gibbs CP, Krischer J, Peckham BM, et al. Obstetric anesthesia: A national survey. Anesthesiology 1986; 65:298.

Leighton BD, Norris MC, Sasis M, et al. Limitations of an epinephrine b epidural anesthesia test dose in laboring patients. Anesthesiology 1987; 66:688.

Reisner LS. Obstetric anesthesia. Anesth Clin North Am 1990; 8:55, 157.

Shnider SM, Levinson G. Anesthesia for obstetrics. Baltimore: Williams & Wilkins, 1987:109, 159.

Youngstrom P, Eastwood D, Patel H, et al. Epidural fentanyl and bupivacaine in labor: Double blind study. Anesthesiology 1984; 62:A414.

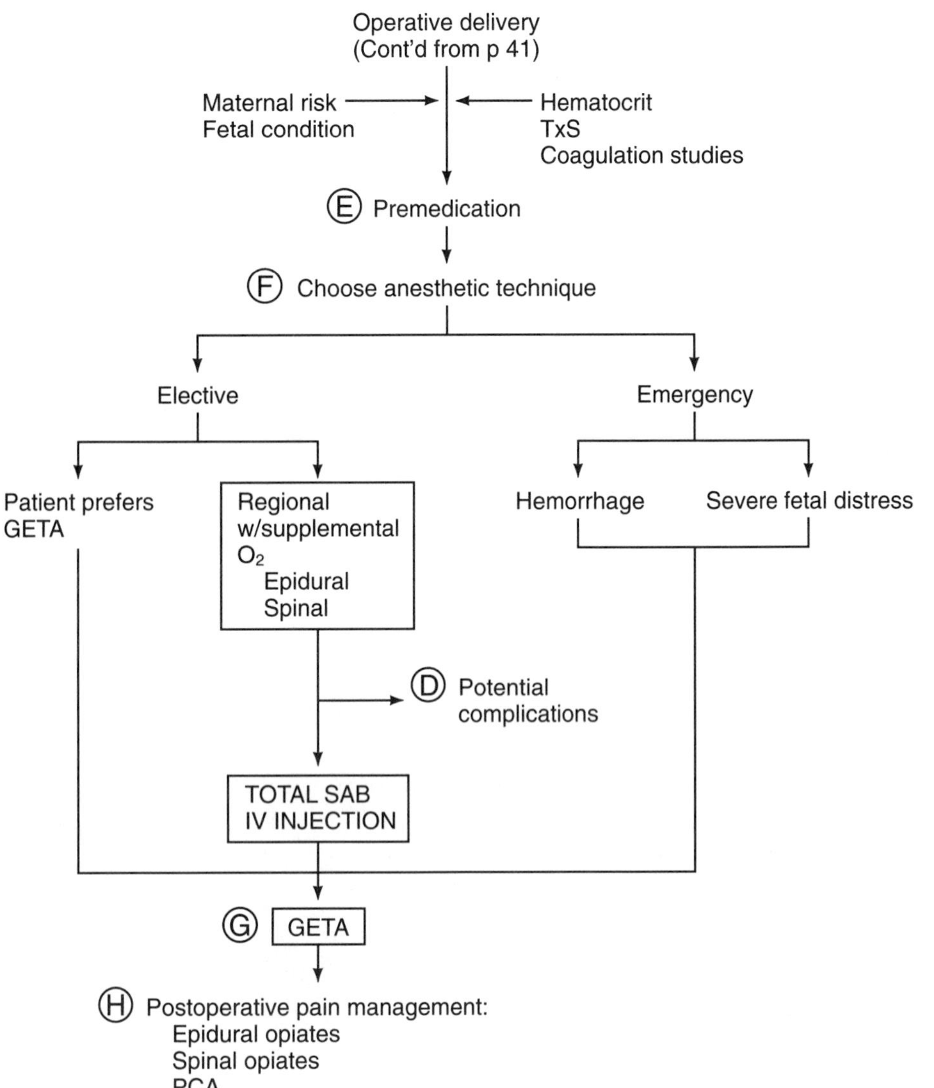
Operative delivery
(Cont'd from p 41)
Maternal risk
Fetal condition
Hematocrit
TxS
Coagulation studies
E Premedication
F Choose anesthetic technique
Elective
Emergency
Patient prefers
GETA
Regional
w/supplemental
O2
Epidural
Spinal
Hemorrhage
Severe fetal distress
D Potential
complications
TOTAL SAB
IV INJECTION
G GETA
H Postoperative pain management:
Epidural opiates
Spinal opiates
PCA

CHRONIC PAIN SYNDROMES

Myofascial Pain Syndromes
Postherpetic Neuralgia
Reflex Sympathetic Dystrophy
Metastatic Cancer Pain
Diabetic Neuropathy
Chronic Pancreatic Pain
Neurogenic Pain
Central Pain Syndrome
Phantom Pain
Pain in the Spinal Cord–Injured Patient
Fibromyositis
Rheumatoid Arthritis
Osteoarthritis
Nonsomatic Pain

MYOFASCIAL PAIN SYNDROMES

Robert D. Culling, D.O.
Laurie G. Kilbourn, M.D.

Myofascial pain (MP) is a descriptive term applied to painful sensations occurring along one or more skeletal muscles and their associated fascia. MP is one of the most common causes of acute and chronic pain and occurs to some extent to almost everyone at some time. It is also one of the most frequently missed diagnoses and inadequately treated conditions. This is unfortunate in view of the fact that it is one of the most effectively treatable pain-producing conditions.

Other terms used to describe MP include muscular rheumatism, myalgia, fibromyalgia, myositis, fibrositis, myofibrositis, and myofasciitis. MP is characterized by the presence of one or more discrete hypersensitive regions (trigger points [TPs]) in the involved muscle or fascia causing local and referred pain.

Travell and Simons postulated that an initial muscle injury or overload results in rupture of the sarcoplasmic reticulum and release of ionized calcium, which in turn results in a sustained contraction. This depletes adenosine triphosphate (ATP) to a critical level and produces ischemia with release of histamine, kinins, and prostaglandins. The nociceptive impulses are carried to the CNS, resulting in increased muscle tension, sympathetic activity, and local ischemia. This can produce a vicious cycle of pain and spasm.

A. The diagnosis of MP involves careful history taking and a complete physical examination. MP may begin acutely with an obvious inciting event or may be insidious in nature from chronic muscle fatigue or overuse. The description of the pain pattern provides an important clue to the location of TPs. Several TP manuals are available for consultation.

B. Myofascial pain may be the primary cause of the pain but may be secondary to other disease processes such as facet dysfunction. Secondary myofascial pain recurs if the primary cause is not identified and treated. Other musculoskeletal disorders (arthritis, bursitis, myopathies) should be excluded from the diagnosis.

C. The typical pain associated with myofascial TPs is usually a constant, deep ache. Active TPs are always tender and on palpation reproduce the referred pain symptoms. Latent TPs do not cause pain during normal daily activities but are tender on palpation.

D. On palpation of a TP with the tip of a finger, a taut band of muscle fibers is appreciated. Application of pressure to an active TP reproduces the referred pain pattern, causes pain in the TP, and often elicits the "jump sign," which consists of an outcry, wince, or jumping on the part of the patient. The sensitivity of a TP can be quantified with a pressure threshold meter, also referred to as an algometer. Standard laboratory, x-ray, and nerve conduction tests and electromyography are not helpful in making the diagnosis of MP.

E. Treatment of MP is aimed at improving patient function, decreasing pain, and preventing disability. The first-line therapy should be the spray and stretch technique described by Travell and Simons. The objective is to inactivate TPs by full stretching of the involved muscles. The vapocoolant decreases the discomfort so that active range of motion exercises can be performed.

F. Penetration of the TP with a needle reproduces the pain pattern. The goal is to disrupt the TP with the needle. Good results have been obtained with dry needling, saline, local anesthetic, and steroid injection. Local anesthesia is commonly used to reduce discomfort and interrupt the pain cycle (p 270). The patient then undergoes stretching and range of motion exercises.

G. Other adjunctive therapies include deep massage, moist hot packs, ultrasonography, ice massage, biofeedback, and transcutaneous electrical nerve stimulation (TENS). The patient should be instructed in stretching exercises in the home.

H. Identification and correction of any perpetuating factors that may be present (correctable or compensatable anatomic inadequacies, poor posture, emotional stress responses, depression) are vitally important for successful treatment. A successful outcome depends on extinguishing chronic pain behavior.

References

Fischer AA. Documentation of myofascial trigger points. Arch Phys Med Rehabil 1988; 69:286.

Fricton JR, Esam AA. Advances in pain research and therapy: Myofascial pain and fibromyalgia. New York: Raven Press, 1990.

Travell JG, Simons DG. Myofascial pain and dysfunction: The trigger point manual. Baltimore: Williams & Wilkins, 1983.

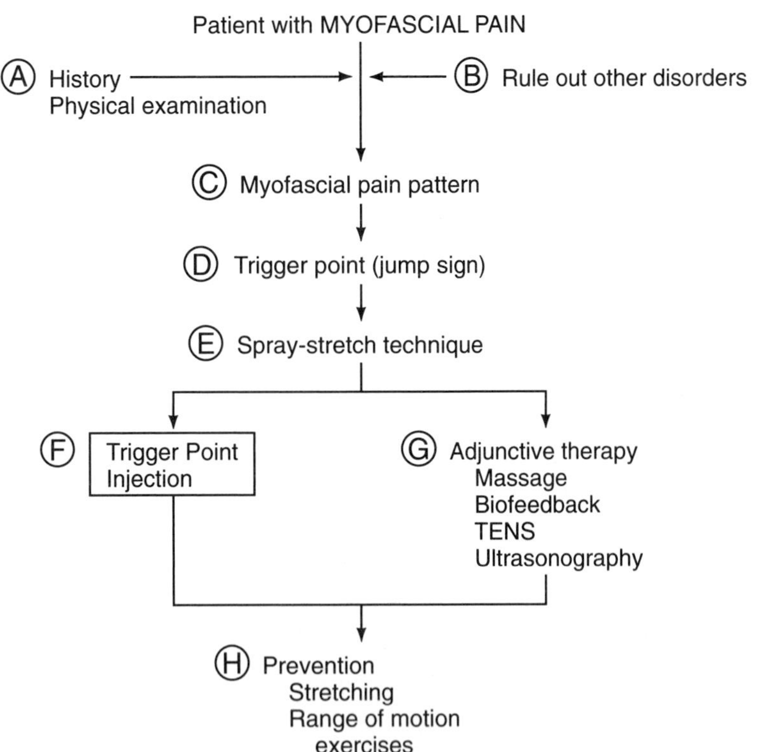
Patient with MYOFASCIAL PAIN
(A) History
Physical examination
(B) Rule out other disorders
(C) Myofascial pain pattern
(D) Trigger point (jump sign)
(E) Spray-stretch technique
(F) Trigger Point Injection
(G) Adjunctive therapy
Massage
Biofeedback
TENS
Ultrasonography
(H) Prevention
Stretching
Range of motion exercises

POSTHERPETIC NEURALGIA

Robert Sprague, M.D.

Postherpetic neuralgia (PHN) is a chronic pain syndrome that develops after acute herpes zoster (HZ). Therapy of PHN is problematic at best, and the most efficacious approach is prevention of PHN by prompt treatment of HZ (p 28). PHN is predominantly a disease of the elderly, who not only may have adverse reactions to therapeutic drugs but also are less able to cope physically and mentally with the disease.

A. A key point in the management of HZ/PHN patients is the delineation of the point at which HZ stops and PHN begins. A reasonable guideline for diagnosis of PHN is hypopigmentation, hypo/hypesthesia, dysesthesia, allodynia, or hyperpathia existing 2 months after the acute vesicular eruption of HZ. As with HZ, physical examination to determine dermatomal distribution is important. A thorough drug history should also be elicited, as many patients who present to the pain clinic are already taking oral analgesics, and some form of addiction may be present. The concomitant diagnosis of myofascial syndrome or reflex sympathetic dystrophy with PHN must always be considered, and appropriate examinations should be performed.

B. Anesthetic approaches in therapy for PHN have had little success. Therapeutic modalities have included sympathetic blockade, somatic blocks, skin infiltration with local anesthetics mixed with steroids, cryoanalgesia, and epidural steroids. The use of anesthetic approaches in PHN has not been supported in the literature, but there have been many anecdotal reports of favorable results.

C. The pharmacologic approach in PHN therapy has been the most rewarding, specifically with tricyclic antidepressants (TCAs) (Table 1). Watson and coworkers showed that amitriptyline in doses not affecting depression scores significantly improved pain scores. The purported mechanism of TCA benefit is an increase in CNS concentrations of serotonin, a neurotransmitter also believed to have central pain inhibitory actions. The sharp, shooting pain component of PHN often is unresponsive to TCAs, and anticonvulsants may be prescribed in that setting. Carbamazepine, valproic acid, clonazepam, and phenytoin have been prescribed with varying rates of success. Topical therapies with capsaicin and with a mixture of lidocaine and alcohol have been investigated, and results have been promising.

TABLE 1 Drug Therapy in Postherpetic Neuralgia

Agent	*Recommended Dosage*	*Remarks*
Amitriptyline	25 mg hs (range 50–150 mg)	First line therapy
Doxepin	25 mg hs (range 50–150 mg)	Fewer side effects
Carbamazepine	100 mg b.i.d.	Anticonvulsants are used for shooting pain of PHN, and not for initial therapy
Valproic acid	125 mg b.i.d.	
Clonazepam	0.5 mg b.i.d.	

D. Neuroaugmentation therapy with the transcutaneous electrical nerve stimulator unit as well as counterirritation methods have been beneficial in PHN. These may be useful as home adjunct therapies. Spinal cord electrical stimulation also has been effective in alleviating the pain (p 224).

E. As with all chronic pain syndromes, the benefits of psychological support and physical therapy cannot be overlooked. Depression and secondary myofascial syndromes are often encountered in PHN.

References

Colding A. The effect of regional sympathetic blocks in the therapy of herpes zoster. Acta Anaesth Scand 1969; 13:133.

Portenoy RK. Postherpetic neuralgia: A workable treatment plan. Geriatrics 1986; 41:34.

Watson CP. Postherpetic neuralgia—208 cases. Pain 1988; 35:289.

Watson CP. Postherpetic neuralgia and topical capsaicin. Pain 1988; 33:332.

Watson CP. Amitriptyline versus placebo in postherpetic neuralgia. Neurology 1982; 32:671.

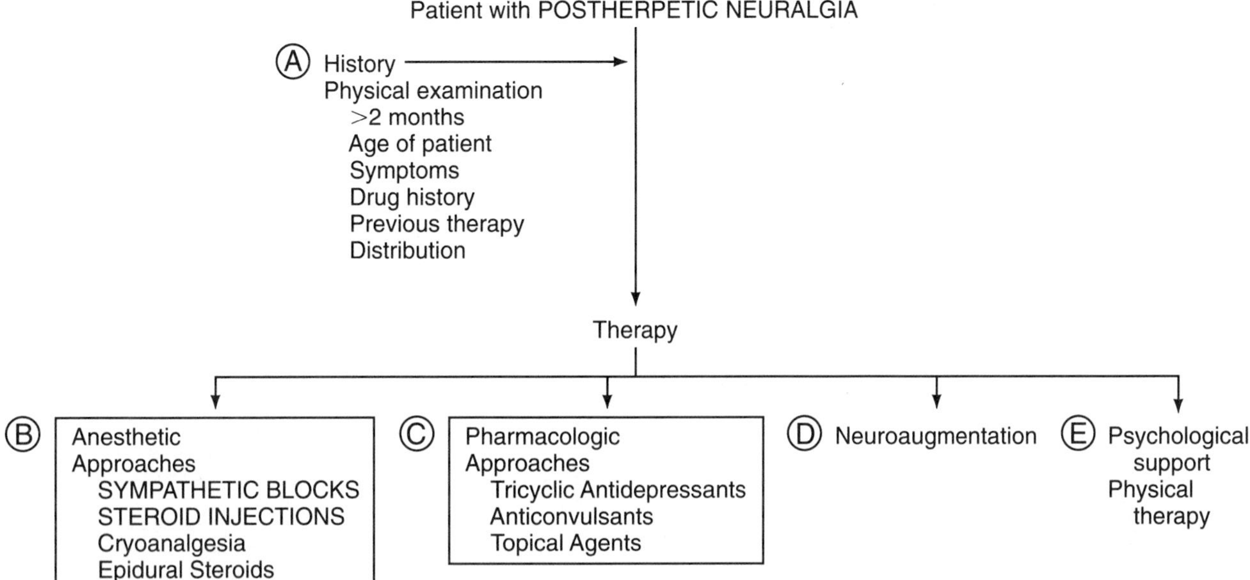
Patient with POSTHERPETIC NEURALGIA
(A) History
Physical examination
>2 months
Age of patient
Symptoms
Drug history
Previous therapy
Distribution
Therapy
(B) Anesthetic Approaches
SYMPATHETIC BLOCKS
STEROID INJECTIONS
Cryoanalgesia
Epidural Steroids
(C) Pharmacologic Approaches
Tricyclic Antidepressants
Anticonvulsants
Topical Agents
(D) Neuroaugmentation
(E) Psychological support
Physical therapy

REFLEX SYMPATHETIC DYSTROPHY

Mark E. Romanoff, M.D.

The clinical entity of causalgia or reflex sympathetic dystrophy (RSD) was first described during the Civil War by Mitchell. Since that time, many theories of the pathophysiology of RSD have been formulated, but none have successfully explained all the symptoms seen in this syndrome.

The International Association for the Study of Pain has defined RSD as a syndrome of pain in an extremity mediated by sympathetic overactivity that does not involve a major nerve. Causalgia is defined as burning pain, allodynia, and hyperpathia of an extremity with partial nerve damage. The more general term introduced by Roberts in 1986, sympathetically mediated pain, should encompass all these clinical entities. In this chapter the generic term RSD is used to label this syndrome.

A. RSD often occurs after major trauma to an extremity but may be seen after a minor injury. Many cases have no precipitating events. The patient's history can help identify the type of injury that occurred and other associated symptoms. The physical examination may reveal signs of nerve damage and muscle atrophy. Changes in blood flow can be seen as a temperature change; edema; or hair, nail, or skin changes. The signs and symptoms of RSD are listed in Table 1. The hallmarks include a burning pain out of proportion to the injury, hyperpathia and/or allodynia, and vasomotor changes. These symptoms are often varied and the stages mentioned in the table may last days or months, which may make the diagnosis difficult. Patients with RSD may present with atypical symptoms. RSD involving the knee or back is often the most difficult to diagnose. The differential diagnosis includes myofascial pain syndrome, Raynaud's disease and syndrome, nerve entrapment, and acrocyanosis.

B. Diagnostic studies may help confirm the diagnosis. Radiography of the area may reveal patchy demineralization (Sudeck's atrophy) induced by chronic ischemia from sympathetic induced vasoconstriction. The triple-phase bone scan is reported to have high specificity and sensitivity in the diagnosis of RSD, but it has a low predictive value in patients with symptoms lasting >6 months. MRI currently has no role in the diagnosis of RSD. Measurements of blood flow (temperature, thermography, Doppler, plethysmography) help establish differences between the normal and affected limb and in following treatment. The best diagnostic test is a sympathetic block (see D). Pain relief with a sympathectomy is pathognomonic of RSD as well as the treatment of choice. It must be remembered that RSD is a *clinical diagnosis*. Despite negative results from tests such as the triple-phase bone scan and Doppler studies, a sympathetic block should be performed if the diagnosis of RSD is suspected.

TABLE 1 Signs and Symptoms of Reflex Sympathetic Dystrophy

Stage	Signs and Symptoms
Stage 1 (acute) Denervation phase	Pain out of proportion to injury Burning pain Hyperpathia, allodynia Increased pain with dependent position Increased temperature commonly Accelerated hair/nail growth Decreased range of motion Edema Sweating (increased or decreased)
Stage 2 (dystrophic) Hypersensitivity phase	Constant pain Decreased temperature Cyanosis (livedo reticularis) Hair loss, ridged and cracked nails Hyperhidrosis Diffuse osteoporosis (Sudeck's atrophy) Continued decreased range of motion Indurated edema Personality changes
Stage 3 (atrophic)	Pain moving proximally, may improve Irreversible tissue damage Atrophic skin, thickened fascia Flexion contractures Bony demineralization Temperature may normalize Sweating (increased or decreased) Muscle wasting Markedly decreased range of motion Continuing personality changes

C. Physical therapy (PT) alone has been shown to improve the outcome. It should include whirlpool therapy, active and passive range of motion exercises, and weightbearing for lower extremities. Most patients cannot participate in PT because of pain, so it needs to be combined with other pain-reducing techniques.

D. Sympathetic nerve blocks are used for diagnosis and treatment. RSD of the head, neck, and upper extremities can be treated with stellate ganglion blocks (p 242). Thoracic RSD is treated with a thoracic sympathetic block (p 244) or an epidural/subarachnoid block. Lumbar sympathetic blocks (p 248) or an epidural/subarachnoid block can be used for lower extremity RSD. It is important to measure the results of the sympathetic block. This is usually done by measuring temperature, thermographic, or sympathogalvanic responses. A 1° to 1.5° C temperature increase indicates a successful sympathectomy.

(Continued on page 52)

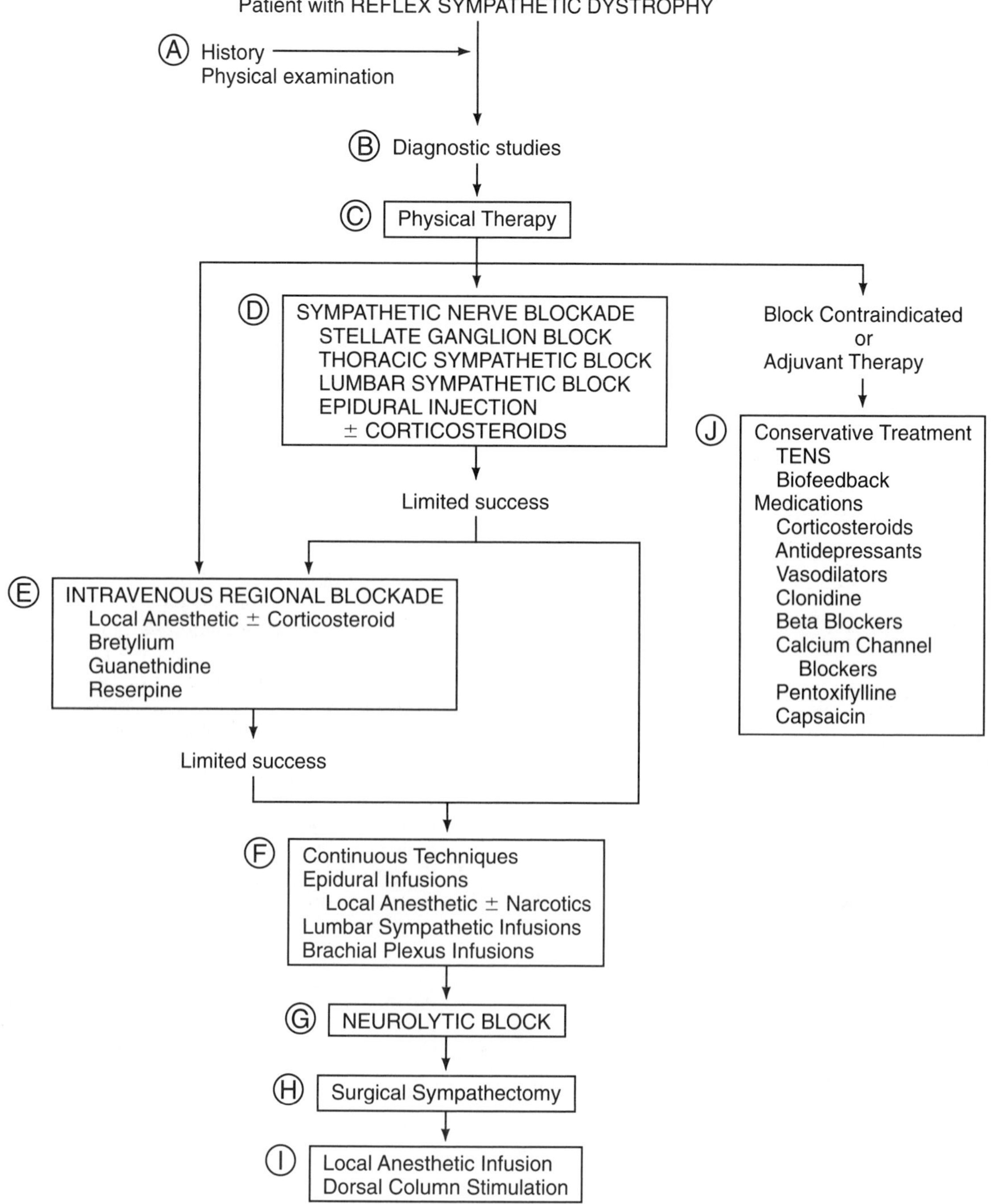

Patient with REFLEX SYMPATHETIC DYSTROPHY
(A) History
Physical examination
(B) Diagnostic studies
(C) Physical Therapy
(D) SYMPATHETIC NERVE BLOCKADE
STELLATE GANGLION BLOCK
THORACIC SYMPATHETIC BLOCK
LUMBAR SYMPATHETIC BLOCK
EPIDURAL INJECTION
± CORTICOSTEROIDS
Block Contraindicated
or
Adjuvant Therapy
(J) Conservative Treatment
TENS
Biofeedback
Medications
Corticosteroids
Antidepressants
Vasodilators
Clonidine
Beta Blockers
Calcium Channel
Blockers
Pentoxifylline
Capsaicin
Limited success
(E) INTRAVENOUS REGIONAL BLOCKADE
Local Anesthetic ± Corticosteroid
Bretylium
Guanethidine
Reserpine
Limited success
(F) Continuous Techniques
Epidural Infusions
Local Anesthetic ± Narcotics
Lumbar Sympathetic Infusions
Brachial Plexus Infusions
(G) NEUROLYTIC BLOCK
(H) Surgical Sympathectomy
(I) Local Anesthetic Infusion
Dorsal Column Stimulation

Local anesthetics are commonly used for sympathetic blockade. Some authors suggest the addition of corticosteroids, but no studies have definitively shown improved efficacy with this practice. Injections are usually performed once to establish the diagnosis and to evaluate the duration of pain relief. Injections given every day to every week have been recommended for up to eight to ten injections. If the duration of pain relief continues to lengthen or if pain does not return, this approach is warranted. If pain relief is only for the duration of the local anesthesia, alternative approaches must be sought.

E. Hannington-Kiff popularized the use of IV regional blockade for treatment of RSD. The original studies used guanethidine, but reserpine and now bretylium have been used successfully. Local anesthetic blocks alone or with corticosteroids have also been reported to improve pain in these patients. These blocks can also be repeated as often as every other day if pain relief is evident.

F. Limited success with single-shot sympathetic blocks or IV regional blocks should be followed by continuous techniques. An intensive PT program should be performed concurrently with the blocks. Brachial plexus, lumbar sympathetic, or epidural catheters may be placed and dosed continuously or intermittently before PT. One study showed excellent results with local anesthetic injections followed by a continuous infusion of narcotics. The narcotics allowed active participation in PT without motor deficits.

G. Neurolytic sympathetic blocks should be considered if sympathetic blocks provide significant pain relief, but only for the duration of the local anesthesia. Stellate ganglion neurolytic blocks are rarely performed because of the potential damage to nearby structures. Lumbar sympathetic neurolytic blocks can be performed easily with little risk of motor weakness from lumbar plexus involvement. Increased pain from partial denervation has been described. Long-term results are promising.

H. Surgical sympathectomy is indicated if neurolytic techniques have failed or if neurolytic blocks are contraindicated. Success rates are quite high if the diagnosis has been confirmed by sympathetic blocks before surgery. One study revealed an 84% success rate after 2 years of follow-up; other studies showed similar rates. A 40% incidence of postsympathectomy neuralgia, although temporary, is disconcerting.

I. IV local anesthetic infusions have reduced the size of the painful area and decreased the intensity of pain in some patients. The availability of oral lidocaine analog (mexiletine, tocainide) allows for maintenance therapy. Dorsal column stimulation has been used for upper and lower extremity RSD. A response rate of >80% is often noted (p 224).

J. Conservative therapy may be used if sympathetic blocks are contraindicated (anatomic abnormalities, anticoagulation status, patient reluctance) or as adjunctive therapy to enhance the effect of sympathetic blocks. Transcutaneous electrical nerve stimulation (TENS) may be most helpful in the initial denervated phase of RSD. Biofeedback can improve blood flow, reverse dystrophic changes, and provide pain relief, but only case reports have been cited in the literature. Medications may also improve pain and function in RSD. Corticosteroids (prednisone up to 200 mg/day) have been reported to provide good to excellent results in up to two thirds of patients. Antidepressants such as amitriptyline have improved the outcome in RSD. Vasodilators such as prazosin, phenoxybenzamine, nifedipine, and labetalol have been used with varied success. Other beta blockers such as propranolol have also been studied. Clonidine, a central alpha-$_2$-agonist that reduces peripheral sympathetic tone, has been studied, revealing limited success. The vasoactive drugs can all have severe side effects such as bradycardia and hypotension, which usually limits their use. Pentoxifylline, a phosphodiesterase inhibitor that makes red blood cell membranes more flexible, allowing improved blood flow in "low-flow" states, has also been shown to be effective in RSD. Case reports have suggested a role for topical capsaicin.

References

Blanchard J, Ramamurthy S, Walsh N, et al. Intravenous regional sympatholysis: A double-blind comparison of guanethidine, reserpine, and normal saline. J Pain Sympt Manag 1990; 5:357.

Cheshire WP, Snyder CR. Treatment of reflex sympathetic dystrophy with topical capsaicin. Pain 1990; 42:307.

Cooper DE, DeLee JC, Ramamurthy S. Reflex sympathetic dystrophy of the knee. Am J Bone Joint Surg 1989; 3:365.

Glazer S, Portenoy RK. Systemic local anesthetics in pain control. J Pain Sympt Manag 1991; 6:30.

Hannington-Kiff JG. Intravenous regional sympathetic block with guanethidine. Lancet 1974; 1:1019.

Kleinert HE, Norberg H, McDonough JJ. Surgical sympathectomy: Upper and lower extremity. In: Omer GE, Spinner M, eds. Management of peripheral nerve problems. Philadelphia: WB Saunders, 1980:285.

Koch E, Hofer HO, Sialer G, et al. Failure of MR imaging to detect reflex sympathetic dystrophy of the extremities. Am J Roentgenol 1991; 156:113.

Mockus MB, Rutherford RB, Rosales C, Pearce WH. Sympathectomy for causalgia. Arch Surg 1987; 122:668.

Robaina FJ, Dominguez M, Rodriquez DM, et al. Spinal cord stimulation for relief of chronic pain in vasospastic disorders of the upper limbs. Neurosurgery 1989; 24:63.

Roberts WJ. A hypothesis on the physiological basis for causalgia and related pains. Pain 1986; 24:297.

Schwartzman RJ, McLellan TL. Reflex sympathetic dystrophy. Arch Neurol 1987; 44:555.

METASTATIC CANCER PAIN

Jeffrey Priest, M.D.

Metastatic cancer pain is a treatable medical condition that deserves immediate attention. Besides being agonizing, the pain is a vivid reminder that the disease is pursuing its natural course. Pain management involves not only control of the pain sensation but also the reassurance that pain control is possible. Opioids are the mainstay of metastatic pain control, and the tendency to overestimate opioid strength, duration, and addictive potential should be kept in mind.

A. Metastatic cancer can produce any type of pain and in any location. A careful history of pain and previous pain control measures should be reviewed. General categories of cancer pain are somatic (well localized), visceral (poorly localized), and deafferentation (paroxysmal and electric pains). Pain should be classified as to its source before a regimen is undertaken. When selecting a regimen, consider the patient's physical status, life expectancy, mobility, quality of life, location and type of pain, inpatient or outpatient status, and desires and expectations.

B. Drug administration routes include oral, rectal, intravenous, subcutaneous, intramuscular, epidural, and intrathecal, but the oral route is by far the most convenient. When pain is mild, an NSAID may be all that is required for patient comfort. Moderate pain may be treated initially with oxycodone, with codeine preparations combined with an NSAID, or with a tricyclic antidepressant. Severe pain should be treated with a strong opioid such as morphine and any adjuvant drugs deemed helpful. Narcotics should be administered on a chronological and breakthrough pain basis. Sustained release opioid compounds are very effective. Oral medications can be supplemented with biofeedback techniques or transcutaneous electrical nerve stimulators. A benzodiazepine may be indicated, as sleep may be as important as pain relief to many patients. Deafferentation pain may respond better to phenytoin or carbamazepine combined with an NSAID and a tricyclic antidepressant than to an opioid-based regimen.

C. Expect to upgrade the opioid doses or potency during treatment, as tolerance is likely to develop and pain is likely to increase. Increase doses in a stepwise fashion until the pain is controlled or until side effects become intolerable. For example, we titrated epidural morphine to 20 mg every 2 hours, without notable side effects, in order for a patient to ambulate without tremendous pain (she died 2 weeks later).

D. Anticipate opioid side effects and treat them promptly. Opioid side effects usually consist of constipation, pruritus, sedation, nausea, urinary retention, respiratory depression, withdrawal, and addiction. Tolerance to respiratory depression occurs early in treatment, whereas constipation may never cease. Constipation can be corrected with stool softeners. Sedation may be ameliorated with dextroamphetamine or methylphenidate. Antiemetics will reduce nausea. Urinary retention is usually transient but may require bladder catheterization in the elderly. Diphenhydramine may lessen the pruritus, but decreasing or changing the opioid is the most effective therapy. Titrated carefully, naloxone will eradicate all opioid side effects with some preservation of pain relief. Regimens that suddenly decrease total systemic opioid concentrations may precipitate acute opioid withdrawal symptoms. Psychological addiction to opioids is rare with metastatic pain. If side effects are intolerable with adjuvant aids, changing the route of administration or dose/schedule is indicated.

E. Continuously administered opioids, neuraxially placed opioids, and neuroablative measures are the three main alternatives to standard outpatient pain control regimens. Continuous delivery systems include transcutaneous fentanyl patches, PCA pumps, intramuscular injections, and implantable pumps with opioid reservoirs. Neuraxial opioids can be placed utilizing epidural or intrathecal catheters on a continuous or intermittent basis and can be permanent or temporary, subcutaneous or extracutaneous. Neuroablative procedures may be chemical or surgical, and effects may be short-lived or permanent and irreversible. These techniques are potentially time-consuming for the physician but may produce superior pain relief.

F. Reevaluate patients frequently once a stable regimen is obtained. Pain relief plateaus are subject to failure because of disease progression and drug tolerance. Generally, patients can be reasonably comfortable with titrated oral medications alone. As terminal conditions draw near or as pain becomes unbearable, more invasive techniques may be preferable.

References

Abrams SE, Burchman SL, Taylor ML, Kettler RE. Management of common cancer pain syndromes. In: Abrams SE, ed. The pain clinic manual. Philadelphia: JB Lippincott, 1990.

Ferrer-Brechner T. Anesthetic techniques for the management of cancer pain. Cancer 1989; 63:2343.

Inturrisi CE. Management of cancer pain: Pharmacology and principles of management. Cancer 1989; 63:2308.

Payne R. Cancer pain: Anatomy, physiology, and pharmacology. Cancer 1989; 63:2266.

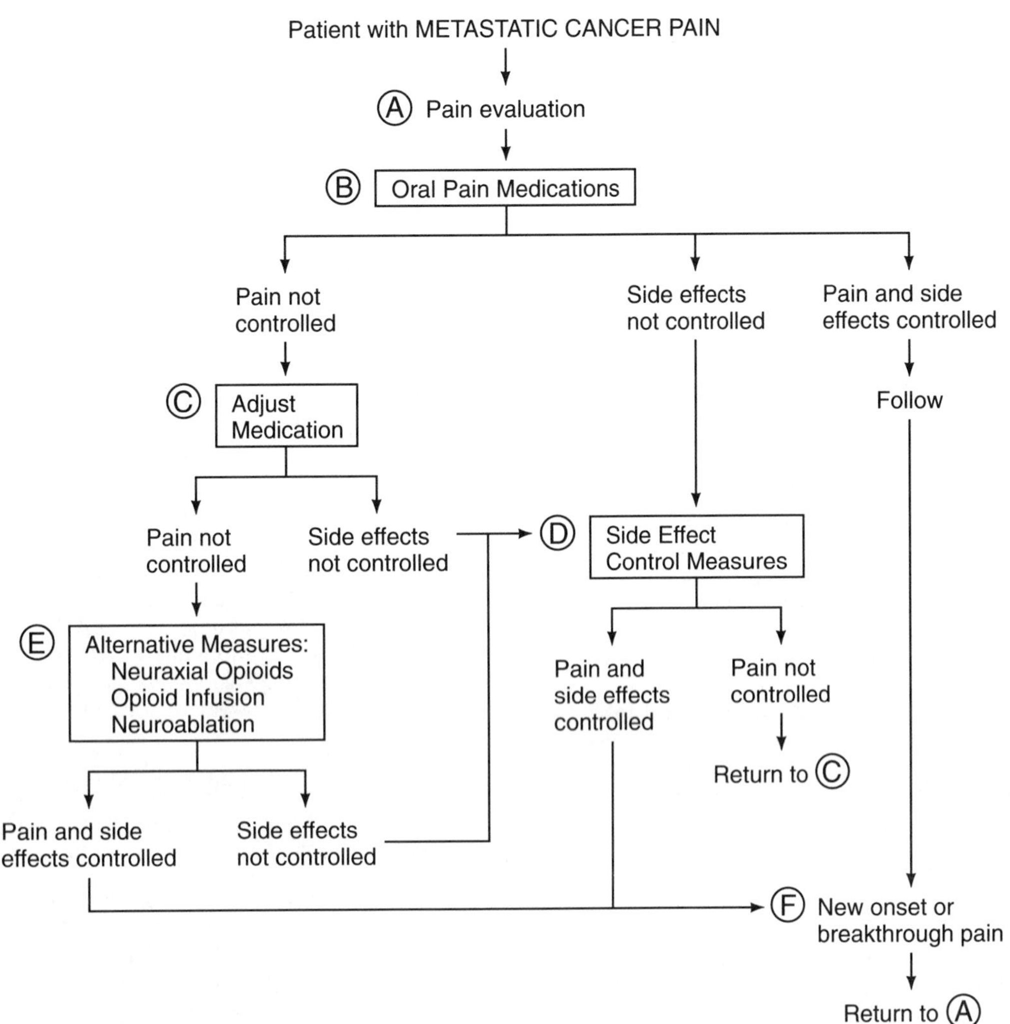

Patient with METASTATIC CANCER PAIN
(A) Pain evaluation
(B) Oral Pain Medications
Pain not controlled
Side effects not controlled
Pain and side effects controlled
(C) Adjust Medication
Follow
Pain not controlled
Side effects not controlled
(D) Side Effect Control Measures
(E) Alternative Measures: Neuraxial Opioids Opioid Infusion Neuroablation
Pain and side effects controlled
Pain not controlled
Return to (C)
Pain and side effects controlled
Side effects not controlled
(F) New onset or breakthrough pain
Return to (A)

DIABETIC NEUROPATHY

Richard Barohn, M.D.

Various types of peripheral neuropathies (PNs) occur in patients with diabetes mellitus (DM) and are often painful. Diabetic PNs are usually treated symptomatically. No specific metabolic therapy has shown any significant clinical benefit. Nevertheless, optimal glucose control is always attempted. PNs associated with DM can broadly be classified into generalized/symmetric and focal/asymmetric types.

A. Compressive mononeuropathies occur frequently in DM and are clinically indistinguishable from those occurring in nondiabetics. Carpal tunnel syndrome is the most common. Initially, it is managed conservatively with NSAIDs and wrist splints. If this fails, surgical decompression may be necessary.

B. Other mononeuropathies, such as those involving cranial nerves (CNs) III, VI, and VII (Bell's palsy), are thought to be due to nerve ischemia and infarction. They tend to recover spontaneously over weeks or months. With CN III palsy, an aneurysm is unlikely if the pupil examination and brain CT scan are normal.

C. Diabetic lumbosacral radiculoplexopathy (DLSRP), or diabetic amyotrophy, consists of profound leg weakness (often more prominent proximally) and severe back and leg pain. DLSRP begins unilaterally but often involves the other leg within weeks. It is presumably due to ischemia of the roots of the lumbosacral (LS) plexus. Weight loss frequently occurs. Therapy consists of reducing the pain with drugs and transcutaneous electrical nerve stimulation (TENS), as listed in G, H, and I, and aggressive physical therapy. Oral narcotics are often required temporarily for the severe pain. Reflex sympathetic dystrophy (RSD) may occur and should be treated appropriately (p 150). The symptoms persist or progress for several months and then may slowly resolve spontaneously. DLSRP is most frequently misdiagnosed as a compressive radiculopathy, but imaging studies of the LS spine are normal. Nevertheless, patients with DLSRP frequently undergo unnecessary LS spine surgery.

D. A limited form of DLSRP can involve isolated thoracic roots, causing severe dermatomal pain in the trunk. The differential diagnosis consists of herpes zoster neuritis, but a rash never develops if diabetes mellitus is the cause. Treatment is as outlined in E, F, and G. Cervical root involvement is very rare.

E. For symptoms of autonomic neuropathy, hypotension can be treated with elastic garments on the lower extremities and oral fludrocortisone (Florinef); gastroparesis can be treated with metoclopramide.

F. Generalized distal symmetric peripheral neuropathy (DSPN) predominantly alters sensory and/or autonomic function. Significant weakness in DSPN is rare, although some motor involvement is usually found on EMG. It usually consists of only numbness and tingling in the toes and fingers. If pain is not present, the medications listed in G should not be used.

G. DSPN may be associated with severe burning pain in the feet and occasionally in the hands. Oral drug therapy for the pain consists of the following options: (1) a tricyclic antidepressant (TCA) (amitriptyline, 75 to 150 mg at bedtime); (2) carbamazepine (600 to 1200 mg a day in three or four divided doses); (3) phenytoin (300 mg at bedtime); or (4) clonazepam (0.5 to 1 mg at bedtime or b.i.d.). If the above are not helpful, adding fluphenazine (Prolixin, 1 mg t.i.d.) to TCA therapy occasionally can relieve pain. Tardive dyskinesia is a potential side effect of fluphenazine.

H. Capsaicin cream (0.025% or 0.075%) applied t.i.d. or q.i.d. may be helpful in painful DSPN.

I. TENS can be a useful nonpharmacologic therapy for pain relief in some patients (p 194).

J. An unusual, purely sensory generalized PN can occur acutely. The burning pain may extend over all the limbs and trunk, and the skin is extremely sensitive to touch. The neuropathy is associated with weight loss, hence the term diabetic neuropathic cachexia. Treatment consists of optimizing diabetic control and the measures outlined in G, H, and I. This PN is self-limited and improves over many months.

References

Archer AG, Watkins PJ, Thomas PK, et al. The natural history of acute painful neuropathy in diabetic mellitus. J Neurol Neurosurg Psychiatry 1983; 46:49.

Barohn RJ, Sahenk Z, Warmolts JR, Mendell JR. The Bruns-Garland syndrome (diabetic amyotrophy). Arch Neurol 1991; 48:1130.

Chokroverty S, Reyes MG, Rebino FA, et al. The syndrome of diabetic amyotrophy. Ann Neurol 1977; 2:181.

Donofrio P, Walker F, Hunt V, et al. Topical capsaicin in painful diabetic neuropathy. Neurology 1990; 40:4 (Suppl 1).

Dyck JD, Thomas PK, Asbury AK, et al. Diabetic neuropathy. Philadelphia: WB Saunders, 1987.

Ellenberg M. Diabetic neuropathic cachexia. Diabetes 1974; 23:418.

Mendel CM, Klern RF, Chappell DA, et al. A trial of amitriptyline and fluphenazine in the treatment of painful diabetic neuropathy. JAMA 1986; 255:637.

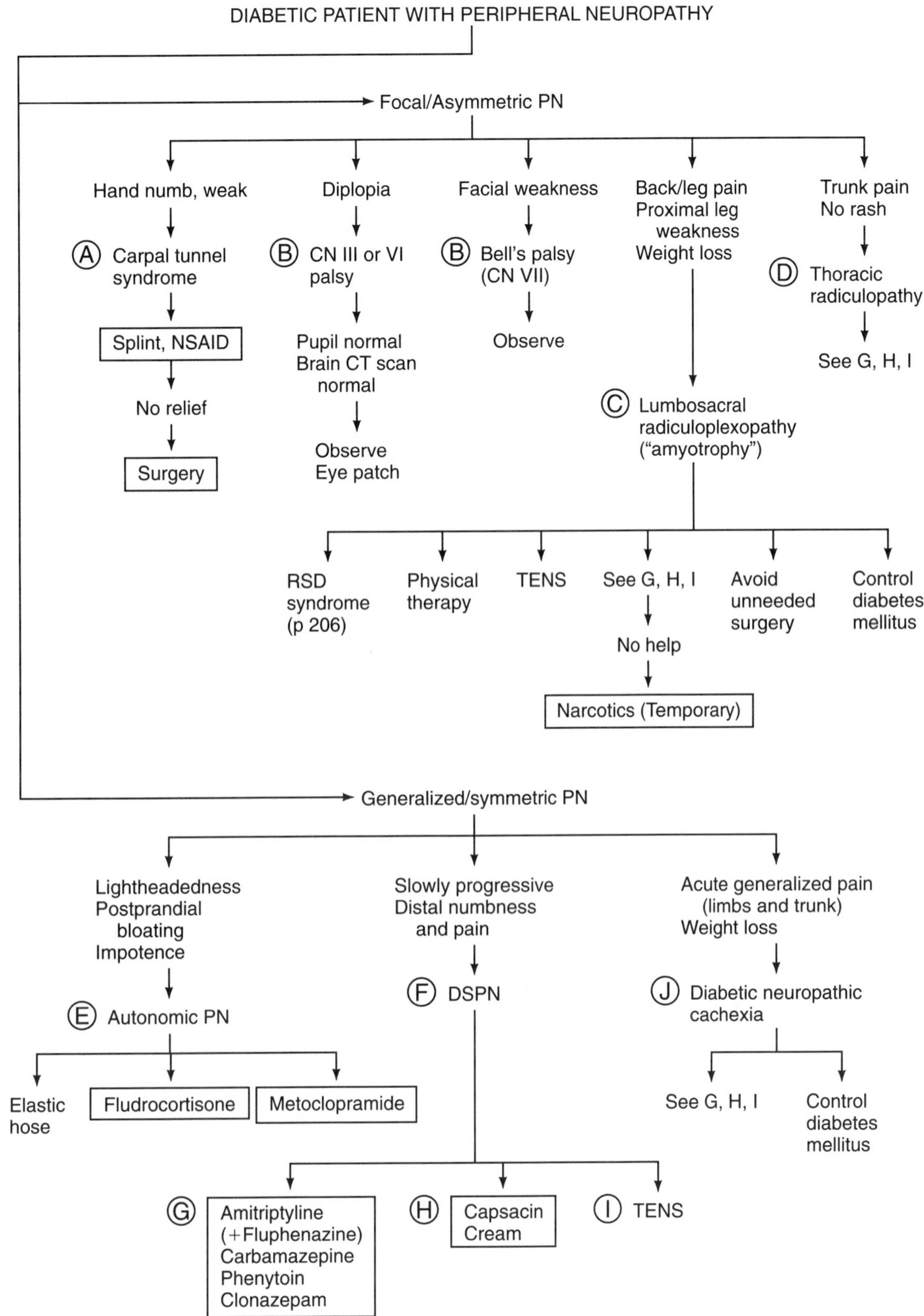
DIABETIC PATIENT WITH PERIPHERAL NEUROPATHY
Focal/Asymmetric PN
Hand numb, weak
A Carpal tunnel syndrome
Splint, NSAID
No relief
Surgery
Diplopia
B CN III or VI palsy
Pupil normal
Brain CT scan normal
Observe
Eye patch
Facial weakness
B Bell's palsy (CN VII)
Observe
Back/leg pain
Proximal leg weakness
Weight loss
C Lumbosacral radiculoplexopathy ("amyotrophy")
Trunk pain
No rash
D Thoracic radiculopathy
See G, H, I
RSD syndrome (p 206)
Physical therapy
TENS
See G, H, I
No help
Narcotics (Temporary)
Avoid unneeded surgery
Control diabetes mellitus
Generalized/symmetric PN
Lightheadedness
Postprandial bloating
Impotence
E Autonomic PN
Elastic hose
Fludrocortisone
Metoclopramide
Slowly progressive
Distal numbness and pain
F DSPN
G Amitriptyline (+Fluphenazine) Carbamazepine Phenytoin Clonazepam
H Capsacin Cream
I TENS
Acute generalized pain (limbs and trunk)
Weight loss
J Diabetic neuropathic cachexia
See G, H, I
Control diabetes mellitus

CHRONIC PANCREATIC PAIN

Robert Sprague, M.D.

Chronic pancreatitis (CP) is a relatively common malady in the United States and most frequently is caused by the excessive and prolonged use of alcohol. Numerous other causes of CP exist, ranging from cystic fibrosis to alpha$_1$-antitrypsin deficiency. The majority of patients complain of a constant, gnawing, boring epigastric pain. The pain may vary in intensity but never subsides entirely. It is often worsened by eating. Narcotic addiction is common.

A. Evaluation consists of a complete physical examination and review of pertinent laboratory data and psychological evaluation with reference to alcohol abuse. The cause of CP should be elicited, and long-standing alcohol abuse must be addressed prior to beginning definitive therapy. Patients also may be addicted to narcotics, as these are commonly prescribed for bouts of acute pancreatitis. Patients should be examined for the possibility of a pancreatic pseudocyst. Various radiologic examinations such as ultrasonography and CT as well as endoscopic pancreatography can be helpful in making this determination. It is important for the consulting anesthesiologist to ascertain whether a pseudocyst is present before performing a celiac plexus block (CPB).

B. Medical therapy of CP is based on enzyme replacement and pancreatic rest via nasogastric suctioning and abstinence from alcohol. Dietary restrictions are also implemented. Narcotics are often used to palliate the pain.

C. Surgical approaches to management of CP consist of local resection with pancreaticojejunostomy. Seventy-five percent of patients will obtain pain relief with this therapy, but most develop pancreatic endocrine and exocrine deficiencies.

D. Anesthetic management of CP consists of CPB. The use of neurolytic CPB is somewhat controversial, as these patients are not terminally ill and may require repeated CPBs, replete with associated complications (Table 1). Neurolytic blocks are by no means permanent and usually afford 4- to 6-month pain-free intervals. A neurolytic CPB will create a "silent abdomen," with lack of visceral sensation to warn of an impending intra-abdominal emergency. Some studies have shown rather dramatic improvement in pain management of CP with neurolytic blocks. The use of steroids with CPB for CP has also been studied but appears to offer no benefit. Left-sided interpleural catheters may be useful in treating acute exacerbations. Performance of CPB is described elsewhere (p 246). 25 cc of 50% alcohol is placed via each needle to effect a neurolytic block. The alcohol may be mixed with 1% lidocaine because the injection of alcohol may be exquisitely painful. The block may take 24 to 48 hours to produce a maximal effect. Radiologic guidance is recommended in the performance of neurolytic CPB.

TABLE 1 Complications of Neurolytic Celiac Plexus Block

Hypotension
Back pain
Accidental subarachnoid/epidural injection
Renal perforation
Pneumothorax
Permanent neurologic damage (due to placement near motor/sensory roots)

References

Bridenbaugh PO, Cousins MJ, eds. Neural blockade in clinical anesthesia and management of pain. 2nd ed. Philadelphia: JB Lippincott, 1988.

Greenberger NJ, Toskes PP. Approach to the patient with pancreatic disease. In Wilson JD, et al (eds): Principles of internal medicine. 12th ed. New York: McGraw-Hill, 1991.

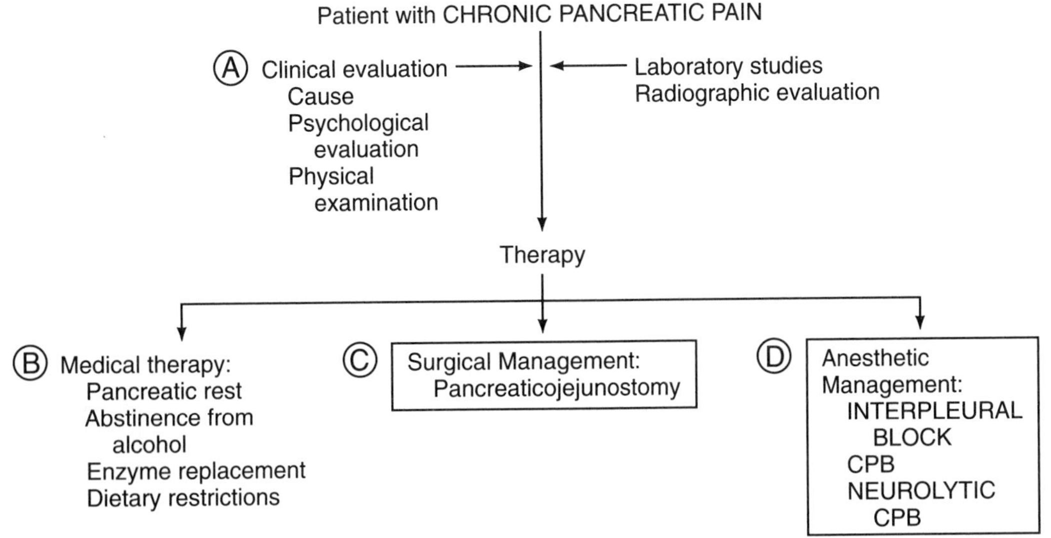
Patient with CHRONIC PANCREATIC PAIN
Ⓐ Clinical evaluation
Cause
Psychological evaluation
Physical examination
Laboratory studies
Radiographic evaluation
Therapy
Ⓑ Medical therapy:
Pancreatic rest
Abstinence from alcohol
Enzyme replacement
Dietary restrictions
Ⓒ Surgical Management:
Pancreaticojejunostomy
Ⓓ Anesthetic Management:
INTERPLEURAL BLOCK
CPB
NEUROLYTIC CPB

NEUROGENIC PAIN

Mark E. Romanoff, M.D.

Neurogenic or neuropathic pain can be defined as non-nociceptive. The pain is thought to originate from trauma or diseases that affect peripheral nerves, the spinal cord, or the brain. The term deafferentation pain (anesthesia dolorosa, phantom limb) is often used interchangeably, but this condition is more appropriately considered as a subset of neurogenic pain. Neurogenic pain encompasses many different and varied pain syndromes such as reflex sympathetic dystrophy (RSD), peripheral neuropathy, plexus avulsion, postherpetic neuralgia, phantom limb pain, trigeminal neuralgia, post-thoracotomy pain, and perhaps postlaminectomy pain. All these syndromes may in part or in whole be caused by neurogenic factors. The pain in these syndromes may not be related to the amount of nerve damage done. The cause of neurogenic pain is as varied as each syndrome. Peripheral mechanisms include neuroma formation after neural trauma, ectopic impulse generation after demyelination, and sympathetic efferent/somatic afferent communications. Spinal cord changes may occur after peripheral nerve injury, including modifications in dorsal horn neurotransmitter concentrations. This may cause either an increase in sensitivity to nociceptors or relaying of non-nociceptive input to nociceptor pathways. The thalamus may also be implicated. Changes in the balance of nociceptive to non-nociceptive information or the loss of inhibition of pain pathways may increase the perception of pain. Some syndromes are a combination of peripheral and central factors.

The signs and symptoms of these syndromes are varied, depending on the location of the lesion. Some hallmarks of neurogenic pain common to most syndromes are sensory loss in the affected area; burning dysesthetic pain; paroxysms of sharp, shooting pain; hyperalgesia; allodynia; and signs of sympathetic hyperactivity. As the causes of these syndromes are varied, diagnostic studies must be individualized. Nociceptive pain is often narcotic sensitive, whereas neurogenic pain is usually not. Sodium thiopental infusions may temporarily relieve neurogenic pain in up to 60% to 80% of patients and are used as part of a diagnostic work-up.

A. Few well-controlled studies have been attempted to determine the efficacy of treatment, and results from those studies are often poor (<50% success rates). The lesions responsible for these syndromes are diverse, so that, as with diagnosis, treatment must be individualized. However, some generalizations can be made. Conservative treatment should include medications, physical therapy, transcutaneous electrical nerve stimulation (TENS), and psychological interventions. Antidepressant medications appear to decrease pain in these patients with or without changes in depressive symptoms. If no success is seen after an adequate trial of antidepressants, an anticonvulsant agent is initiated. Phenytoin, carbamazepine, or clonazepam is commonly used; the drug is added to, not substituted for, the antidepressant medication. Anticonvulsants usually have little effect on the burning pain but can improve the sharp, shooting pain. A therapeutic level or significant side effects should be obtained before these medications are deemed ineffective. Neuroleptic agents such as fluphenazine and haloperidol can be substituted for anticonvulsant medications for further pain control, but their side effects (tardive dyskinesia, extrapyramidal symptoms, neuroleptic malignant syndrome) commonly limit their use. Physical therapy should be initiated early in the course of treatment if it can be tolerated. TENS has decreased pain in some patients (p 194). Worsened pain with TENS treatment has also been observed. Hypnosis, behavioral therapy, and other psychological techniques are suggested (p 198).

B. Nerve blocks alone usually do not alleviate all the symptoms, because they usually affect only one aspect of the pain (burning or lancinating). The predominant type of pain should direct which type of fibers should be blocked, sympathetic or somatic.

C. Sympathetic blockade often alleviates or ameliorates vasomotor symptoms, hyperpathia, and burning pain. Syndromes responding well to sympathetic blocks include causalgia, RSD, postherpetic neuralgia, and post-traumatic pain. Despite the low success rate with other syndromes, patients with signs or symptoms consistent with increased sympathetic activity should undergo a trial of sympathetic blocks. This avoids overlooking any RSD patient who might benefit from sympatholysis (p 50). Oral sympatholytic agents may also be helpful.

D. Permanent sympathectomy may be helpful for patients exhibiting a limited or temporary response to sympathetic blocks. Pain relief with a permanent sympathectomy may last only 6 months to 1 year. Subsequent attempts at sympathectomy are often of limited value. A permanent sympathectomy can be performed percutaneously by the anesthesiologist with phenol or absolute alcohol solutions or by a surgical approach. Pain from long-standing peripheral vascular disease may also respond to this treatment.

E. Pain can often be relieved with somatic blocks. The response is often short-lived (duration of the local anesthesia) but may last longer than the duration of blockade. A series of blocks (often three to seven) or continuous blockade (p 208) may be necessary to break the cycle of pain. Conditions that may respond well to these blocks include stump pain, failed laminectomy syndrome, and post-thoracotomy syndrome.

F. Neurolytic somatic blocks should be used with caution. Side effects are common (numbness in the affected area, motor loss or increased pain from neuralgia). Some recent work suggests that previous somatic blockade may not predict the response to neurolytic procedures. This may be due to an IV or CNS effect of the local anesthetic used in the block.

(Continued on page 62)

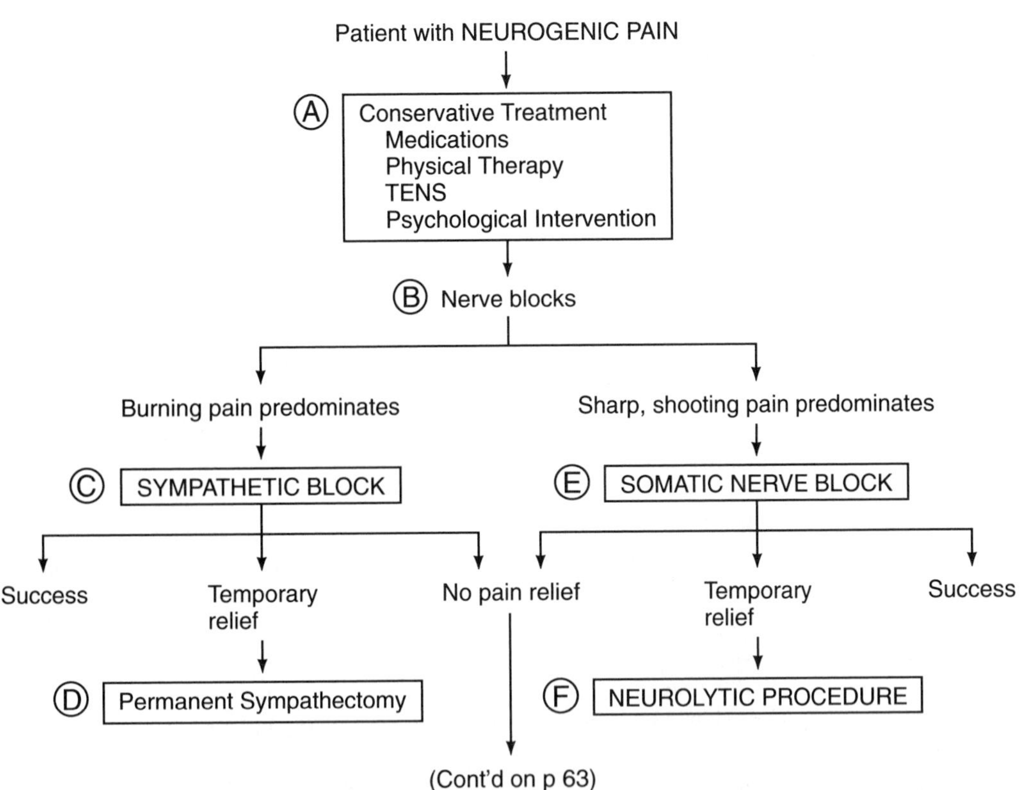
Patient with NEUROGENIC PAIN
A
Conservative Treatment
Medications
Physical Therapy
TENS
Psychological Intervention
B Nerve blocks
Burning pain predominates
Sharp, shooting pain predominates
C SYMPATHETIC BLOCK
E SOMATIC NERVE BLOCK
Success
Temporary relief
No pain relief
Temporary relief
Success
D Permanent Sympathectomy
F NEUROLYTIC PROCEDURE
(Cont'd on p 63)

G. If pain relief is not satisfactory with the types of blocks chosen, a reappraisal of the diagnosis or syndrome may be helpful. If sympathetic blocks were performed initially, somatic blocks can be tried. A differential block may help delineate the pain problem more fully. Placebo responders or central pain mechanisms may then be identified. Conservative treatment should be continued or reinstituted and may have increased efficacy after a series of blocks.

H. Further medication trials based on the results of the differential blocks can be begun. The use of narcotics is controversial. Most authors consider neurogenic pain to be opioid insensitive. However, newer work suggests that because neurogenic pain is diverse, there is a spectrum of narcotic sensitivity. Narcotic trials can be expanded to intrathecal/epidural delivery in patients with severe pain that appears sensitive to opioids. IV local anesthetic infusions (2-chloroprocaine, lidocaine) have had limited success in patients with neurogenic pain (p 18). The mechanism of action may be peripheral (a decrease in spontaneous firing of neuromas) or central (selective afferent block in the spinal cord or thalamus). If these are successful, maintenance therapy with mexiletine or tocainide can be given. Blood levels should be followed.

I. Gratifying results can be seen in some patients after neurosurgical pain-reducing procedures. Dorsal root entry zone (DREZ) lesions can be effective for avulsion injuries, RSD, postherpetic neuralgia, spinal cord damage, and occasionally phantom limb pain. DREZ lesions usually have no effect on post-thoracotomy pain. Patients with trigeminal neuralgia may respond to trigeminal ablation in >85% of cases (p 256). Cordotomy can be attempted in patients with unilateral sharp pain of spinal cord origin or cauda equina syndrome. Pain relief is often temporary (<6 months in duration). Dorsal column stimulation may be helpful in patients with peripheral vascular disease, plexus lesions, postherpetic neuralgia, post-traumatic pain, and thalamic pain (p 224). A dorsal rhizotomy is usually ineffective for these syndromes. Deep brain stimulation has been performed in patients with anesthesia dolorosa, phantom limb pain, and failed laminectomy syndrome, with approximately 50% pain relief.

References

Arner S, Lindblom U, Meyerson BA, Molander C. Prolonged relief of neuralgia after regional anesthetic blocks. A call for further experimental and systematic clinical studies. Pain 1990; 43:287.

Arner S, Meyerson BA. Lack of analgesic effects of opioids on neuropathic and idiopathic forms of pain. Pain 1988; 33:11.

Edwards TW, Habib F, Burney RG, Begin G. Intravenous lidocaine in the management of various chronic pain states. A review of 211 cases. Reg Anesthesia 1985; 10:1.

Max MB. Towards physiologically based treatment of patients with neuropathic pain. Pain 1990; 42:131.

McMahon S, Koltzenburg M. The changing role of primary afferent neurons in pain. Pain 1990; 43:269.

Mucke L, Maciewicz R. Clinical management of neuropathic pain. Neurol Clin 1987; 5:649.

Portenoy RK, Foley KM, Inturrisi CE. The nature of opioid responsiveness and its implications for neuropathic pain: New hypotheses derived from studies of opioid infusions. Pain 1990; 43:273.

Tasker RR, Dostrovsky FO. Deafferentation and central pain. In: Wall PD, Melzack R, eds. Textbook of pain. 2nd ed. New York: Churchill Livingstone, 1990:154.

Taub A, Collins WF. Observations on the treatment of denervation dysesthesia with psychotropic drugs: Postherpetic neuralgia, anesthesia dolorosa, peripheral neuropathy. In: Bonica JJ, ed. Advances in neurology. New York: Raven Press, 1974:309.

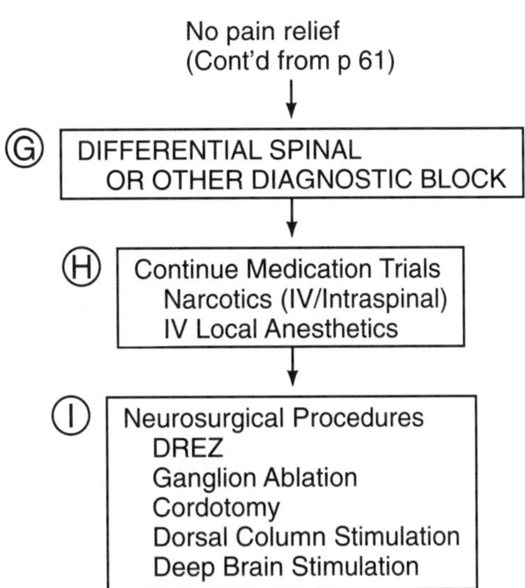
No pain relief
(Cont'd from p 61)
G
DIFFERENTIAL SPINAL
OR OTHER DIAGNOSTIC BLOCK
H
Continue Medication Trials
Narcotics (IV/Intraspinal)
IV Local Anesthetics
I
Neurosurgical Procedures
DREZ
Ganglion Ablation
Cordotomy
Dorsal Column Stimulation
Deep Brain Stimulation

CENTRAL PAIN SYNDROME

David Vanos, M.D.

Central pain syndrome (CPS) is defined as pain arising as a result of a CNS lesion, at the level of either the brain or the spinal cord, or both. The CNS lesion may be of virtually any cause, such as tumor, trauma, arteriovenous malformation, stroke, or surgery. Thus, for CPS, we consider spinal cord lesions (e.g., syringomyelia), cordotomy, stroke, brain tumor, spinal cord tumor, or CNS trauma. Thalamic or pseudothalamic pain syndromes are a subset of this and can occur after a lesion to the ventroposterolateral and/or ventroposteromedian regions of the thalamus. At one time considered synonymous with CPS, it is the most common form. The incidence of CPS is 1 per 50,000 with stroke, 5% with cordotomy, and 20% with spinal cord injury.

The pain is usually described as diffuse, unilateral, and burning with allodynia, hypesthesia, hypalgesia, hyperpathia, dysesthesia. There may be signs of neurologic damage to structures that supply the affected region. Usually the spinothalamic tract or thalamus is involved in the lesion. Onset is generally 2 weeks to 2 years after the lesion has occurred. The pain may have spontaneous, continuous, burning, stabbing, and aching components. Severity is wide, ranging from mild to intolerable. Nonnoxious stimuli may elicit or trigger the pain, even auditory stimuli, visual stimuli, or visceral activity (e.g., urination). Other associated problems (e.g., hemiparesis) occur secondary to the damage of structures proximal to the lesions. Vasomotor and sudomotor atrophy may occur. Anxiety and depression are common associated features. Some mechanisms offered to explain CPS are listed in Table 1.

TABLE 1 CPS Mechanisms

Activation of previously ineffective synapses
Increased effect of surviving synapses
New aberrant connections
Chemical hypersensitivity to neurotransmitters and neuromodulatory substrates
Ephaptic connections
Spontaneous activity generated at site of injury
Altered somatotopic representation of one or more sensory modalities
Loss of inhibitory connections
Altered ascending or descending inhibitory pathways
Desensitization of pattern-generating systems
Spontaneous activity in denervated neurons

A. Evaluation should include a thorough history, especially any previous neurologic incidents. A complete neurologic examination is important to identify any peripheral cause for the pain. CT or MRI scans may help localize the lesion. A psychological evaluation, along with differential blocks, can help identify psychogenic pain originating at the cortical level as a result of processes such as psychosis, conversion, personality disorders, hysteria, and magnification (p 6).

B. Centrally active medications such as tricyclic antidepressants (TCAs) and phenothiazines have proved effective, especially in patients with depression and anxiety. Phenytoin and carbamazepine are useful for the lancinating type of pain. IV naloxone with oral naltrexone maintenance therapy may be considered for certain types of central pain (e.g., thalamic syndrome).

C. Peripheral sympathetic blocks may be useful for certain subsets of CPS that produce chronic pain and hyperpathia, and reportedly even for lesions of the thalamus.

D. Transcutaneous electrical nerve stimulation (TENS) of peripheral nerves has proved ineffective for medullary and thalamic lesions. Dorsal column nerve stimulation (DCNS) and surgery, including rhizotomy, cordotomy, and stereotactic operations, have been disappointing in terms of long-term success. Deep brain stimulation of the thalamic area of the brain is available at only a few centers and its efficacy has yet to be established.

E. Psychological support is beneficial in most CPS patients and should be offered.

References

Budd K. The use of the opiate antagonist, naloxone, in the treatment of intractable pain. Neuropeptides 1985; 5:419.

Cousins MJ, Bridenbaugh PO. Neural blockade in clinical anesthesia and management of pain. 2nd ed. Philadelphia: JB Lippincott, 1988:759.

Loh L, Nathan PW, Schott GD. Pain due to lesions of the central nervous system removed by sympathetic block. Br Med J 1981; 282:1026.

Pagin CA. Central pain due to spinal cord and brain stem damage. In: Wall PD, Melzack R, eds. Textbook of pain. New York: Churchill Livingstone, 1989.

Tasker RR. Neurostimulation and percutaneous neural destructive techniques. In: Cousins MJ, Bridenbaugh PO, eds. Neural blockade in clinical anesthesia and management of pain. 2nd ed. Philadelphia: JB Lippincott, 1988:1086.

Wall PD, Melzack R. Textbook of pain. New York: Churchill Livingstone, 1984:641.

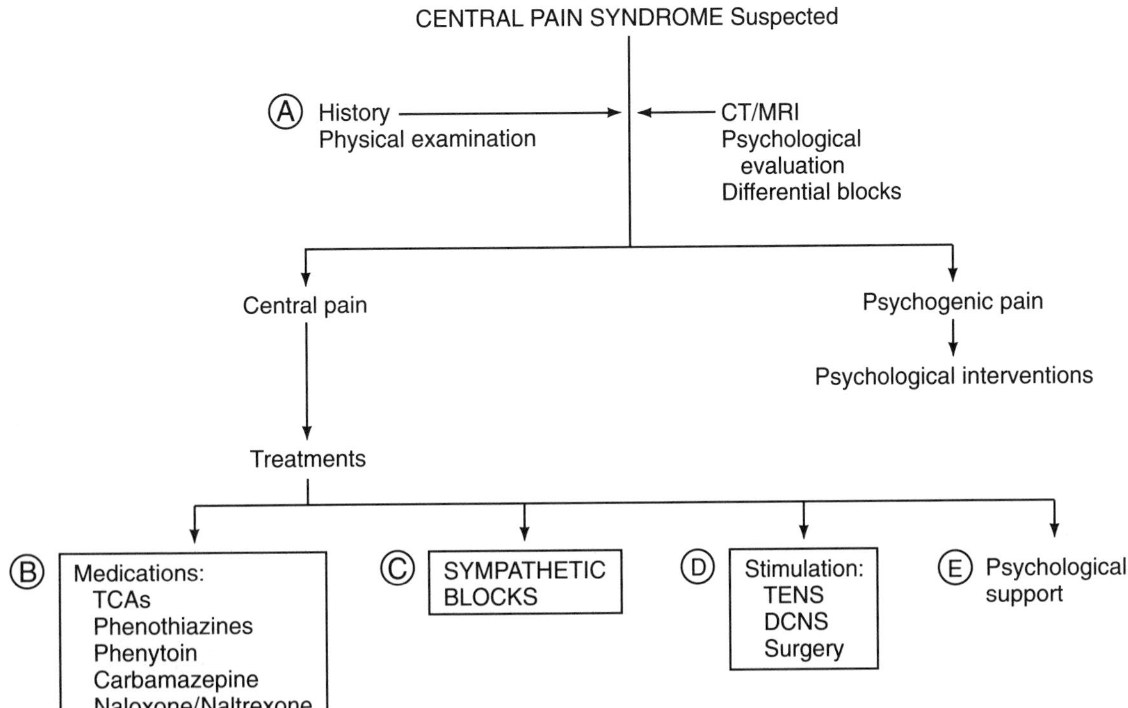
CENTRAL PAIN SYNDROME Suspected
(A) History
Physical examination
CT/MRI
Psychological evaluation
Differential blocks
Central pain
Psychogenic pain
Psychological interventions
Treatments
(B) Medications:
TCAs
Phenothiazines
Phenytoin
Carbamazepine
Naloxone/Naltrexone
(C) SYMPATHETIC BLOCKS
(D) Stimulation:
TENS
DCNS
Surgery
(E) Psychological support

PHANTOM PAIN

Norman G. Gall, M.D.

Phantom pain is pain in the part of a limb that is no longer there. It must be differentiated from phantom sensation, which is the sensation that the amputated part is still there (only parts of the amputated limb may be felt to be present); and stump pain, which is pain that is specifically located in, and does not extend beyond, the stump. Phantom pain is more frequently present in rapid-onset situations requiring amputation (such as trauma) and is relatively rare in slow-onset situations such as diabetic arteriosclerotic peripheral vascular disease. Recent philosophy is that stump pain and phantom pain with similar characteristics may have closely related physiologic mechanisms that may respond to similar effective treatment interventions.

A. Presurgical or immediate postsurgical warning to the patient that phantom sensation and pain are possible, along with successful fitting of and ambulation with a prosthesis, are the most successful interventions in preventing phantom pain. Upper extremity phantom pain is often more recalcitrant to prosthetic fitting, since functional replacement of the upper extremity by an artificial device is more difficult. Before treatment regimens for phantom pain are initiated, the second line of defense should be an attempt to use phantom exercises. These can be effective only if the patient can move the phantom limb. In the lower extremity, these consist of isometric exercises at the ankle to the count of ten in plantar flexion, dorsiflexion, inversion, and eversion, followed by toes curled down and toes flared up. This often provides sufficient night phantom pain relief to allow a return to sleep.

B. Patients with burning phantom pain may exhibit decreased blood flow to the stump similar to the situation in reflex sympathetic dystrophy. Biofeedback and relaxation techniques may prove helpful. Transcutaneous electrical nerve stimulation (TENS) or nitropaste applied to the stump also may relieve pain. If these measures do not help, sympathetic blockade may be necessary (p 248). A differential block may be necessary to rule out a central pain syndrome.

C. Cramping pain may respond to a phantom exercise program and biofeedback. Muscle relaxants have been used but should be discontinued if they offer no help after a 4-week trial period. TENS can also be useful.

D. Lightning pain may be the result of a neuroma. Examine the stump closely; if a neuroma is present it can be injected with a bupivacaine-steroid solution. If results are only temporary, a neurolytic injection or surgical resection may be needed to provide long-term relief.

E. Trigger point–induced phantom pain can present with any kind of symptoms; however, it is elicited most frequently with motion. Examine the residual limb as well as the back and neck to identify any trigger points that reproduce the phantom pain. Spray and stretch, trigger point injections, and a Medcosonolator may prove helpful. Use of any agent for >14 days is a waste of time, in my opinion.

F. Psychological components of phantom pain, like all other chronic pain, are more common if the pain has occurred for $\geqq 1$ year. Adjunct interventions, including counseling, behavior modification, and drug therapy for anxiety, stress, depression, etc., should be used along with other major forms of treatment. The prosthesis should be constantly evaluated for lack of fit and alignment. A team approach to treatment works best.

References

Sherman RA. Published treatments of phantom limb pain. Am J Phys Med 1980; 59:232.

Sherman RA. Stump and phantom limb pain. Neurol Clin 1989; 7:249.

Sherman RA, Gall N, Gormley J. Treatment of phantom limb pain with muscular relaxation training to disrupt the pain-anxiety-tension cycle. Pain 1979; 6:47.

Sherman RA, Sherman CJ, Gall NG. A survey of current phantom limb pain treatment in the United States. Pain 1980; 8:85.

Sherman RA, Tippens JK. Suggested guidelines for treatment of phantom limb pain. Orthopedics 1982; 5:1595.

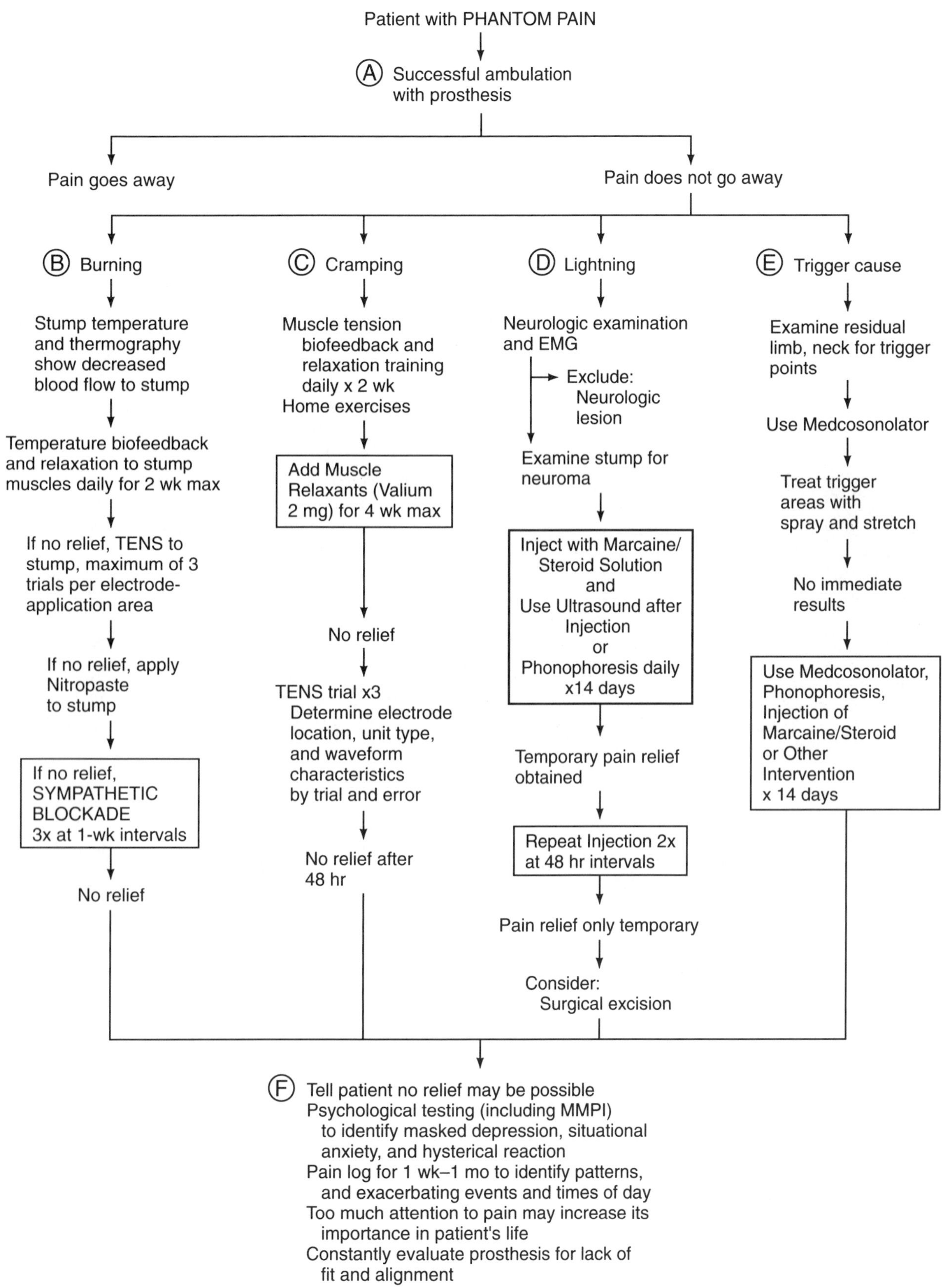

Patient with PHANTOM PAIN
(A) Successful ambulation with prosthesis
Pain goes away
Pain does not go away
(B) Burning
Stump temperature and thermography show decreased blood flow to stump
Temperature biofeedback and relaxation to stump muscles daily for 2 wk max
If no relief, TENS to stump, maximum of 3 trials per electrode-application area
If no relief, apply Nitropaste to stump
If no relief, SYMPATHETIC BLOCKADE 3x at 1-wk intervals
No relief
(C) Cramping
Muscle tension biofeedback and relaxation training daily x 2 wk
Home exercises
Add Muscle Relaxants (Valium 2 mg) for 4 wk max
No relief
TENS trial x3
Determine electrode location, unit type, and waveform characteristics by trial and error
No relief after 48 hr
(D) Lightning
Neurologic examination and EMG
Exclude: Neurologic lesion
Examine stump for neuroma
Inject with Marcaine/ Steroid Solution and Use Ultrasound after Injection or Phonophoresis daily x14 days
Temporary pain relief obtained
Repeat Injection 2x at 48 hr intervals
Pain relief only temporary
Consider: Surgical excision
(E) Trigger cause
Examine residual limb, neck for trigger points
Use Medcosonolator
Treat trigger areas with spray and stretch
No immediate results
Use Medcosonolator, Phonophoresis, Injection of Marcaine/Steroid or Other Intervention x 14 days
(F) Tell patient no relief may be possible
Psychological testing (including MMPI) to identify masked depression, situational anxiety, and hysterical reaction
Pain log for 1 wk–1 mo to identify patterns, and exacerbating events and times of day
Too much attention to pain may increase its importance in patient's life
Constantly evaluate prosthesis for lack of fit and alignment

PAIN IN THE SPINAL CORD–INJURED PATIENT

Douglas Barber, M.D.

Estimates of the prevalence of chronic pain in spinal cord–injured (SCI) patients range from 27% to 77%. The percentage of SCI patients with chronic pain so severe that it interferes with the activities of daily living has been reported to range from 5% to 44%. Patients with cauda equina injuries often experience the most severe pain seen in SCI patients. A careful history, including a review of the mechanisms of injury, the time of onset of the pain, and the distribution of the pain, is necessary in evaluating these patients. In patients with lesions above T8, one must consider referred pain from an acute abdomen.

A. Radicular pain is particularly amenable to anticonvulsant therapy. Radiography, electrodiagnostic tests, and diagnostic/therapeutic epidural steroid injections may be of benefit in identifying the cause of the pain. If an identifiable anatomic lesion is demonstrated on radiologic imaging, neurosurgical intervention may be warranted.

B. Hypersensitivity of the sympathetic nervous system may result in a reflex sympathetic dystrophy (RSD) syndrome. Diagnosis is made with sympathetic blocks and triple-phase bone scan. RSD is typically treated by sympathetic blockade via stellate ganglion block (upper extremity) or lumbar sympathetic block (lower extremity), or with IV regional techniques. Typically, a series of blocks is indicated. An aggressive program of physical therapy to the affected extremity should be carried out in concert with the injection therapy.

C. Central deafferentation pain is thought to be a result of loss of inhibition or augmentation of ascending excitatory pathways and/or descending pathways from the periaqueductal/periventricular gray matter. A denervation hypersensitivity phenomenon has been implicated. Tricyclic antidepressants and behavioral techniques are believed to be the most effective agents in treating this pain phenomenon. Neurosurgical techniques, particularly dorsal root entry zone (DREZ) thermal ablation, may be considered in patients who are refractory to conservative therapy.

D. Post-traumatic cystic myelopathy (syringomyelia) may develop in up to 7% of patients with complete quadriplegia. The average time from injury to the appearance of symptoms is approximately 4 years in those with complete lesions and 10 years in those with incomplete lesions. The mode of presentation varies; the most common initial complaint is pain. Pain is usually aggravated by straining, coughing, or sitting. Loss of motor function generally appears late. Definitive treatment consists of neurosurgical shunting of the cyst to the subarachnoid space or peritoneum. However, the indications for surgery must relate to the functional consequences of the disabilities relating to loss of motor function and to pain.

E. The pain associated with neuroma formation may be treated with anticonvulsants or tricyclic antidepressants in combination with transcutaneous electrical nerve stimulation (TENS).

F. Vertebral column injury, especially if unstable, may require neurosurgical intervention. Orthotics provide particular benefit by decreasing mechanical stress at the injury site and by distributing weight-bearing forces across a greater area.

G. Use tricyclic antidepressants with caution in the SCI patient. Choose those with the least anticholinergic side effects.

References

Bedrock GM, ed. Lifetime care of the paraplegic patient. New York: Churchill Livingstone, 1985.

Ingberg H, Prust F. The diagnosis of abdominal emergencies in patients with spinal cord lesions. Arch Phys Med Rehabil 1968; 49:343.

Ozer MN, Schmitt JK, eds. State of the art reviews: Medical complications of spinal cord injury. Philadelphia: Hanley & Belfus, August, 1987.

Whiteneck G, Lammertse DP, Manley S, Menter R, eds. The management of high quadriplegia. New York: Demos, 1989.

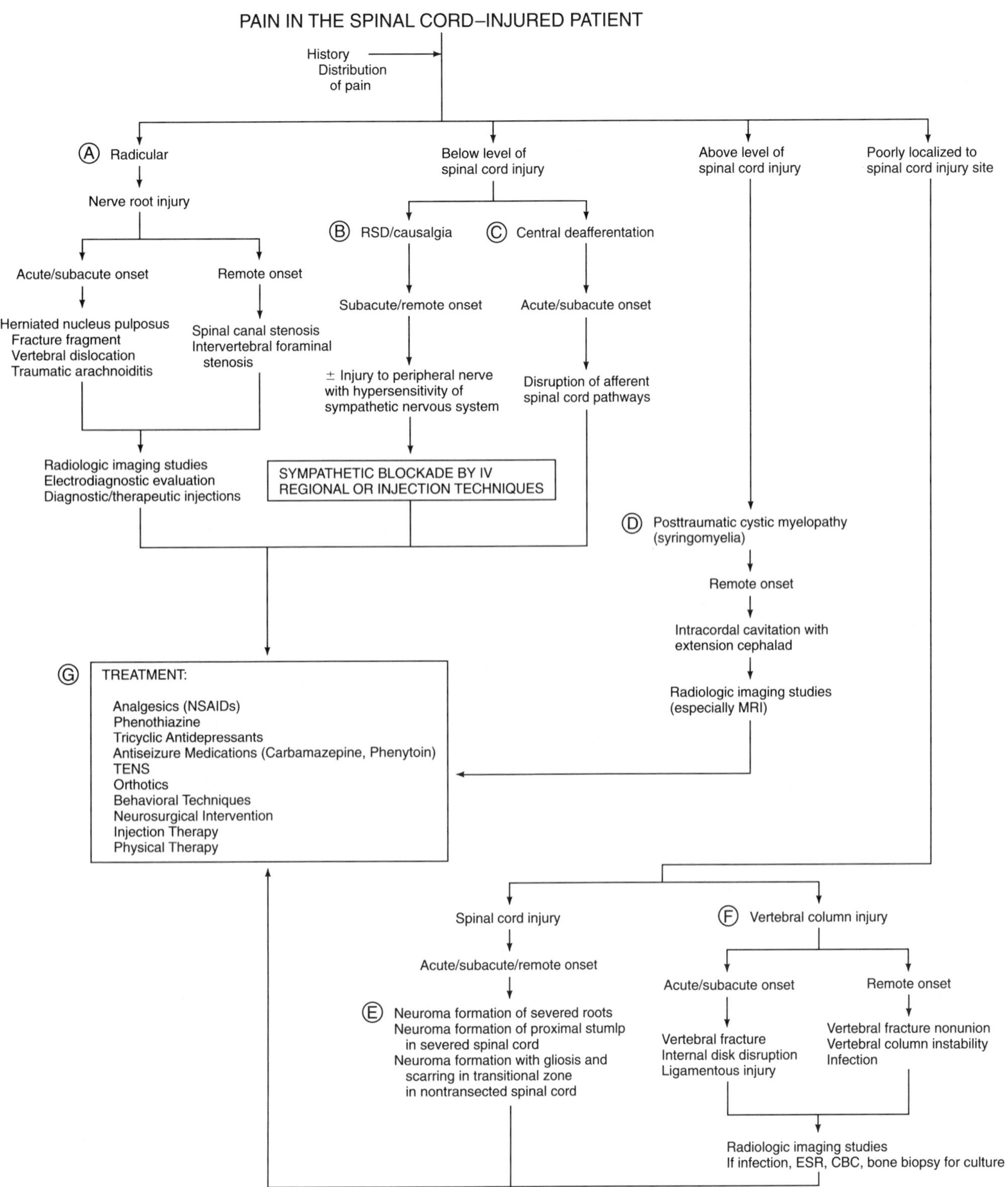
PAIN IN THE SPINAL CORD–INJURED PATIENT
History
Distribution of pain
(A) Radicular
Nerve root injury
Acute/subacute onset
Remote onset
Herniated nucleus pulposus
Fracture fragment
Vertebral dislocation
Traumatic arachnoiditis
Spinal canal stenosis
Intervertebral foraminal stenosis
Radiologic imaging studies
Electrodiagnostic evaluation
Diagnostic/therapeutic injections
Below level of spinal cord injury
(B) RSD/causalgia
(C) Central deafferentation
Subacute/remote onset
Acute/subacute onset
± Injury to peripheral nerve with hypersensitivity of sympathetic nervous system
Disruption of afferent spinal cord pathways
SYMPATHETIC BLOCKADE BY IV REGIONAL OR INJECTION TECHNIQUES
Above level of spinal cord injury
(D) Posttraumatic cystic myelopathy (syringomyelia)
Remote onset
Intracordal cavitation with extension cephalad
Radiologic imaging studies (especially MRI)
Poorly localized to spinal cord injury site
(G) TREATMENT:
Analgesics (NSAIDs)
Phenothiazine
Tricyclic Antidepressants
Antiseizure Medications (Carbamazepine, Phenytoin)
TENS
Orthotics
Behavioral Techniques
Neurosurgical Intervention
Injection Therapy
Physical Therapy
Spinal cord injury
Acute/subacute/remote onset
(E) Neuroma formation of severed roots
Neuroma formation of proximal stumlp in severed spinal cord
Neuroma formation with gliosis and scarring in transitional zone in nontransected spinal cord
(F) Vertebral column injury
Acute/subacute onset
Remote onset
Vertebral fracture
Internal disk disruption
Ligamentous injury
Vertebral fracture nonunion
Vertebral column instability
Infection
Radiologic imaging studies
If infection, ESR, CBC, bone biopsy for culture

FIBROMYOSITIS

Jeffery E. Stedwill, M.D.

The appropriate diagnosis to assign the patient with chronic aching muscles continues to be an area of much controversy. The term *fibrositis* has fallen into relative disuse in recent years, whereas the terms *myofascial pain syndrome* for localized ailments and *fibromyalgia* for more global complaints have been adopted. Recently myofascial pain and fibromyalgia have been considered opposite ends of a spectrum, with a large number of cases of myalgia falling somewhere in the middle. We refer to this spectrum as fibromyositis. Myofascial pain is a regional painful condition with tender points and taut bands of muscle that refer pain to distant sites upon palpation. Fibromyalgia has been defined as a chronic condition characterized by diffuse tender points (>3 anatomic sites for >3 months), morning stiffness, daytime fatigue, and sleep disturbance. The etiology of fibromyositis has thus far eluded investigators. Recent reports have demonstrated abnormal muscle histology and immunoglobin deposition on basement membranes, reduced high-energy phosphates, increased serum concentrations of specific peptides proportionate to the disease impact, and elevated CSF levels of substance P. Arousal disturbances in sleep have been found to induce disease symptoms when artificially induced in asymptomatic volunteers. The psychological makeup of fibromyositis sufferers has been studied extensively, and psychopathology is not considered an etiologic factor, but increased incidence of significant anxiety and depression are believed to be probable exacerbating factors.

A. Evaluation includes a thorough history and physical examination. Laboratory studies, including EMG, EEG, radiography, and biopsy, may be needed, as well as neuropsychiatric testing. Rheumatoid arthritis, polymyalgia rheumatica, hypothyroidism, polymyositis, and widespread osteoarthritis must be ruled out during initial evaluations.

B. If the initial evaluation fails to reveal a specific pathology the diagnosis is based on characteristic manifestations and exclusion of underlying causes. Pain should be present within muscles or their attachments (especially parascapular, paracervical, paralumbar, and gluteal sites) rather than in joints. No abnormalities such as leg length discrepancy or postural abnormality should be present. Evaluate patients for associated symptoms of nonrestorative sleep, daytime fatigue, evidence of psychological distress, and aggravation of symptoms by physical inactivity or overactivity. Ask questions about family members experiencing similar symptoms, as the possibility of an autosomal dominant inheritance pattern has been suggested.

C. Treatment rests on a foundation of education and reassurance and on scrupulous avoidance of physician-imposed disability in response to the pain complaint. Inform the patient that he or she has a well-recognized condition (to allay fears that the pain is "all in the head"), that it is nonprogressive, and that physical exertion, although possibly causing short-term exacerbation of symptoms, is not harmful and may actually contribute to remission.

D. Motor dysfunction from chronic muscle misuse (e.g., habitual concentration, abnormal postural stress, and inactivity or overuse) must be corrected. Other perpetuating factors, such as vitamin C and folate deficiencies and a cold, damp environment, should be eliminated. Hot packs combined with high-frequency, high-intensity transcutaneous electric nerve stimulation (TENS) and deep massage are helpful. Gentle self-stretching while in a hot shower has been advocated. Symptoms can be further relieved with progression to an aerobic conditioning program. When psychological stress is a contributing factor, stress management courses and EMG biofeedback may be useful. Treatments advocated for specific painful sites include trigger/tender point injections and Vapocoolant spray and stretch techniques.

E. Treat sleep disorders aggressively with low-dose amitriptyline (10–50 mg). Alternative medications reported to be useful in treating sleep and other disease symptoms are cyclobenzaprine, fluoxetine, and clonidine. Various NSAIDs and benzodiazepines frequently are used but have not been proven effective.

F. Unrecognized or inadequately treated fibromyositis can cause significant disability and pronounced suffering. Maintain a high index of suspicion when evaluating patients with symptoms of this common disorder. Referral to an inpatient pain management program may prove beneficial.

References

Bengtsson A, Henriksson KJ, Larson J. Reduced high-energy phosphate levels in the painful muscles of patients with primary fibromyalgia. Arthritis Rheum 1986; 29:817.

Campbell SM, Gatter RA, Clark S: A double blind study of cyclobenzaprine in patients with primary fibrositis. Arthritis Rheum. 28:S40, 1985.

Caro XJ. Immunofluorescent detection of IgG at the dermal-epidermal junction in patients with apparent primary fibrositis syndrome. Arthritis Rheum. 1984; 27:1174.

Geller SA. Treatment of fibrositis with fluoxetine hydrochloride (Prozac). Am J Med 1989; 87:594.

Goldenberg DL. Fibromyalgia syndrome: An emerging but controversial condition. JAMA 1987; 257:2782.

Graff-Radford SB, Reeves JL. Effects of transcutaneous electrical nerve stimulation on myofascial pain and trigger point sensitivity. Pain 1989; 37:1.

Jacobsen S, Jensen LT: Primary fibromyalgia: Clinical parameters in relation to serum procollagen type III aminoterminal peptide. Br J Rheum 1990; 29:174.

McCain GA, Bell DA, Mai FM, Halliday PD. A controlled study of the effect of the supervised cardiovascular fitness

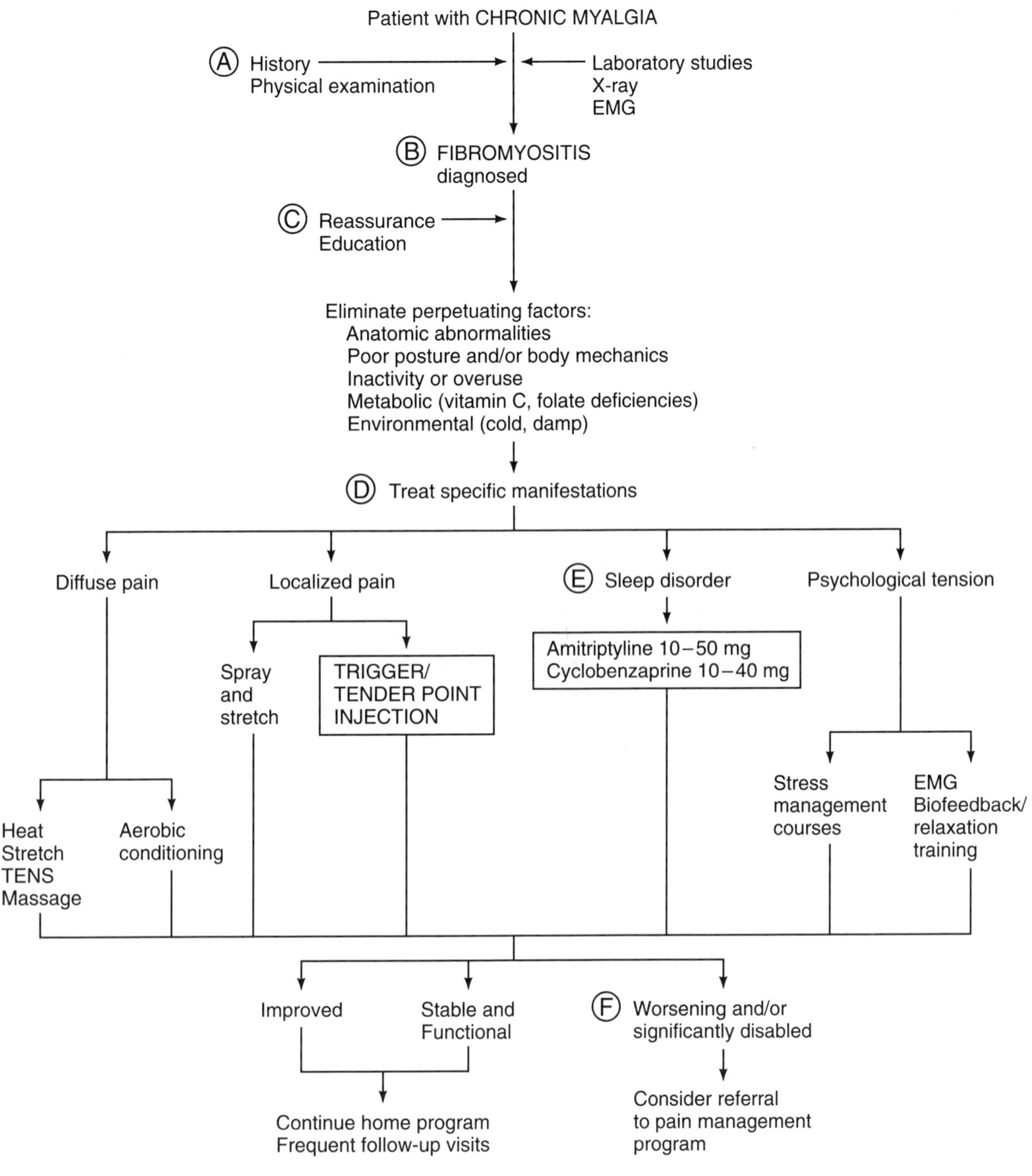

training program on the manifestations of primary fibromyalgia. Arthritis Rheum 1988; 31:1135.

Moldofsky H. Sleep and fibrositis syndrome. Rheum Dis Clin North Am 1989; 15:91.

Pellegrino MJ, Waylonis GW, Sommer A. Familial occurrence of primary fibromyalgia. Arch Phys Med Rehabil 1989; 70:61.

Thompson JM. Tension myalgia as a diagnosis at the Mayo Clinic and its relationship to fibrositis, fibromyalgia and myofascial pain syndrome. Mayo Clin Proc 1990; 65:1237.

Uveges MJ, Parker JC. Psychological symptoms in primary fibromyalgia syndrome: Relationship to pain, life stress, and sleep disturbance. Arthritis Rheum 1990; 33:1279.

Vaeroy H, Helle R. Elevated CSF levels of substance P and high incidence of Raynaud phenomenon in patients with fibromyalgia: New features for diagnosis. Pain 1988; 32:21.

Yunus MB. Primary fibromyalgia syndrome and myofascial pain syndrome: Clinical features and muscle pathology. Arch Phys Med Rehabil 1988; 69:451.

RHEUMATOID ARTHRITIS

Ellen Leonard, M.D.

Rheumatoid arthritis (RA) is a systemic disease that affects both axial and peripheral joints. Joints exhibit inflammation, pain, and deformity. RA affects all ethnic groups. Treatment must be orchestrated to balance pharmacotherapy with environmental, psychological, rehabilitative, and surgical factors.

A. Aspirin is used initially in the pharmacologic management of RA. If symptoms persist or side effects occur, the next drug of choice is an NSAID. Because there are many classes of these drugs, multiple trials with different classes may need to be undertaken. A trial should last 2 to 3 weeks. If there is no improvement at this point in the management, refer the patient to a rheumatologist, as other medications may be required to reduce the inflammation in the joints.

B. RA is a chronic disease with typical associated psychological problems. The patient and family require counseling and education concerning the disease process and its effects on everyday life. Areas that need to be examined include sexuality, self-image, family interactions, avocation, and vocation.

C. Surgery is an important part of treatment. Refer the patient to an orthopedist for intractable pain, severe deformity, or joint instability.

D. Rehabilitation is an ongoing and constantly changing portion of treatment. A balance of therapies is used to aid in maintaining function, reducing pain, and decreasing inflammation.

E. To maintain function, a variety of areas need to be examined. The patient must be instructed in exercises to prevent atrophy and to maintain range of motion (ROM) of the joints. The joints must be protected from overuse by the application of assistive devices and orthotics. Orthotics can also increase comfort. Because the general physical condition of the patient is of the utmost importance, exercise and leisure activities should be evaluated. Swimming is an excellent activity, especially in warm water.

F. Pain is an ongoing problem. Various physical modalities can be used to aid in its control. Superficial heat is useful because it elevates the pain threshold, increases circulation, decreases muscle spasm, and increases stretch. Heat applied in the form of hydrotherapy also provides relaxation. Cold can be applied to decrease pain and muscle spasm. Transcutaneous electrical nerve stimulation (p 194) is also useful in managing pain.

G. Inflammation is reduced in concert with pharmacotherapy by using cold, rest, and selected injection of corticosteroids. Rest can be of the joint only or can be systemic. A specific body part can be rested using orthotics. Patients need at least 8 hours of sleep at night in addition to periods of rest during the day. Prolonged bed rest is detrimental.

References

Delisa J, ed. Rehabilitation medicine: Principles and practice. Philadelphia: JB Lippincott, 1988.

Katz W. Modern management of rheumatoid arthritis. Am J Med 1985; 79:24.

Rodman G. Primer on the rheumatic diseases. Atlanta: Arthritis Foundation, 1983.

Wall P.D. Textbook of pain. 2nd ed. New York: Churchill Livingstone, 1989.

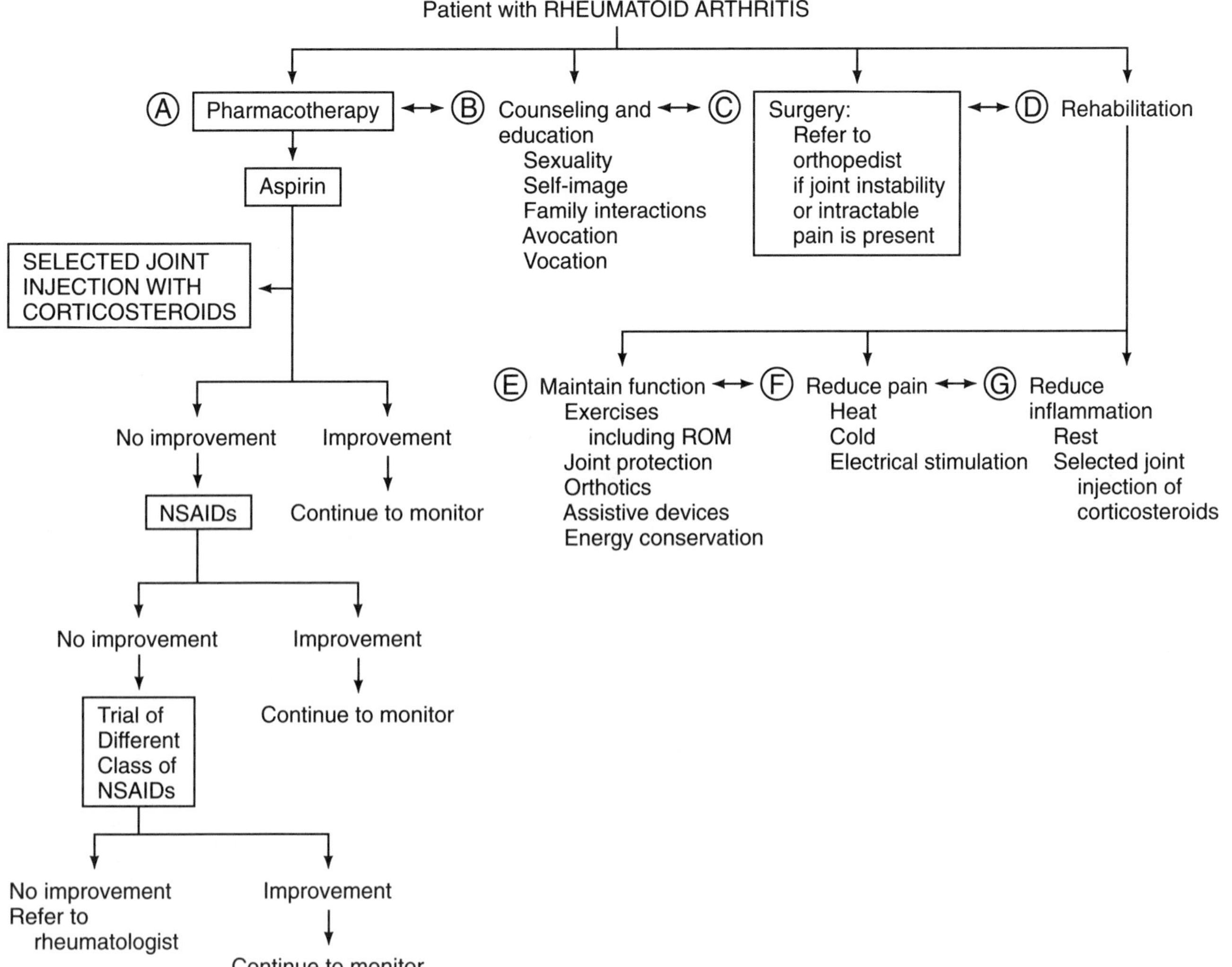

Patient with RHEUMATOID ARTHRITIS
Ⓐ Pharmacotherapy
Aspirin
SELECTED JOINT INJECTION WITH CORTICOSTEROIDS
No improvement
Improvement
NSAIDs
Continue to monitor
No improvement
Improvement
Trial of Different Class of NSAIDs
Continue to monitor
No improvement Refer to rheumatologist
Improvement
Continue to monitor
Ⓑ Counseling and education
Sexuality
Self-image
Family interactions
Avocation
Vocation
Ⓒ Surgery:
Refer to orthopedist if joint instability or intractable pain is present
Ⓓ Rehabilitation
Ⓔ Maintain function
Exercises including ROM
Joint protection
Orthotics
Assistive devices
Energy conservation
Ⓕ Reduce pain
Heat
Cold
Electrical stimulation
Ⓖ Reduce inflammation
Rest
Selected joint injection of corticosteroids

OSTEOARTHRITIS

Ellen Leonard, M.D.

Osteoarthritis (degenerative joint disease) is the most common joint disease of the axial and peripheral skeleton. It is classified as primary or secondary and as generalized or localized. Pain in osteoarthritis is not correlated with the severity of the disease. The etiology of osteoarthritis is unclear.

A. A detailed history and physical examination help to determine the source of the pain and a logical approach to treatment. Possible sources are cartilage, bone, synovial membrane, joint capsule, ligaments, and tendons.

B. X-ray and laboratory data are useful in excluding other joint diseases. X-ray abnormalities correlate poorly with amount of pain.

C. The patient requires reassurance and education regarding the basis and progression of his or her disease. Weight reduction is crucial in obese patients. Instruct the patient about modification of activities to protect joints and about an exercise and rest program.

D. Patients with pain benefit from a physical therapy program using (1) heat to decrease pain, (2) range of motion (ROM) exercises to maintain or increase range, and (3) strengthening of muscles to improve function. Analgesics can be used selectively on an intermittent basis. Aspirin and other NSAIDs are more beneficial than narcotics.

E. Joint stability can be augmented by selective bracing. Bracing decreases the strain on ligamentous structures and decreases further damage to the joints.

F. Inflammation can be intra-articular and periarticular. Anti-inflammatory drugs such as aspirin and NSAIDs can reduce inflammation and pain. Intra-articular injection should be used judiciously; it is occasionally useful in the carpometacarpal joint. Periarticular injections can abolish pain in instances of point tenderness of the capsule and ligaments.

G. Consider surgery for patients with intractable pain or significant deformity that cannot be controlled by conservative means.

References

Brandt Kenneth. Nonsteroidal anti-inflammatory drugs in treatment of osteoarthritis. Clin Orthop 1986; 213:84.

Delisa J, ed. Rehabilitation medicine: Principles and practice. Philadelphia: JB Lippincott, 1988:765.

Rodman Gerald. Primer on the rheumatic diseases. Atlanta: Arthritis Foundation, 1983:104.

Wall PD. Textbook of pain. New York: Churchill Livingstone, 1984:215.

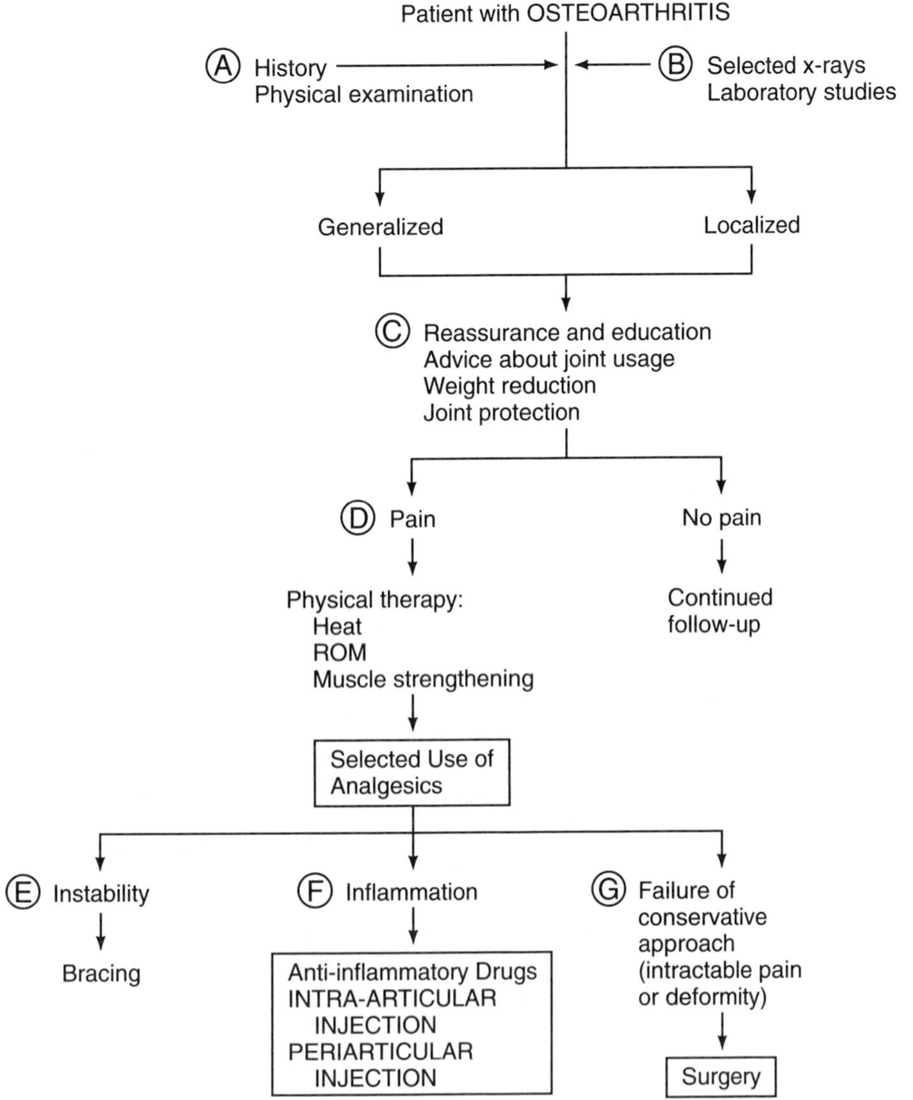
Patient with OSTEOARTHRITIS
(A) History
Physical examination
(B) Selected x-rays
Laboratory studies
Generalized
Localized
(C) Reassurance and education
Advice about joint usage
Weight reduction
Joint protection
(D) Pain
No pain
Physical therapy:
Heat
ROM
Muscle strengthening
Continued
follow-up
Selected Use of
Analgesics
(E) Instability
(F) Inflammation
(G) Failure of
conservative
approach
(intractable pain
or deformity)
Bracing
Anti-inflammatory Drugs
INTRA-ARTICULAR
INJECTION
PERIARTICULAR
INJECTION
Surgery

NONSOMATIC PAIN

Lawrence S. Schoenfeld, Ph.D.

Treatment for chronic pain can be planned effectively only after distinguishing between patients whose pain has a primarily peripheral (somatic) etiology and those with nonperipheral (nonsomatic) pain. By further differentiating the nonsomatic pain patients into primary subgroups (malingering, somatoform, depression, and drug-seeking), target psychological-social-economic issues can be resolved. Although this protocol has limitations and is costly, it helps to reduce unwarranted somatic interventions, iatrogenic injury, and abnormal illness behavior. Etiology is quickly established through a collaborative evaluation with an anesthesiologist and mental health professional (psychologist).

A. Two diagnostic techniques (diagnostic epidural opioid and pentothal) are helpful in identifying the patient with chronic nonsomatic pain. The diagnostic epidural opioid technique may identify chronic patients with pain primarily under operant control. In the nonsomatic pain patient, the pentothal pain test often dramatically demonstrates absence of a pain response under pentothal, using maneuvers that had demonstrated significant pain behavior pre–pentothal induction (p 16).

B. A pain-psychological evaluation investigates motivation, cognition, and affect associated with the chronic pain condition. Under amytal sedation, conflict areas can be further explored. Low dose amytal produces relaxation and improvement in patients with somatoform disorders and a worsening of pain complaints (with increased anxiety) in malingerers. With moderate amytal, the patient with a somatoform disorder demonstrates significant physical improvement, often with spontaneous abreaction, whereas the malingerer often complains about the test, demonstrates guarding behavior, and may become hostile.

C. Inform malingering patients that there is nothing significantly wrong with them physically or psychologically. Encourage a return to normal activities. Primary gains should not be supported by medical attention, treatment, or through medical excuses.

D. A somatoform pain disorder (psychogenic pain) may develop in response to a variety of conflicts, including difficulties dealing with sexuality, marital dysfunction, and job-related stress. An interdisciplinary pain management program provides a setting in which pain patients usually are able to accept psychological intervention.

E. Depression often continues after an injury or peripheral illness has resolved, resulting in further disuse and associated chronic pain. Mobilizing the patient's coping strategies with antidepressant medication, activity programs, and psychotherapy results in a successful treatment outcome.

F. Drug-seeking behavior should be confronted openly and detoxification programs offered (p 188). Successful treatment requires periodic drug screening and supportive psychological therapies.

References

Cherry DA, Gourlay GK, McLachlan M, Cousins MJ. Diagnostic epidural opioid blockade and chronic pain. Pain 1985; 21:143.

Ellis J, Ramamurthy S, Schoenfeld LS, Walsh N, Hoffman J. Diagnostic epidural opioid technique. Clin Pain 1989; 5:211.

Schoichet RP. Sodium amytal in the diagnosis of chronic pain. Can Psychiatr Assoc J 1978; 23:219.

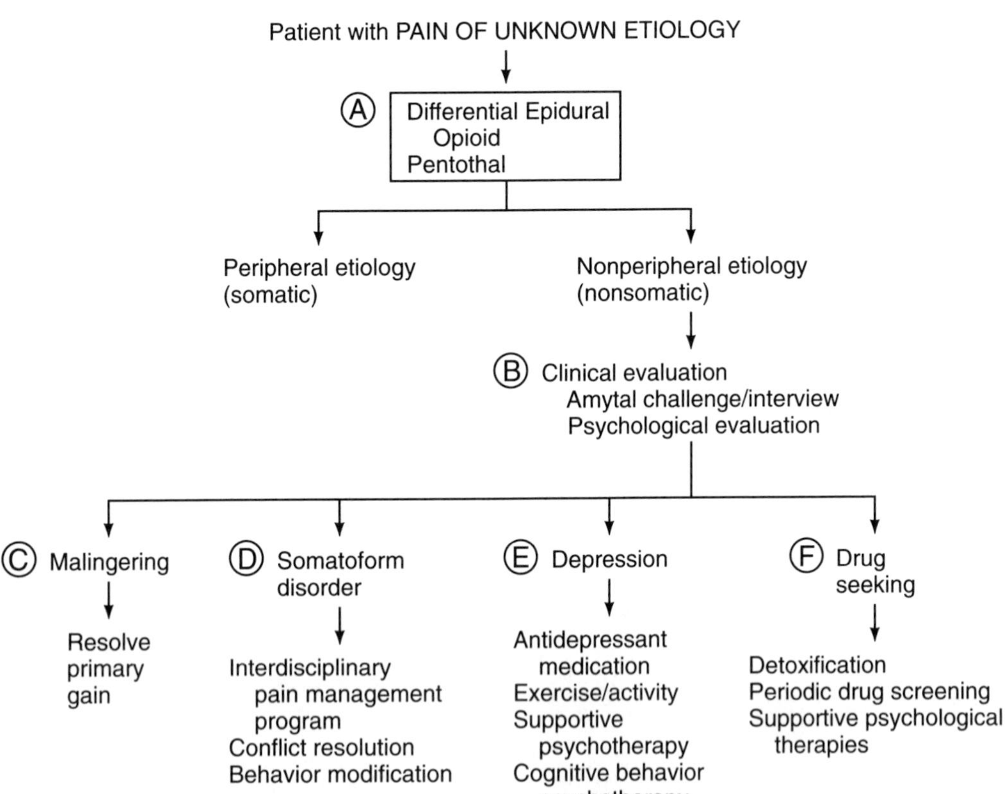
Patient with PAIN OF UNKNOWN ETIOLOGY
(A) Differential Epidural Opioid Pentothal
Peripheral etiology (somatic)
Nonperipheral etiology (nonsomatic)
(B) Clinical evaluation
Amytal challenge/interview
Psychological evaluation
(C) Malingering
Resolve primary gain
(D) Somatoform disorder
Interdisciplinary pain management program
Conflict resolution
Behavior modification
(E) Depression
Antidepressant medication
Exercise/activity
Supportive psychotherapy
Cognitive behavior psychotherapy
(F) Drug seeking
Detoxification
Periodic drug screening
Supportive psychological therapies

HEAD AND NECK PAIN

APPROACH TO THE PATIENT WITH HEADACHE

Richard Barohn, M.D.

A. In approaching the patient with headache (HA), first establish whether it is due to a serious intracranial pathologic process. Symptoms that suggest a nonbenign HA include (1) no prior history of HA, (2) age over 60, (3) "worst HA of my life," (4) worsening of HA with position change, (5) focal weakness or sensory symptoms, (6) diplopia, (7) recent personality change, and (8) brief episodes (seconds) of visual loss (due to increased intracranial pressure). Signs suggesting a nonbenign HA include (1) an abnormal neurologic examination, (2) abnormal mental status examination, (3) papilledema, (4) fever, (5) stiff neck (meningismus), and (6) significantly elevated blood pressure. Patients with any of these features need further neurologic evaluation, usually beginning with CT of the brain, to rule out a mass lesion. A lumbar puncture may be needed to diagnose meningitis, subarachnoid hemorrhage, or pseudotumor cerebri.

B. Any patient over 60 years of age with new-onset unilateral frontal HA should have an erythrocyte sedimentation rate (ESR) to screen for temporal arteritis. If the ESR is elevated, refer the patient for temporal artery biopsy.

C. For most benign HAs, no further evaluation is needed beyond the history and neurologic examination.

D. Benign HA is divided into 3 broad groups: (1) tension (muscle contraction) HA, (2) vascular HA, and (3) benign HA due to less common etiologies (e.g., sinus, dental, temporomandibular joint [TMJ], or ocular disease).

E. Most vascular HAs are characterized by throbbing pain with nausea and vomiting (p 82).

F. Tension HAs are holocranial in location but frequently are most severe in the occipital-cervical region. The pain associated with tension HA has a tight pressure or squeezing quality and is frequently exacerbated by stress.

G. Treatment for benign HAs consists of abortive therapy at the time of the pain, and prophylactic therapy to reduce the frequency and severity of HAs in the future. Abortive therapy consists of a mild NSAID. If there is significant cervical muscle tenderness, a mild relaxant such as methocarbamol or chlorzoxazone (Parafon Forte) may be useful. Abuse of such drugs should be avoided, however, and patients need to be warned about excessive sedation.

H. Prophylactic therapy for tension HA involves controlling external stresses that precipitate HAs or modifying reaction to stress. Self-relaxation techniques such as biofeedback may be useful in this regard (p 202).

I. Many patients with tension HAs are depressed. Treatment of the underlying depression with a tricyclic antidepressant (e.g., amitriptyline, nortriptyline) can be beneficial. Some patients with chronic tension HA, who are not obviously depressed, may also receive benefit from these drugs.

J. HAs due to abnormalities of the sinus, dentition, TMJ, or eyes are less common than tension and vascular HAs. They are characterized by focal pain in the area of pathology. Most patients who believe they have "sinus" HA or HA because they "need glasses" actually have vascular or tension HA.

References

Pennon H. The relaxation response. New York: Van Books, 1976.

Raskin NH. Headache. 2nd ed. New York: Churchill Livingstone, 1988.

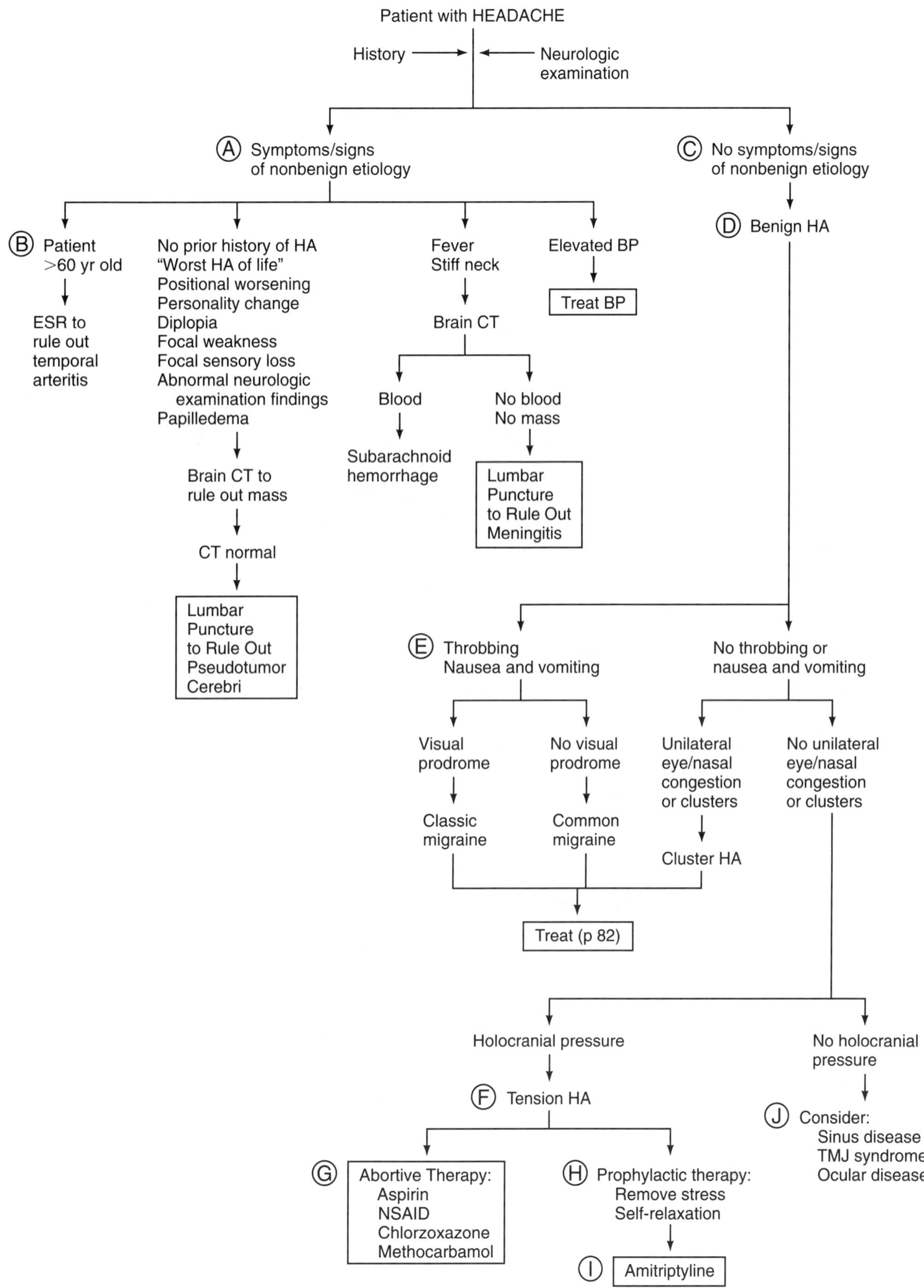
Patient with HEADACHE
History
Neurologic examination
(A) Symptoms/signs of nonbenign etiology
(C) No symptoms/signs of nonbenign etiology
(B) Patient >60 yr old
ESR to rule out temporal arteritis
No prior history of HA
"Worst HA of life"
Positional worsening
Personality change
Diplopia
Focal weakness
Focal sensory loss
Abnormal neurologic examination findings
Papilledema
Brain CT to rule out mass
CT normal
Lumbar Puncture to Rule Out Pseudotumor Cerebri
Fever
Stiff neck
Brain CT
Blood
Subarachnoid hemorrhage
No blood
No mass
Lumbar Puncture to Rule Out Meningitis
Elevated BP
Treat BP
(D) Benign HA
(E) Throbbing
Nausea and vomiting
Visual prodrome
Classic migraine
No visual prodrome
Common migraine
No throbbing or nausea and vomiting
Unilateral eye/nasal congestion or clusters
Cluster HA
No unilateral eye/nasal congestion or clusters
Treat (p 82)
Holocranial pressure
(F) Tension HA
(G) Abortive Therapy:
Aspirin
NSAID
Chlorzoxazone
Methocarbamol
(H) Prophylactic therapy:
Remove stress
Self-relaxation
(I) Amitriptyline
No holocranial pressure
(J) Consider:
Sinus disease
TMJ syndrome
Ocular disease

VASCULAR HEADACHE

Richard Barohn, M.D.

Vascular headaches (HAs) are common, and the prevalence may be as high as 30% of women and 17% of men ages 21 to 34. Less commonly, children can experience vascular HAs. One should be cautious about diagnosing vascular HA in someone over age 50 who has no prior history of the disorder. Vascular HAs can be separated into two broad groups: migraine and cluster. Migraines are much more common.

A. Migraine HAs are throbbing, are often unilateral, and are usually associated with nausea and vomiting. There is often a family history of migraine HA.

B. If a visual prodrome precedes the migraine HA (flashing, sparkling, occasionally zig-zag lights, or an enlarging scotoma or field defect in one or both eyes), it is classified as a classic migraine. Common migraine has no visual prodrome. This distinction is not critical because both types of migraine HA are treated in the same manner.

C. Abortive therapy for migraine HA consists of (1) sleeping or resting in a dark, quiet room, (2) applying a cold, moist towel to the forehead, and (3) oral Midrin (isometheptene mucate, acetaminophen, dichloralphenazone) or an ergotamine tartrate (ET) preparation when the visual prodrome occurs or at the onset of the HA. Midrin can be repeated every hour (no more than 5 capsules in 12 hours). ET is available in oral (PO), sublingual (SL), and rectal (PR) preparations that contain 1 or 2 mg of ET per dose. An aerosolized inhaler is also available. ET can be repeated hourly up to a total of 6 mg per HA (no more than 10 mg/week). Sumatriptan, a specific serotonin agonist for cerebral vasculature, has been shown to be effective in aborting both migraine and cluster headaches.

D. Nausea and vomiting frequently occur with migraine HA. Therefore, we use promethazine (Phenergan), 25 mg PO or PR, at the onset of the HA, along with Midrin or an ET preparation. ET can cause nausea in some patients.

E. If the migraine HA is severe enough to bring the patient to the emergency room, dihydroergotamine (DHE) can be given IM (1 mg) or IV (0.5 to 0.75 mg).

F. Avoid oral and parenteral narcotics or sedatives if possible. For patients with confirmed migraine HAs in whom the likelihood of drug abuse is low, occasionally we use an oral sedative, butalbital (Fiorinal), or a mild narcotic (codeine or propoxyphene) if the aforementioned drugs are not effective.

G. Prophylactic therapy for migraine HA should be considered if more than two severe HAs occur per month. Four groups of medications are used: (1) beta blocking drugs, (2) tricyclic antidepressant drugs (amitriptyline or nortriptyline, 50 to 150 mg daily), (3) calcium channel blocking drugs (verapamil, 80 mg b.i.d.), and (4) methysergide, 2 mg t.i.d. Each drug should be used daily for at least 2 months before it is considered ineffective. We use the drugs in the order listed.

H. If beta blocking drugs are used, those that can be taken once (long-acting propranolol, nadolol) or twice (metoprolol) a day are preferred. We begin with Inderal LA, 80 mg once a day. Monitor blood pressure and pulse for hypotension and bradycardia.

I. In cluster headache (CHA), the pain is sharp, hemicranial, and associated with ipsilateral lacrimation, conjunctival erythema, rhinorrhea, and occasionally Horner's syndrome. Daily CHAs occur once or twice a year for periods of 30 to 60 days. During a CHA, patients tend to pace around the room.

J. Abortive therapy for CHA consists of (1) ET (the inhaler form may be particularly effective), (2) 100% oxygen therapy (7 L/minute for 15 minutes), and (3) 1 ml of 4% topical lidocaine applied intranasally (drops or aerosol) in the nostril ipsilateral to the CHA.

K. Once the daily CHAs begin, prophylactic therapy to lessen the severity or duration of the HA can consist of (1) cyproheptadine, 4 mg q.i.d.; (2) ET, PO or PR, 1 mg b.i.d. (skip 1 day/week); (3) prednisone, 60 mg/day for 1 week, then taper over 1 week; (4) methysergide; and (5) lithium, 300 mg b.i.d. to t.i.d.

References

Callaham M, Raskin NH. A controlled study of dihydroergotamine in the treatment of acute migraine headache. Headache 1986; 26:168.

Couch JR, Ziegler DK, Hassanein R. Amitriptyline in the prophylaxis of migraine. Neurology 1976; 26:121.

Diamond S, Solomon GD, Freitag FG, Megta ND. Long-acting propranolol in the prophylaxis of migraine. Headache 1987; 27:70.

Markley HG, Cheronis JCD, Piepho RW. Verapamil in prophylactic therapy of migraine. Neurology 1984; 34:973.

Raskin NH. Headache. 2nd ed. New York: Churchill Livingstone, 1988.

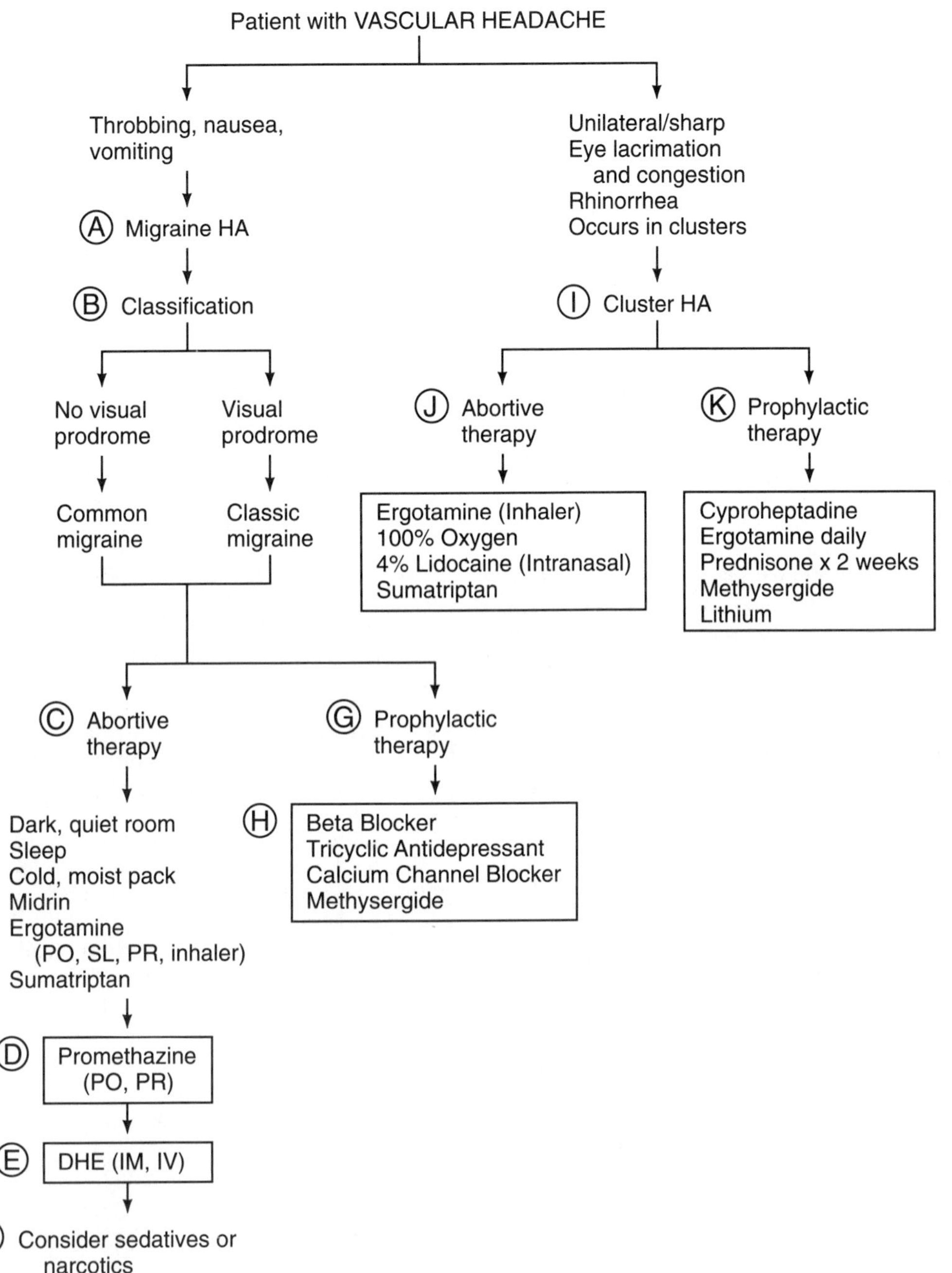

Patient with VASCULAR HEADACHE
Throbbing, nausea, vomiting
Ⓐ Migraine HA
Ⓑ Classification
No visual prodrome
Visual prodrome
Common migraine
Classic migraine
Ⓒ Abortive therapy
Dark, quiet room
Sleep
Cold, moist pack
Midrin
Ergotamine (PO, SL, PR, inhaler)
Sumatriptan
Ⓓ Promethazine (PO, PR)
Ⓔ DHE (IM, IV)
Ⓕ Consider sedatives or narcotics
Ⓖ Prophylactic therapy
Ⓗ Beta Blocker
Tricyclic Antidepressant
Calcium Channel Blocker
Methysergide
Unilateral/sharp
Eye lacrimation and congestion
Rhinorrhea
Occurs in clusters
Ⓘ Cluster HA
Ⓙ Abortive therapy
Ergotamine (Inhaler)
100% Oxygen
4% Lidocaine (Intranasal)
Sumatriptan
Ⓚ Prophylactic therapy
Cyproheptadine
Ergotamine daily
Prednisone x 2 weeks
Methysergide
Lithium

TRIGEMINAL NEURALGIA

Richard Barohn, M.D.

Facial pain due to trigeminal neuralgia (TN), also known as tic douloureux, has the following features: (1) brief, paroxysmal, intense, lancinating or shock-like pain; (2) unilateral; (3) confined to the distribution of the fifth cranial nerve (CN-V), with the mandibular and maxillary divisions affected more often than the ophthalmic; and (4) provocation by minimal stimuli (chewing, talking, brushing teeth, cold wind on the face). TN occurs most often in the sixth and seventh decades. The etiology is unknown, although some physicians, principally led by Janetta, believe that the cause is external compression of the trigeminal nerve roots in the posterior fossa by arteries or veins.

A. Patients with TN do not complain of numbness, and examination of all cranial nerves (including CN-V) is normal, as is the entire neurologic examination. If these are abnormal, TN is unlikely, and a search for a mass lesion (intrinsic to the pons, cerebellopontine angle, or cavernous sinus) or chronic meningitis needs to be conducted. MRI of the brain and posterior fossa is indicated, followed by a lumbar puncture if the MRI is normal.

B. Occasionally patients with connective tissue disease (Sjögren's disease, systemic lupus erythematosus, scleroderma) can present with trigeminal neuropathy. Usually the serum antinuclear antibody assay (ANA) is positive.

C. Patients with continuous unilateral aching pain are often diagnosed with atypical facial pain. If all possible causes have been eliminated (including dental and temporomandibular joint disease), treatment is difficult. Occasionally tricyclic antidepressants can be useful.

D. Herpes zoster can involve CN-V, usually in the ophthalmic division. The characteristic rash will eventually erupt. The pain is burning and constant and can persist after the rash has resolved (postherpetic neuralgia, p 48).

E. If TN occurs in a patient 20 to 40 years old and the pain is bilateral, the possibility of multiple sclerosis should be considered.

F. Medical therapy for TN consists of the following options: (1) carbamazepine (CARB), (2) baclofen, and (3) phenytoin. Each drug should be tried for at least 2 to 3 weeks before it is considered ineffective.

G. CARB is the drug of choice for TN; however, the drug dose needs to be increased gradually to avoid unpleasant side effects (nausea, ataxia, confusion). Begin with 200 mg daily and increase by 200 mg every 2 to 3 days (in three divided doses). A dose adequate to relieve pain may not be reached for 4 to 7 days.

H. If the patient is in so much pain that the delay needed to reach an effective CARB dose is not advisable, phenytoin can be administered IV at the same time that oral CARB therapy is begun. The phenytoin IV dose (18 mg/kg) must be given slowly (50 mg/min), and the blood pressure and heart rate need to be closely monitored while the drug is being administered. Pain relief often is immediate and may last for several days until the oral CARB becomes effective.

I. If all of the medical therapies fail, consider more invasive interventions. The following approaches may relieve pain in 80 to 90% of patients: (1) retrogasserian glycerol injection as described by Hakanson, (2) percutaneous radiofrequency rhizotomy of the trigeminal ganglion, and (3) microvascular decompression via posterior craniotomy. Unfortunately, about 8% of patients develop a dysesthetic pain syndrome (anesthesia dolorosa) following percutaneous rhizotomy. Microvascular decompression, the third option, has a surgical morbidity and mortality rate of 7% and 1%, respectively. The invasive procedure of choice varies from institution to institution. We employ percutaneous rhizotomy initially, as it is less invasive and has a very good success rate in medically refractory TN. If this fails or pain recurs, the more invasive microvascular decompression is done.

References

Hagen NA, Stevens JC, Michet CJ Jr. Trigeminal sensory neuropathy associated with connective tissue diseases. Neurology 1990; 40:891.

Janetta PJ. Microsurgical management of trigeminal neuralgia. Arch Neurol 1985; 42:800.

Morley TP. Case against microvascular decompression in the treatment of trigeminal neuralgia. Arch Neurol 1985; 42:801.

Raskin NH. Headache. 2nd ed. New York: Churchill Livingstone, 1988.

Sweet WH. The treatment of trigeminal neuralgia (tic douloureux). N Engl J Med 1986; 315:174.

Sweet WH. Percutaneous methods for the treatment of trigeminal neuralgia and other faciocephalic pain: Comparison with microvascular decompression. Semin Neurol 1988; 8:272.

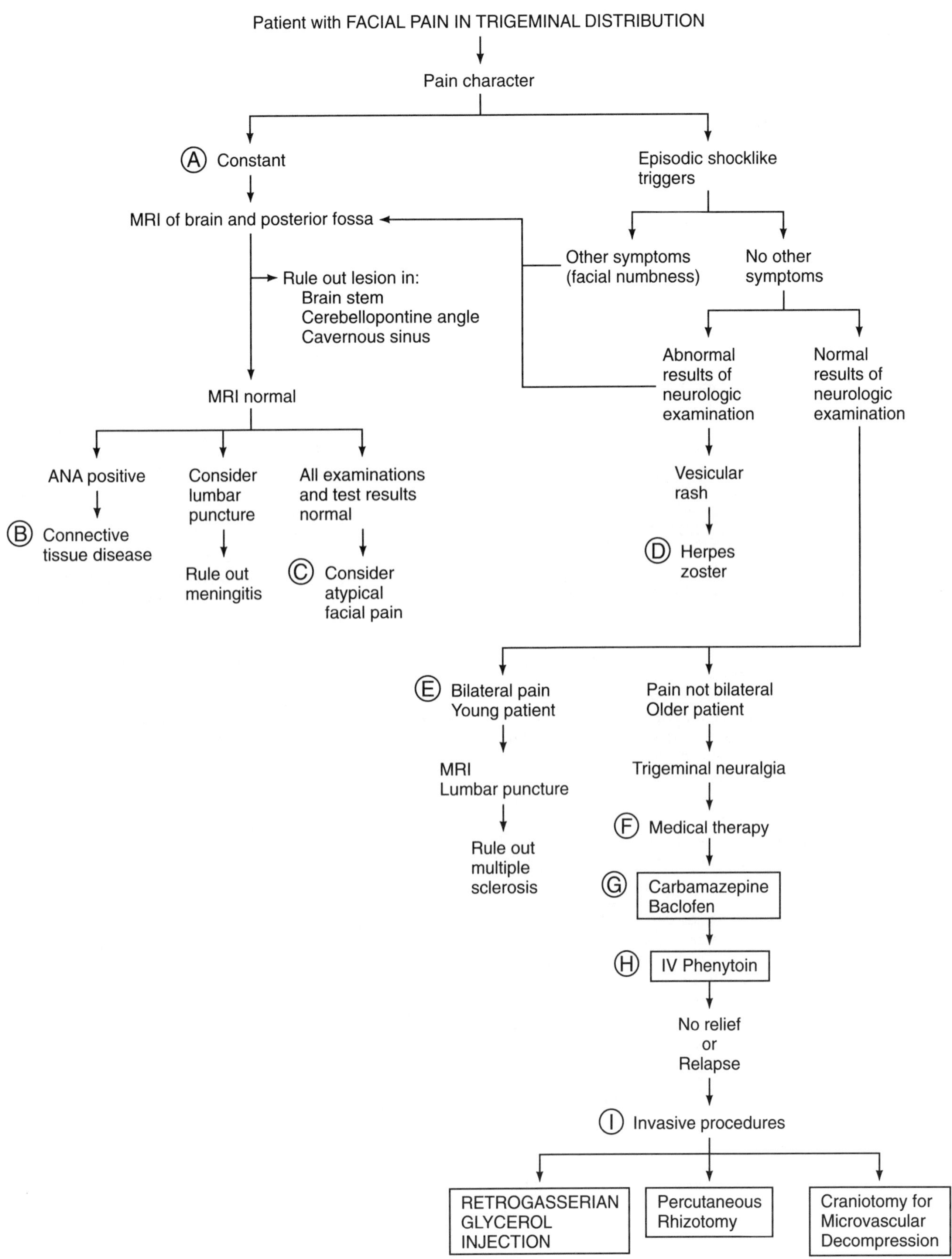
Patient with FACIAL PAIN IN TRIGEMINAL DISTRIBUTION
Pain character
(A) Constant
Episodic shocklike triggers
MRI of brain and posterior fossa
Rule out lesion in:
Brain stem
Cerebellopontine angle
Cavernous sinus
Other symptoms (facial numbness)
No other symptoms
Abnormal results of neurologic examination
Normal results of neurologic examination
MRI normal
ANA positive
(B) Connective tissue disease
Consider lumbar puncture
Rule out meningitis
All examinations and test results normal
(C) Consider atypical facial pain
Vesicular rash
(D) Herpes zoster
(E) Bilateral pain
Young patient
MRI
Lumbar puncture
Rule out multiple sclerosis
Pain not bilateral
Older patient
Trigeminal neuralgia
(F) Medical therapy
(G) Carbamazepine
Baclofen
(H) IV Phenytoin
No relief
or
Relapse
(I) Invasive procedures
RETROGASSERIAN GLYCEROL INJECTION
Percutaneous Rhizotomy
Craniotomy for Microvascular Decompression

CRANIOMANDIBULAR DISORDERS

John S. McDonald, D.D.S., M.S., F.A.C.D.
James C. Phero, D.M.D., F.A.C.D.
W. Corbett Holmgreen, D.D.S., M.D.

Craniomandibular disorder (CMD) is a collective term that includes clinical problems involving the masticatory musculature, the temporomandibular joint (TMJ), or both. The term is synonymous with TMJ disorder. CMD is the major reason for nondental pain in the orofacial region and is a subclass of musculoskeletal disorders.

A. The most common presenting symptom is pain, usually localized in the muscles of mastication, the preauricular area, and/or the TMJ. The pain is usually aggravated by chewing or other jaw functions. Historically, CMD signs and symptoms were thought to be related to occlusal irregularities and dysfunctional occlusal contacts. Current theory goes beyond occlusion to encompass the musculature and the mechanics of joint function, including dysfunction, adaption, and degeneration, as factors in CMD. It has been estimated that approximately 15% of the population suffers from CMD. Statistics show that it affects females more frequently than males, by as much as 4:1. The average age range of CMD patients is between the second and fourth decades. The signs and symptoms of CMD generally increase in frequency and severity over time. During evaluation, patient history should include discussion of pain onset and nature, TMJ noise and locking, previous head and neck trauma, previous treatment, and relevant social history. Physical examination should encompass mandibular movement, including interincisal measurement; dental evaluation; muscle tenderness; and TMJ sounds. Radiographic evaluation should not be limited to the TMJ and may include transpharyngeal and transorbital views, Panorex, tomography, arthrotomography, CT, and MRI.

B. Various facial pain syndromes can produce pain that mimics CMD. Some of the more common of these are trigeminal neuralgia; vascular headache, including migraine and cluster headache and temporal arteritis; postherpetic pain; stylohyoid (Eagle's) syndrome; carotidynia; and pathology related to the CNS, nasopharynx, and/or oropharynx.

C. Myofascial pain dysfunction (MPD) syndrome is the most common painful disorder of CMD. MPD is a regional muscle pain disorder characterized by muscle tenderness, slightly limited range of motion, and local and referred pain. The cardinal sign is muscle spasm, manifested by muscle tenderness. This condition responds to conservative management including pharmacotherapy, topical therapy, diet, and occlusal splint therapy. When more advanced treatment is indicated, invasive therapy may include occlusal equilibration, orthodontics, and subcondylar osteotomy.

D. Internal derangement of the TMJ is defined as an abnormal relationship of the articular disk to the mandibular condyle, fossa, and articular eminence. The most common internal derangement involves an anteromedial displacement of the disk with the retrodiscal tissues, specifically in the bilaminar zone over the head of the condyle. The diagnostic triad of significant internal derangement includes pain, clicking of the joint (currently or formerly), and limitation of opening or a history of such limitation. Pain may be noted around the TMJ capsule or in the masticatory musculature. The type of clicking most frequently encountered is the reciprocal click, in which the opening click signifies repositioning of the displaced disk over the condylar head, allowing normal jaw opening, followed by a closing click, which signifies repeat anterior dislocation of the disk before occlusion of the teeth. The clicking may spontaneously cease and be followed by a period of limited jaw opening or "closed lock," at which time the meniscus is permanently dislocated anteriorly and mechanically blocks condylar opening movement.

When definitive intra-articular CMD disease has been verified by appropriate conservative means, the pain specialist may wish to support the use of TMJ arthroscopy to further define the depth of the problem and in certain instances correct the pathologic condition. After arthroscopy, open joint surgery may be necessary for further correction of pathology when symptoms persist. The U.S. insurance industry is reluctant to cover open joint TMJ surgery, especially when reconstruction appears to be indicated. The Proplast-coated Vitek implant disaster has intensified "third party carrier" hesitation to authorize this type of surgery. Unfortunately, patients who received the Proplast-coated Vitek TMJ implants are at significant risk for serious sequelae including asymptomatic implant failure, giant cell tumor reaction, and bone degeneration. It is imperative that evaluation of patients who have undergone TMJ surgery include verification of the nature of the surgery and the type of implant placed, if any.

E. Degenerative joint disease (DJD), or osteoarthritis, is an organic degeneration of the articular surfaces of the joint. DJD is usually unilateral and related to trauma. Crepitus is a prominent feature. Rheumatoid arthritis, in contrast to DJD, first involves the synovial membrane rather than the articular cartilage. Thus, destruction of the osteoarthritic condyle begins at the periphery and extends toward the center. Rheumatoid changes are generally bilateral and crepitus is characteristic.

True ankylosis is a bony or fibrous fusion of the condyle to the temporal bone at the TMJ. False

Patient with CRANIOMANDIBULAR DISORDER

(A) History
Physical examination

(B) Rule out nonarticular problems mimicking CMD

Extra-articular CMD

(C) MPD

May present as
Jaw pain
Frontal or frontotemporal headache
Toothache
Otologic manifestation
Sinus pain
Pre- or postauricular pain
Sore throat
Periorbital pain

May present with
Pain (muscle tenderness)
Limitation and/or deviation of jaw movement
Trismus

Intra-articular CMD

(D) Rule out extra-articular cause of jaw limitation (e.g., mass)

Intra-articular dysfunction developing concomitant with or subsequent to MPD

CMD that begins in joint and is limited to it

Articular disk displacement
With reduction
Without reduction

Dislocation

Inflammatory conditions

(E) Arthritides

Ankylosis

(F) Interdisciplinary Therapy

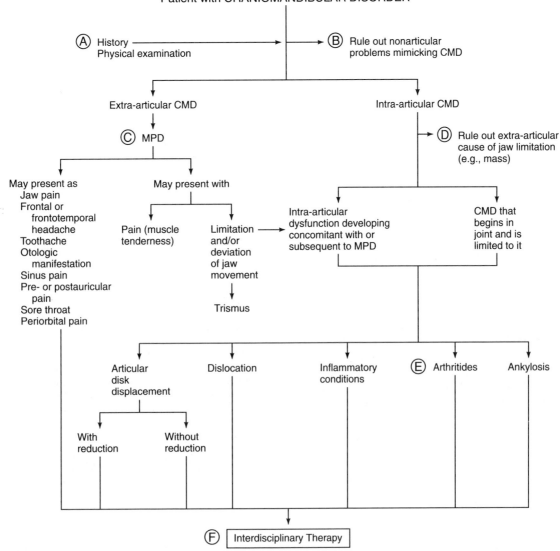

ankylosis relates to conditions outside the joint that result in lack of mandibular movement. A minimal amount of mandibular movement may be observed, even in cases of complete bony fusion, owing to flexing of the mandibular ramus and angle. Clinically, an opening ≦5 mm indicates complete bony fusion. In open lock, the mouth is opened so widely by yawning, or similar action, that the condyle subluxes out of the glenoid fossa into a position anterior to the articular eminence. Spasm of the masticatory musculature then locks the condyle in this position. In the case of TMJ arthritis, conservative management may involve pharmacotherapy, including NSAIDs and physical therapy. Invasive therapy in these patients may include intra-articular corticosteroid injections and open joint surgery, including reconstruction.

F. CMD therapy is best addressed in an interdisciplinary manner. Conservative multimodal treatment strategies to control pain include teaching the patient to reduce oral habits, stress, and anxiety; applying physical therapy and exercises to restore function; pharmacotherapy, including NSAIDs, for control of pain and inflammation; and intraoral occlusal splint therapy.

References

Clark GT, Seligman DA, Solberg WK, Pullinger AG. Guidelines for the treatment of temporomandibular disorders. J Craniomandib Dis Facial Oral Pain 1990; 4:80.

FDA notifies physicians and patients about risks of TMJ implants. FDA Medical Bulletin 1991; 21:2.

Friction JR. Recent advances in temporomandibular disorders and orofacial pain. J Am Dent Assoc 1991; 122:25.

Gangarosa LP, Mahan PE, Ciarlone AE. Pharmacologic management of temporomandibular joint disorders and chronic head and neck pain. J Craniomandib Pract 1991; 9:328.

Hampf G. A new clinical approach to the treatment of temporomandibular dysfunction and orofacial dysesthesia: Natural history and comparisons with similar chronic pain conditions. J Craniomandib Dis Facial Oral Pain 1992; 6:56.

Just JK, Perry HT, Greene CS. Treating TM disorders: A survey on diagnosis, etiology and management. J Am Dent Assoc 1991; 122:55.

McNeill C, ed. Craniomandibular disorders—guidelines for evaluation, diagnosis, and management. The American Academy of Craniomandibular Disorders. Chicago: Quintessence Publishing, 1990.

FACIAL PAIN

Jeffery T. Summers, M.D.
Emil J. Menk, M.D.

The difficulties in the diagnosis and management of facial pain were well described by Yair Sharav: "Diagnosis and treatment of orofacial pain is complicated by the density of anatomical structures in the area, mechanisms of referred pain and the important psychological meaning attributed to the face and the oral cavity."

A. Several neurologic disorders can manifest as facial pain, including intracranial pathology (multiple sclerosis, infection, neoplasm, infarction, neuromas, and infection or inflammation of nerve tissue). Neoplasms, abscesses, and other masses can expand to impinge on nerves in the facial region and cause facial pain. The dense concentration of nerves in this area and the possibility of referred pain from a remote site often complicate the neurologic examination. An abnormal neurologic examination necessitates a consultation with a neurologist.

B. Myofascial pain is characterized by a steady, deep, aching pain with a hyperirritable focus within a band of skeletal muscle that, when palpated, can produce a sudden jolt of pain. Treatment includes stretching exercises and trigger point injections (p 270).

C. Herpes zoster or "shingles" pain is described variably as dull, sharp, aching, burning, and shooting and usually precedes the outbreak of the lesions by 4 to 5 days. The pain typically is unilateral and localized to the dermatome distribution of one or more divisions of the trigeminal nerve or cervical nerve roots. Treatment includes antiviral agents, corticosteroids, analgesics, and sympathetic nerve blocks. Postherpetic neuralgia usually develops in elderly patients after an outbreak of shingles, and pain may persist for months to years after the lesions have healed (pp 28 and 48).

D. Causalgia and reflex sympathetic dystrophy (RSD) are sympathetic in origin and may result from any traumatic nerve injury (including surgery). Sympathetic pain is classically described as having a superficial burning component with a deeper aching, stabbing, or crushing pain. The pain is aggravated by any stimulus that increases sympathetic outflow to the affected area. In the early stages the involved skin is often warm, dry, and erythematous. Later, trophic changes develop, and the skin may appear thin, brittle, and shiny (p 50).

E. Atypical facial pain usually affects young adults and often is preceded by facial trauma, although there can be a lack of objective findings on physical examination. The pain is usually described as burning, aching, or boring and is frequently accompanied by sensory loss in the area of the pain. Patients with this disorder commonly have significant behavioral and psychological dysfunction that may predate the onset of facial pain. The pain may be unilateral or bilateral and often does not follow specific dermatomes. Treatment involves antidepressants, anticonvulsants, and psychotherapy.

F. Temporal arteritis is a febrile condition usually occurring in persons over age 60. It is characterized by a burning pain caused by inflammation of the temporal artery and may be accompanied by a throbbing temporal headache and hyperalgesia of the scalp. The pain may be worsened by jaw movements (e.g., chewing). Often it is accompanied by visual loss, which constitutes a medical emergency. The pain is usually exacerbated by digital pressure over the involved artery but may be lessened by this maneuver. Corticosteroids are the treatment of choice.

G. Trigeminal neuralgia, or tic douloureux, is characterized by brief, lancinating, electric shock–like pains, with pain-free intervals when the patient is completely asymptomatic. Attacks occur and terminate abruptly, although the patient may experience background burning pain between "shocks." The pain attacks are unilateral and can be triggered by a nonpainful stimulus. The stimulus is commonly in the perioral or nasal region and may be remote from the painful area. The stimulus may be tactile, a nonspecific activity such as chewing or talking, or exposure to wind or temperature changes. Most patients with this condition are over 50 years of age; when it occurs in a young person, multiple sclerosis should be considered. Recurrences usually involve the same area of the face but spread to involve a wider area over time. Episodes can be months to years apart, but it is common for the intervals to become shorter with time. The painful episodes can be totally debilitating and may lead to suicide if not treated (p 84).

H. Vascular facial pain is intermittent, usually occurring in clusters, and may last 30 minutes to hours. It is characteristically described as throbbing or burning. Vascular facial pain is usually sited around the orbit, upper face, or temples and is associated with injection of the eye on the affected side, lacrimation, and nasal congestion (p 82).

I. Facial pain that is not related to any of the common etiologies described above can result from a variety of conditions. Sinus disease, oral pathology (dental or peridontal) and neurologic disorders can all cause facial pain. The treatment for pain related to these disorders entails treating the underlying condition and is probably best managed by physicians experienced in the management of the condition.

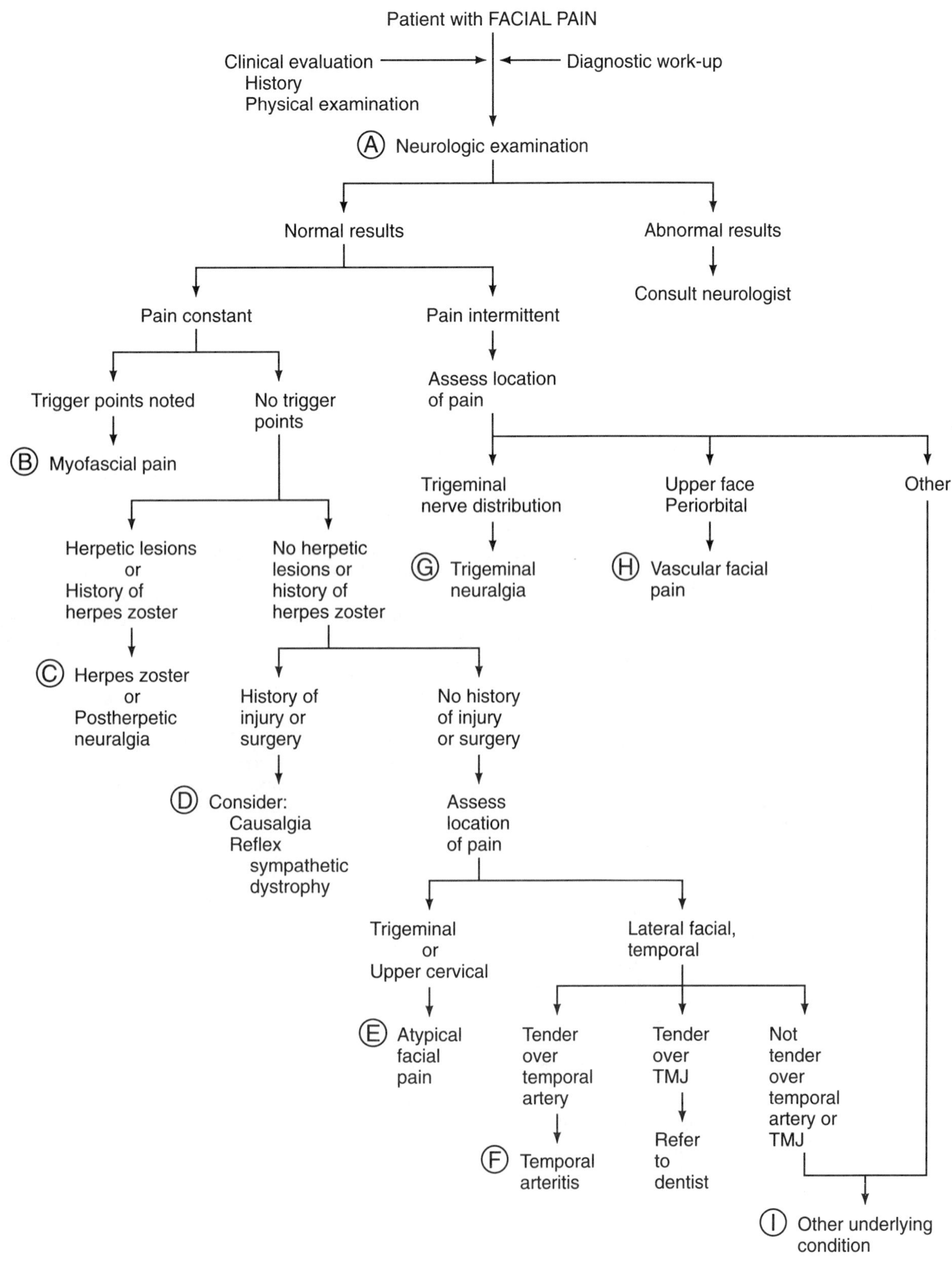

References

Dalessio DF. Headache. In: Wall PD, Melzack R, eds. Textbook of pain. New York: Churchill Livingstone, 1986:282.

Loeser JD. Tic douloureux and atypical facial pain. In: Wall PD, Melzack R, eds. Textbook of pain. New York: Churchill Livingstone, 1986:426.

Phero JC, McDonald JS, Green DB, Robins GS. Orofacial pain and other related syndromes. In: Raj PP, ed. Practical management of pain. 2nd ed. St. Louis: Mosby–Year Book, 1992:226.

Sharav Y. Orofacial pain. In: Wall PD, Melzack R, eds. Textbook of pain. New York: Churchill Livingstone, 1986:338.

TORTICOLLIS

Eric B. Lefever, M.D.

Torticollis is a "twisted neck" that results from a severe state of contracture of the nuchal musculature. The sternocleidomastoid muscle invariably is involved, and additional muscles may act together to produce concomitant neck flexion (antecollis) or extension (retrocollis). It is almost always unilateral. Severe and chronic forms produce permanent contracture and fibrosis and result in scoliotic and degenerative changes of the cervical spine. Pain associated with the condition occurs in the vast majority of cases and is a source of significant morbidity and suffering.

A. Congenital, or pediatric, torticollis is the most common form. It is related to mechanical or local factors such as muscular, postural, or paracervical irritation and is largely benign with a self-limited course. Similarly, in adults local factors such as trauma and degenerative or mechanical defects involving cervical structures may precipitate acute "wry neck."

B. Idiopathic spasmodic torticollis is the most common focal dystonia; it is rarely associated with segmental and generalized dystonia. Onset is usually in the fourth decade of life. Women are affected three times more frequently than men, and the etiology is uncertain. Local trauma, infection, neurovascular compression, and CNS lesions involving the basal ganglia and the brain stem have been reported as initiating factors.

C. Various treatment modalities have been utilized with inconsistent results. This probably reflects the unknown pathophysiology of the disorder, as well as the spontaneous remission rate of 15%. Physical therapy is the cornerstone of any effective treatment program. Its goals are to decrease pain, maintain flexibility of the cervical spine, and prevent fixed postures and contractures. Passive and active range of motion exercises, massage, manual stretching, ultrasonography, and the use of soft or firm collars on an intermittent basis may all prove beneficial.

D. Historically torticollis was considered a psychogenic or hysterical phenomenon. Although a psychogenic etiology has largely been disclaimed, psychological factors do impact on the disorder. Emotional distress invariably exaggerates the condition, and the patient's physical appearance may contribute to depression and lead to social withdrawal. Psychotherapy, stress management, hypnosis and other relaxation techniques, and biofeedback may be beneficial.

E. Measures to relax the contracted muscles may provide symptomatic relief and allow the evaluation of fibrotic and bony changes. These include blocking the spinal accessory nerve with a local anesthetic (p 262). If improvement results, neurolytic block of the accessory nerve may be considered. If more extensive musculature is involved, cervical plexus block may be necessary. Chemical denervation of the muscles involved is also effective. Botulinum toxin acts presynaptically to prevent the release of acetylcholine at the neuromuscular junction. Injection of minute amounts of this toxin into the affected muscles has had good results. Infiltration of a dilute neuromuscular relaxant also has been reported as useful.

F. Beneficial pharmacologic agents include high-dose anticholinergics, tricyclic antidepressants, and haloperidol. Benzodiazepines, although not recommended for routine use, may be beneficial in carefully selected patients.

G. Surgical approaches generally should be reserved for refractory cases, because some degree of disability is unavoidable and therapeutic results are inconsistent and often disappointing. Cervical rhizotomy, surgical denervation, muscular tenotomy, thalamotomy, and dorsal column stimulation are the procedures most commonly utilized.

References

Cremonesi E, Murata KN. Infiltration of a neuromuscular relaxant in diagnosis and treatment of torticollis. Anesth Analg 1986; 65:1077.

Duane DD. Spasmodic torticollis. Adv Neurol 1988; 49:135.

McDowell FH, Cedarbaum JM. The extrapyramidal system and disorders of movement. In: Joynt RJ, ed. Clinical neurology. Vol 3. Philadelphia: JB Lippincott, 1989:46.

Ramamurthy S, Akkineni SR, Winnie AP. A simple technique for block of the spinal accessory nerve. Anesth. Analg. 1978; 57:591.

Tsui J, Eisen A, Calne DB: Botulinum toxin in spasmodic torticollis. Adv Neurol 1988; 50:593.

Wolfort FG, Kanter MA, Miller LB. Torticollis. Plast Reconstr Surg 1989; 84:682.

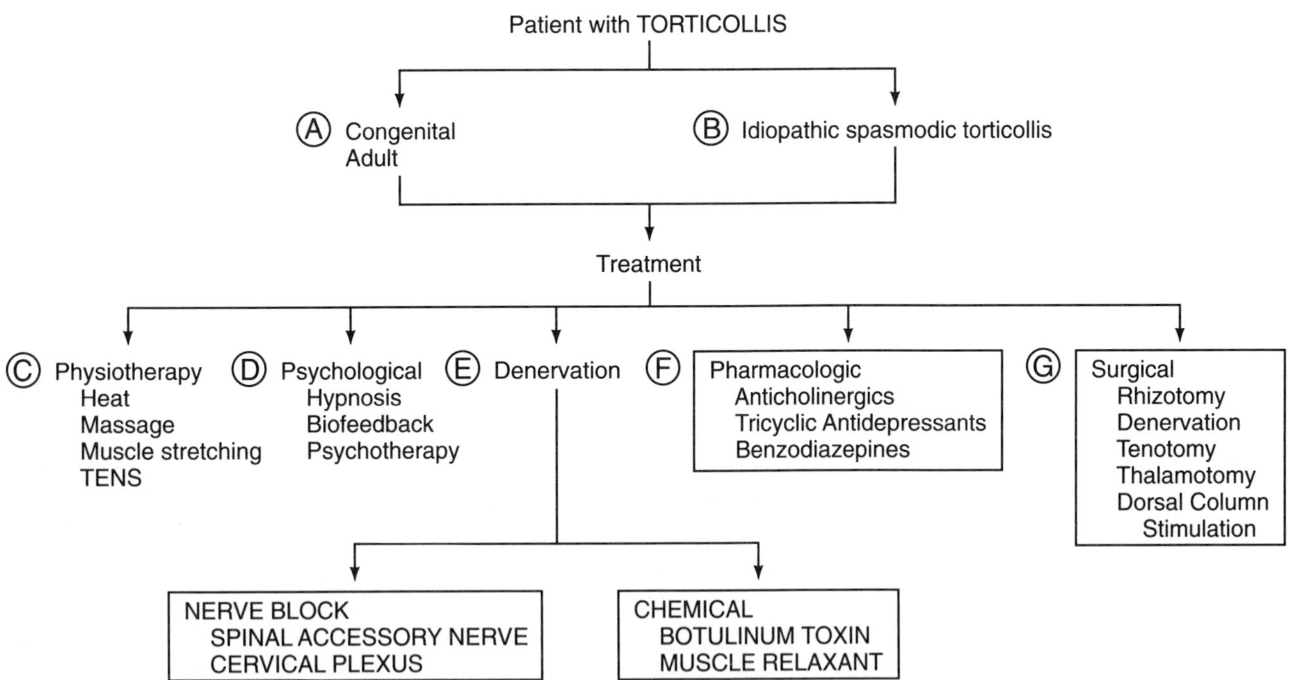

Patient with TORTICOLLIS
(A) Congenital
Adult
(B) Idiopathic spasmodic torticollis
Treatment
(C) Physiotherapy
Heat
Massage
Muscle stretching
TENS
(D) Psychological
Hypnosis
Biofeedback
Psychotherapy
(E) Denervation
(F) Pharmacologic
Anticholinergics
Tricyclic Antidepressants
Benzodiazepines
(G) Surgical
Rhizotomy
Denervation
Tenotomy
Thalamotomy
Dorsal Column
Stimulation
NERVE BLOCK
SPINAL ACCESSORY NERVE
CERVICAL PLEXUS
CHEMICAL
BOTULINUM TOXIN
MUSCLE RELAXANT

WHIPLASH

Paul Dreyfuss, M.D.

Whiplash injury implies a hyperextension of the head upon the shoulders followed by flexion, usually associated with rear-end collisions in a motor vehicle.

A spectrum of injuries from fracture dislocation to mild soft tissue injury is associated with whiplash. With extension, the anterior elements are strained and the posterior elements compressed. The reverse occurs with flexion. Structures that have been involved in pain generation either clinically or experimentally in the neck include the disk, supporting ligaments of the spine, muscles of the neck and shoulder, vertebral body and end plate, esophagus, facet and its capsule, temporomandibular joint, and sympathetic chain and trunks.

Symptoms can be complex and bizarre and include pain in the neck, shoulders, and scapulae; headaches; visual aberrations; tinnitus; dizziness; vertigo; cognitive abnormalities; numbness; dysphagia and hoarseness; radicular pain; nausea; jaw pain; sympathetic dysfunction; neck stiffness; and low back pain.

A. Examine the cervical spine carefully for localized tenderness. A neurologic examination is important. Radiography performed should include AP, odontoid, and lateral views. If no obvious instability is present but there is a possibility of ligamentous instability, take supervised flexion-extension lateral views. If further osseous information is needed, a CT scan is necessary.

B. Treatment is usually empirical, because most patients have soft tissue dysfunction. A soft collar should be weaned from the patient after about 1 week. Initially, heat should be avoided and ice massage recommended to decrease pain, inflammation and spasm. NSAIDs should be used early. A cervical pillow helps keep the neck in a neutral position or in slight flexion when sleeping.

C. After the acute inflammatory phase, patients can tolerate and deserve more aggressive but conservative therapy to avoid the sequelae of immobility and disuse. Depending on the severity of the initial injury, this may begin as soon as 5 to 7 days after the insult. A variety of techniques should be employed. The goal is to decrease inflammation while increasing range of motion (ROM) and preventing soft tissue contraction or restriction of motion segments. An orderly sequence is needed, because aggressive stretching or exercises introduced too early will only exacerbate the patient's complaints. Heat is usually given before and concurrent with the stretching and flexibility program. Ice can be continued if the patient receives benefit. Exercise should begin with gentle isometrics and progress to resistive isotonics up to the patient's toleration level. Aggressive treatment of muscle dysfunction is indicated through a variety of techniques. Traction has been suggested to assist in freeing adhesions, distraction of articular surfaces within the facet joint, relief of nerve root compression, decompression of the disk, relief of spasm, and passive muscle stretching. Traction should not be given in the acute inflammatory phase: it will only exacerbate the symptoms. Cervical spine films, including flexion-extension views if indicated, should be taken before traction is started. Manual traction can be performed before mechanical traction to determine tolerance.

D. Although soft tissue dysfunction and the spectrum of myofascial pain and fibromyalgia represent the greatest portion of impairment, other pathologic entities can exist. There is at times overlap between these entities, and an eclectic approach is most helpful. Conservative intervention should be continued with emphasis on the soft tissue.

E. Entities such as inflammatory arthritis may have been pre-existent before the whiplash and may need separate, specialized treatment.

(Continued on page 94)

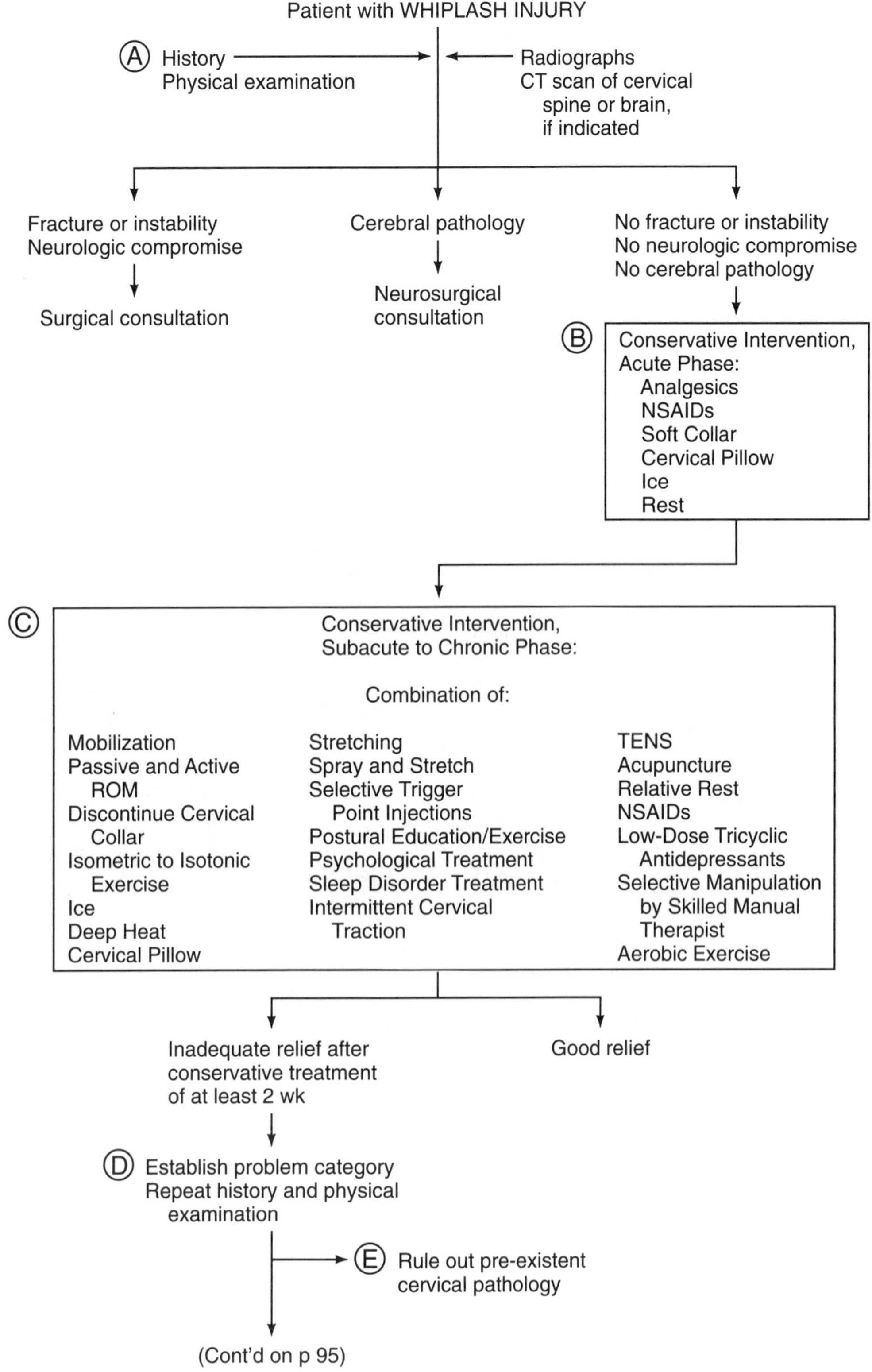
Patient with WHIPLASH INJURY
Ⓐ History
Physical examination
Radiographs
CT scan of cervical spine or brain, if indicated
Fracture or instability
Neurologic compromise
Surgical consultation
Cerebral pathology
Neurosurgical consultation
No fracture or instability
No neurologic compromise
No cerebral pathology
Ⓑ Conservative Intervention, Acute Phase:
Analgesics
NSAIDs
Soft Collar
Cervical Pillow
Ice
Rest
Ⓒ Conservative Intervention, Subacute to Chronic Phase:
Combination of:
Mobilization
Passive and Active ROM
Discontinue Cervical Collar
Isometric to Isotonic Exercise
Ice
Deep Heat
Cervical Pillow
Stretching
Spray and Stretch
Selective Trigger Point Injections
Postural Education/Exercise
Psychological Treatment
Sleep Disorder Treatment
Intermittent Cervical Traction
TENS
Acupuncture
Relative Rest
NSAIDs
Low-Dose Tricyclic Antidepressants
Selective Manipulation by Skilled Manual Therapist
Aerobic Exercise
Inadequate relief after conservative treatment of at least 2 wk
Good relief
Ⓓ Establish problem category
Repeat history and physical examination
Ⓔ Rule out pre-existent cervical pathology
(Cont'd on p 95)

F. Forms of sympathetically mediated pain have been described and may benefit from sympathetic blockade such as a stellate ganglion block (p 242). Sympathetic dysfunction has been implicated in vertigo, tinnitus, headache, nausea, and facial dysesthesias.

G. Cervical lesions within the territory of C1-3 spinal nerves have been shown to refer pain to the head. Possible sources include C1-2 joint pathology, C2-3 and C3-4 facets or their capsules, and the soft tissue structures within that area. Irritation of the C2 ganglia and the greater occipital nerve has been shown to cause cervical headaches. If conservative treatment fails, patients may benefit from a greater occipital nerve injection at the occipital notch, C2 ganglia blockade, or selective blockade of the atlantoaxial joint or C2-3 or C3-4 facet joints.

H. Postconcussive syndrome with its complex symptoms requires specialized treatment.

I. Cervical disks can be a source of pain without a frank disk herniation and radiculopathy. Annular tears, disk compression, and end-plate avulsions may occur and be a significant source of pain. MRI or CT/discography is necessary to identify annular tears. Pre-existent disk disease may exacerbate symptoms. Adequate conservative treatment, including cervical epidural steroids (p 212), should be considered before surgery.

J. Radiculopathy after whiplash secondary to a herniated disk is relatively rare. Cervical spondylosis may predispose to osseous foraminal encroachment without frank disk herniation. Adequate conservative treatment with cervical traction and epidural steroids should be given before surgical consultation, unless there are absolute surgical indications. Pseudoradicular pain can emanate from irritated soft tissues.

K. Cervical spondylosis may predispose to disk and facet dysfunction, with resultant pain syndromes. Patients may need evaluation to rule out cervical stenosis, vertebral-basilar compromise, or myelopathy/radiculopathy if suspicion arises.

L. Facet joint or capsule dysfunction may occur. In whiplash the C4-5, C5-6, and C6-7 facets are usually implicated (p 96). Look carefully for occult facet fracture or dislocation before treatment.

M. Aggressive treatment is indicated for soft tissue dysfunction, using an eclectic approach with emphasis on restoring ROM and function.

N. Symptoms such as vertigo, nausea and vomiting, dysarthria, nystagmus, and partial facial paralysis especially aggravated by neck extension and rotation should alert one to the possibility of vertebral artery compromise.

References

Bland JH. General management methods. In: Bland JH, ed. Disorders of the cervical spine: Diagnosis and medical management. Philadelphia: WB Saunders, 1987.

Bogduk N. The anatomy and pathophysiology of whiplash. Clin Biomech 1986; 1:92.

Cicala R. Long-term results of cervical epidural steroid injections. Clin J Pain 1989; 5:143.

Croft A. Soft-tissue injury: Long and short term effects. In: Foreman S, Croft A, eds. Whiplash injuries: The cervical acceleration-deceleration syndrome. Baltimore: Williams & Wilkins, 1988:271.

LaBan M. "Whiplash"; its evaluation and treatment. Phys Med Rehabil 1990; 4:293.

Liebermann J. Cervical soft tissue injuries and cervical disc disease. In: Leek J, Gershwin ME, Fowler WM Jr, eds. Principles of physical medicine and rehabilitation in musculoskeletal diseases. Orlando: Grune & Stratton, 1986:263.

Murphy M. Non-operative treatment of cervical spine pain. Cervical Spine Research Society Editorial Committee, 1989:670.

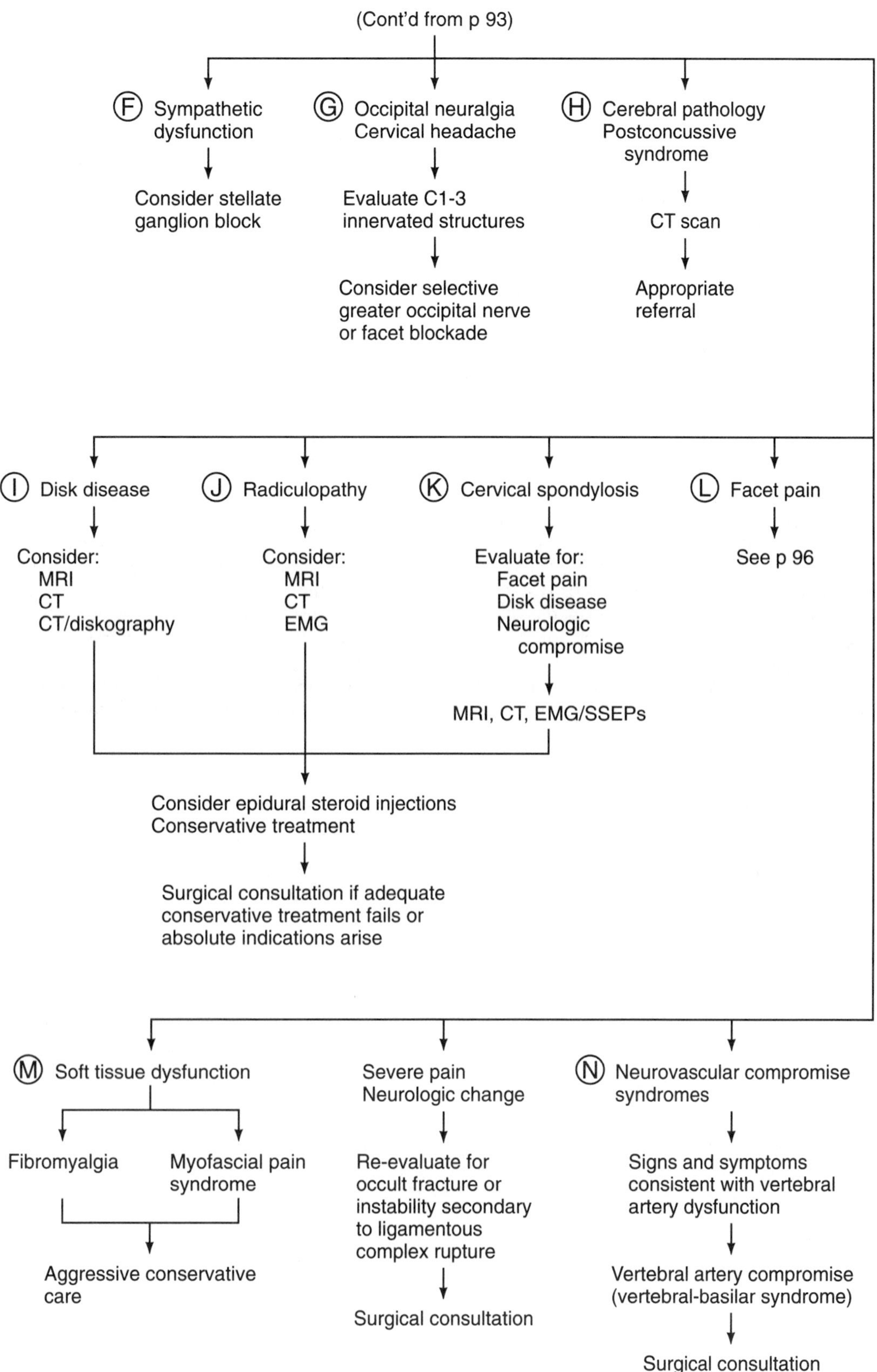
(Cont'd from p 93)
(F) Sympathetic dysfunction
Consider stellate ganglion block
(G) Occipital neuralgia Cervical headache
Evaluate C1-3 innervated structures
Consider selective greater occipital nerve or facet blockade
(H) Cerebral pathology Postconcussive syndrome
CT scan
Appropriate referral
(I) Disk disease
Consider: MRI CT CT/diskography
(J) Radiculopathy
Consider: MRI CT EMG
(K) Cervical spondylosis
Evaluate for: Facet pain Disk disease Neurologic compromise
MRI, CT, EMG/SSEPs
(L) Facet pain
See p 96
Consider epidural steroid injections Conservative treatment
Surgical consultation if adequate conservative treatment fails or absolute indications arise
(M) Soft tissue dysfunction
Fibromyalgia
Myofascial pain syndrome
Aggressive conservative care
Severe pain Neurologic change
Re-evaluate for occult fracture or instability secondary to ligamentous complex rupture
Surgical consultation
(N) Neurovascular compromise syndromes
Signs and symptoms consistent with vertebral artery dysfunction
Vertebral artery compromise (vertebral-basilar syndrome)
Surgical consultation

CERVICAL FACET PAIN

Paul Dreyfuss, M.D.

The cervical zygapophyseal (facet) joints have been implicated as pain-generating structures like the lumbar facet joints. The cervical facet joints lie in a plane 30° to 45° from the horizontal and face backward and upward. They are smaller than their lumbar counterparts, and the capsule usually accepts no more than 2 ml of fluid. The articular planes are relatively flat.

A. Suggestive history includes posterior neck pain with referred pain from the head to the infraspinous fossae. Pain is usually dull and aching in quality, although it can be sharp and localized. C2-3 pain is localized to the upper cervical region, C3-4 pain is posterolateral in the neck, C4-5 pain extends from the posterolateral neck to the spine of the scapula, C5-6 pain extends from the midcervical area to the spine of the scapula, and C6-7 pain enters the supra- and infraspinous fossae. C1-2 and C2-3 joints are commonly associated with headaches. Cervical facet pain is usually unilateral. Physical examination is performed with the patient prone or supine, with the head off the table and cradled in the examiner's hands. These positions better relax the musculature of the neck. Palpate the articular pillars and facets approximately 1.5 cm off midline. Quadrant load the facets with extension and oblique positioning. This may reproduce the pain. The patient with facet pain rarely presents with a neurologic deficit, and a detailed neurologic examination is therefore required to identify any neurologic deficits that could be indicative of other cervical pathology. Facet pain, however, can exist with other entities that cause neurologic changes. Local soft tissues should be evaluated. Cervical facet pain can exist in patients who have solid cervical fusions. Radiographs may or may not show facet arthropathy; the pillar view is best to evaluate the facets.

B. Conservative treatment encompasses a variety of methods, no one technique being superior; a combination is usually employed. Selective trigger point injections (TPIs) may be beneficial, these areas arising secondarily to the underlying irritation. Muscular stretching is very important. Traction can be used both for muscle and facet capsule/joint stretch. Lower weight will stretch the surrounding musculature only. Sixteen pounds is needed to lift the head off the shoulders; approximately 20 to 35 pounds is needed for minimal facet capsule distraction.

(Continued on page 98)

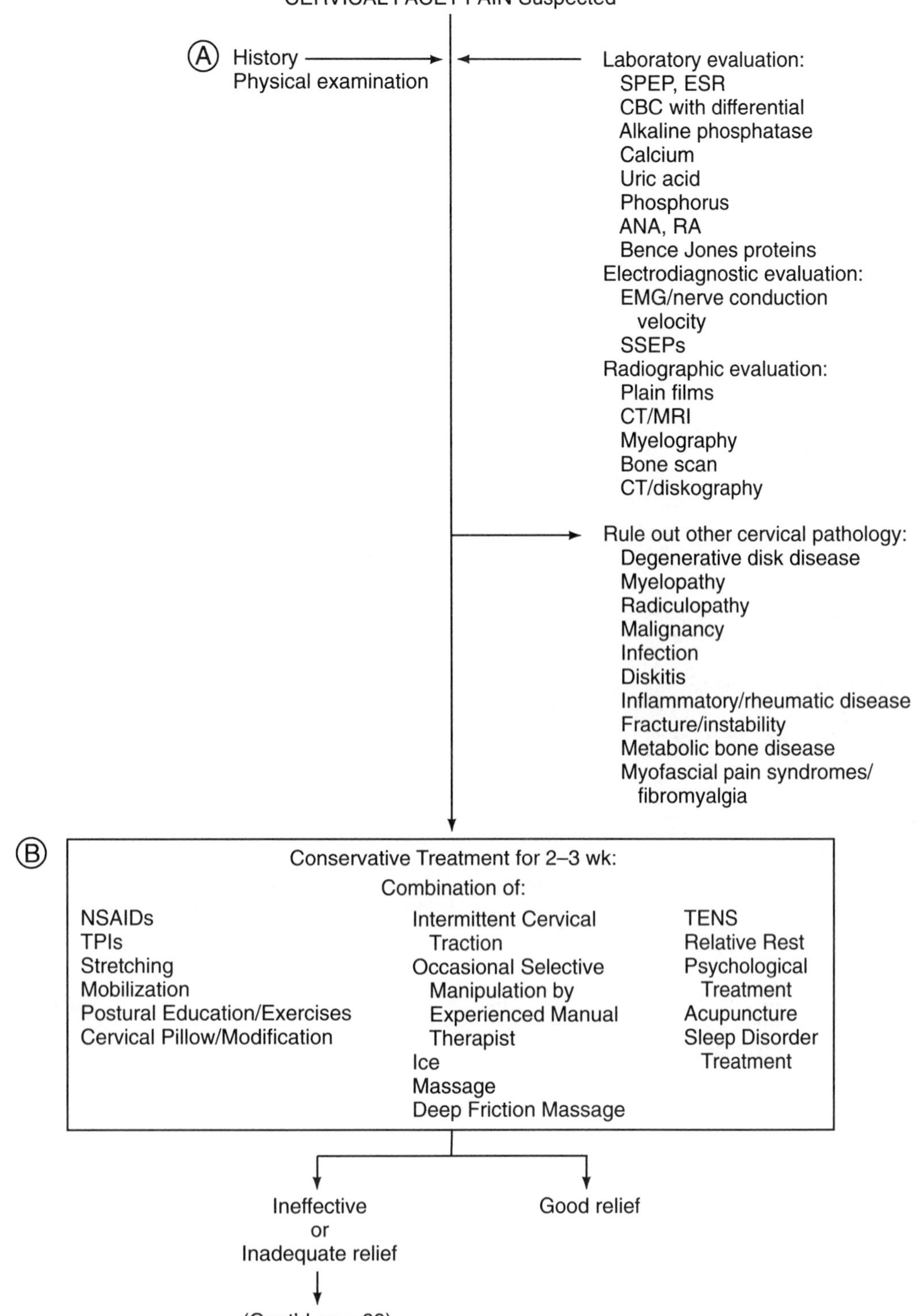
CERVICAL FACET PAIN Suspected
Ⓐ History
Physical examination
Laboratory evaluation:
SPEP, ESR
CBC with differential
Alkaline phosphatase
Calcium
Uric acid
Phosphorus
ANA, RA
Bence Jones proteins
Electrodiagnostic evaluation:
EMG/nerve conduction velocity
SSEPs
Radiographic evaluation:
Plain films
CT/MRI
Myelography
Bone scan
CT/diskography
Rule out other cervical pathology:
Degenerative disk disease
Myelopathy
Radiculopathy
Malignancy
Infection
Diskitis
Inflammatory/rheumatic disease
Fracture/instability
Metabolic bone disease
Myofascial pain syndromes/ fibromyalgia
Ⓑ Conservative Treatment for 2–3 wk:
Combination of:
NSAIDs
TPIs
Stretching
Mobilization
Postural Education/Exercises
Cervical Pillow/Modification
Intermittent Cervical Traction
Occasional Selective Manipulation by Experienced Manual Therapist
Ice
Massage
Deep Friction Massage
TENS
Relative Rest
Psychological Treatment
Acupuncture
Sleep Disorder Treatment
Ineffective or Inadequate relief
Good relief
(Cont'd on p 99)

C. Each C3-4 to C7/T1 facet receives its innervation from the medial branch of the posterior rami nerve at a level above and below the joint. The anatomic location of this medial branch is consistently at the waist of the articular pillar of each cervical vertebra. The block is performed under fluoroscopic guidance with the patient prone. A 22-gauge needle is directed until it rests on the lateral margin of the silhouette of the articular pillar at its waist. At this point 0.5 to 1.5 ml of 0.5% bupivicaine is injected over the underlying nerve. Relief of pain is diagnostic of facet pain. The C2-3 joint is innervated by the third occipital nerve as it crosses behind the joint. To block this nerve, the needle is directed to the lower half of the lateral margin of the C2-3 facet joint. Numbness will occur over the suboccipital region with a successful block. It has been suggested that if precise localization of the symptomatic facet is uncertain, one should first block the C5 and C6 medial branches in lower cervical pain followed by C4 or C7 if the pain is not relieved. For upper cervical pain, a third occipital nerve block is done followed by a C3 or C4 medial branch block.

D. Facet joint injections are made by first entering the skin from several segments below the joint. A 22-gauge needle is advanced upward to the inferior margin of the joint; AP and lateral screening under fluoroscopy is needed to ensure that the needle is advanced only to the joints' midpoint. Previous studies have used 1.5 to 2.0 ml of equal mixtures of 0.5% bupivacaine and depot methylprednisolone. Facet injection is made easier with the patient's neck flexed and head turned to the opposite side, because this helps to open up the facet joint. Avoid anterior needle placement, since the neural foramina, epidural space, and vertebral artery are intimately related to the joint's anterior surface.

E. Percutaneous radiofrequency neurotomy has gained increased attention for the treatment of cervical pain. The procedure aims at interrupting the cervical facet pain by coagulating the nerves that supply it. The target nerves are determined as those that gave relief when anesthetized. Recently, it has been recommended to place the radiofrequency electrodes parallel rather than perpendicular to the nerve to achieve better coagulation. Unless meticulous technique and precise anatomic location is obtained, the radiofrequency electrode placed perpendicular to the nerve may not coagulate it. With fluoroscopic placement a small stimulating current is used (usually less than 4 V) to ensure proper placement and reproduction of the pain. It is important to observe for muscle twitching or gross limb movement, which would indicate placement too close to the anterior rami. The electrode tip is raised to a temperature of 80° to 85° from one 90-second stimulation to three 1-minute stimulations. The effects usually last 3 to 6 months, repeated denervation being equally successful in patients who initially had an excellent response. To ensure adequate denervation, paraspinal electromyography (EMG) in the lumbar spine 30 to 45 days after rhizotomy has been suggested. The degree of denervation found on EMG has correlated well with the adequacy of the rhizotomy and pain relief. It seems logical to extend this hypothesis to cover the cervical spine.

References

April C. Cervical zygapophyseal joint pain patterns 2: A clinical evaluation. Spine 1990; 15:458.

Bogduk N. The cervical zygapophyseal joints as a source of neck pain. Spine 1988; 13:610.

Bogduk N. Technical limitations to the efficacy of radiofrequency neurotomy for spinal pain. Neurosurgery 1987; 20:529.

Bogduk N. Percutaneous lumbar medial branch neurotomy. A modification of facet denervation. Spine 1980; 5:193.

Hildebrandt J. Percutaneous cervical facet denervation. Manual Med 1983; 21:45.

Ouderhoven R. Paraspinal electromyography following facet rhizotomy. Spine 1977; 2:299.

Rashbaum R. Radiofrequency facet denervation. Orthop Clin North Am 1983; 14:569.

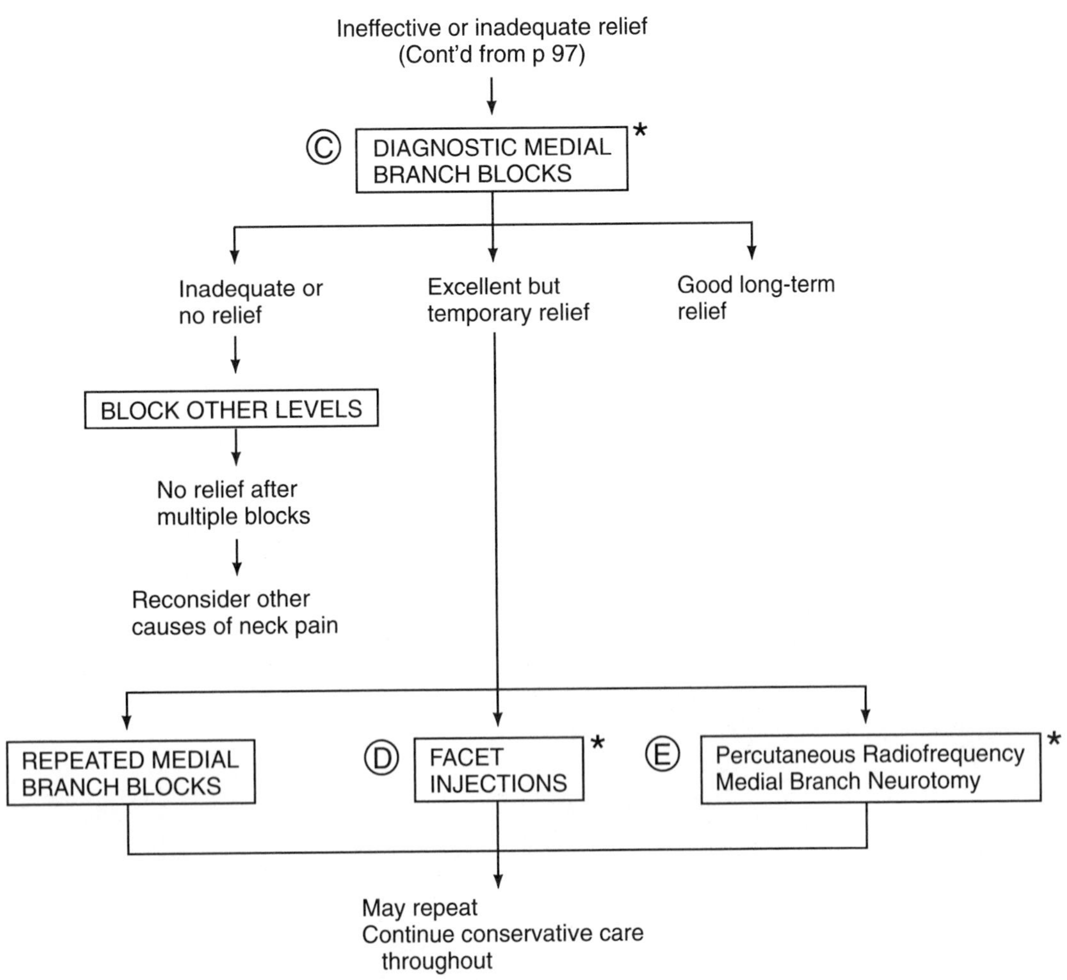
Ineffective or inadequate relief
(Cont'd from p 97)
C DIAGNOSTIC MEDIAL BRANCH BLOCKS *
Inadequate or no relief
Excellent but temporary relief
Good long-term relief
BLOCK OTHER LEVELS
No relief after multiple blocks
Reconsider other causes of neck pain
REPEATED MEDIAL BRANCH BLOCKS
D FACET INJECTIONS *
E Percutaneous Radiofrequency Medial Branch Neurotomy *
May repeat
Continue conservative care throughout
* To be performed only by an experienced physician under fluoroscopic guidance.

UPPER EXTREMITY PAIN

REFLEX SYMPATHETIC DYSTROPHY OF THE HAND

Dominique Schiffer, M.D.

A. Chronic hand pain is diagnosed by eliciting a comprehensive history and performing a thorough physical examination. The exact location of the pain and its quality, intensity, pattern of radiation, and temporal characteristics should be noted, as well as the response to cold, heat, activity, and rest. The history should include questions about accidental or surgical trauma, microtrauma or macrotrauma associated with occupation or diseases such as diabetes, neuromuscular disorders, connective tissue disorders, and malignancy. The physical examination should include inspection, palpation, and evaluation of motor and neurologic function.

B. Mechanical and inflammatory conditions of the hands should be identified during the history and physical examination. Peripheral neuropathies from nerve entrapment, diabetes, uremia, amyloidosis, malnutrition, toxins, and drugs also should be ruled out.

C. Early diagnosis of reflex sympathetic dystrophy (RSD) is important not only because the pain causes disability but also because early treatment gives more promising results and a greater likelihood of cure. RSD has numerous precipitating factors. The most common is trauma secondary to an accidental injury (dislocation, fracture, crush injury of fingers, contusions, or minor injury). Iatrogenic injury that develops from a complication of surgical or medical therapy (ganglia excision, tight casts, intramuscular injections, accidental needle insertion into a nerve) may also be a factor. Various neurologic, musculoskeletal, and visceral diseases may also produce RSD. Examples are myocardial infarction, cerebrovascular accident, multiple sclerosis, and carcinoma.

D. A diffuse, burning, aching, throbbing pain unrelieved by rest is characteristic of RSD. Allodynia is usually present. It may be thermal, mechanical, or both. Cold allodynia is more common than heat allodynia. Hyperpathia, hyperesthesia, and dysesthesia are almost always present. The symptoms may be aggravated by physical and emotional stimuli.

E. The three stages of RSD can be differentiated based on signs and the time since injury. Each stage may last 3 to 6 months. Table 1 describes the physical signs of RSD.

TABLE 1 Physical Signs of Reflex Sympathetic Dystrophy

Sign	*Stage 1*	*Stage 2*	*Stage 3*
Edema	↑ ↑	↑	↓
Vasomotor	↑	↑	↑/↓
Temperature	Warm	Cold	↑/↓
Hidrosis	Hypo-	Hyper-	Normal
Muscle	Hypertonic	Atrophy	Atrophy
Hair	Normal	Decreased	Increased/normal
Nails	Normal	Brittle	Resumed growth
Color	Dusky red/cyanotic	Cyanotic	Normal
Osteopenia	↑	↑ ↑	↑ ↑

F. Vasomotor changes may be documented using thermography, which provides information about the differences in blood flow between the affected and unaffected hand. Sudomotor disturbances can be diagnosed by evaluating the sympathogalvanic reflex. This is manifested by a transient elevation of skin conductivity following a stimulus that evokes a sympathetic response. Cold allodynia and hyperalgesia may be tested for with a drop of acetone. Von Frey's hair test can be used to test for mechanical allodynia. Plain radiography may reveal bony demineralization and osteoporosis. A three-phase technetium bone scan may have predictive value for RSD. However, this can be affected by the duration of symptoms and the patient's age. A sympathetic block usually provides prompt and complete pain relief and modifies the signs associated with RSD. The block results in increased temperature of the hand, disappearance of cyanosis, decreased swelling, and improved function.

G. A sympathetic block may be achieved using techniques such as a stellate ganglion block (p 242), interpleural catheter placement (p 250) to deliver a local anesthetic, or IV regional blockade with guanethidine or reserpine. Because of the technical difficulties that may be encountered with these procedures, three attempts of any one technique should be undertaken before concluding that no therapeutic benefit has been obtained. Transcutaneous electrical nerve stimulation (TENS) (p 194) and dorsal column stimulation (p 224) have been reported to be effective therapies for RSD; however, they are rarely employed as a sole form of treatment. In some studies, topical capsaicin has given complete but temporary pain relief. Oral pharmacologic therapy with propranolol, phenoxybenzamine, corticosteroids, nifedipine, naloxone, or tricyclic antidepressants is an effective adjuvant in the treatment of RSD.

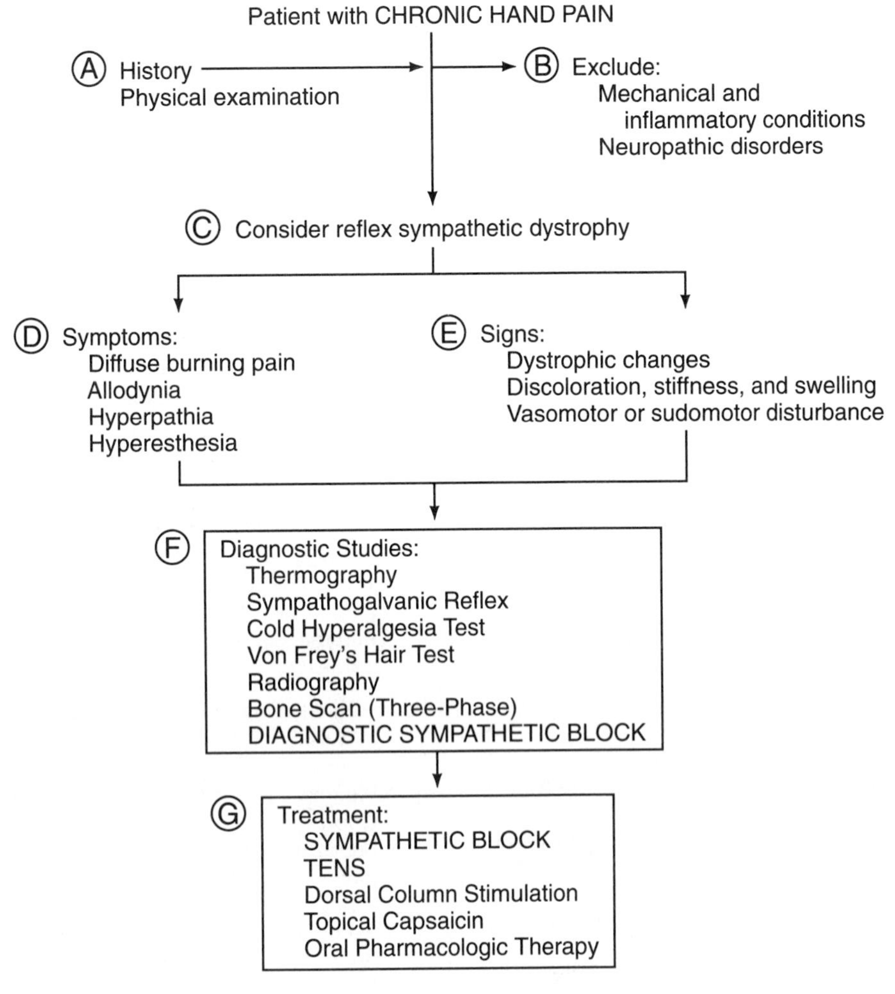

References

Almquist EE, Bonica JJ. Painful conditions of the forearm, wrist and hand. In: Bonica JJ, ed. The management of pain. 2nd ed. Philadelphia: Lea and Febiger, 1990:924.

Bonica JJ. Causalgia and other reflex sympathetic dystrophies. In: Bonica JJ, ed. The management of pain. 2nd ed. Philadelphia: Lea and Febiger, 1990:220.

Cheshire WP, Snyder CR. Treatment of reflex sympathetic dystrophy with topical capsaicin. Pain 1990; 42:307.

Reistad F, McIlvaine WB, Kvalheim L, et al. Interpleural analgesia in treatment of upper extremity reflex sympathetic dystrophy. Anesth Analg 1989; 69:671.

Rothschild B. Reflex sympathetic dystrophy. Arthritis Care Res 1990; 3:144.

Werner R, Davidoff G, Jackson D, et al. Factors affecting the sensitivity and specificity of the three-phase technetium bone scan in the diagnosis of reflex sympathetic dystrophy syndrome in the upper extremity. J Hand Surg 1989; 14:520.

SHOULDER-HAND SYNDROME

Mark E. Romanoff, M.D.

Shoulder-hand syndrome (SHS) was first described by Steinbrocker in 1947, but the term was coined by Dr. Richard H. Freyberg in the same article. It appears to be a form of reflex sympathetic dystrophy (p 50). It has been associated with many factors, which are listed in Table 1.

A. Three stages of SHS have been identified. Stage 1 lasts approximately 3 to 6 months. Initial symptoms include shoulder, hand, and finger pain and tenderness. Shoulder disability and osteoporosis of the shoulder, humeral head, and wrist are evident. Vasomotor and skin changes are also seen. Hand and finger hyperesthesia and swelling are noted. The second stage lasts 3 to 6 months. Muscles atrophy, and early dystrophy may occur. The pain and disability may either continue or actually lessen during this period. Vasodilation and swelling usually abate and the resulting vasospasm causes atrophic changes in the hair, nails, and skin. Osteoporosis continues into the third stage, which can last for years and is characterized by less pain and more disability. Dystrophic changes and contractures occur in the shoulder, hand, and fingers. Ultimately a "frozen shoulder" may be evident. As these dystrophic changes occur, they appear irreversible. SHS is unilateral in 75% of cases. Elbow involvement is rare. This syndrome is seen more frequently in women and in patients >50 years old.

B. A wide range of syndromes should be considered in the differential diagnosis. Referred visceral pain should be excluded early in the course. Abdominal visceral pain can be referred to the shoulder. Myocardial ischemic pain may also be referred to the shoulder (right or left) and may not be associated with chest pain. History taking, physical examination, and ECG should be performed to rule out this entity in the population at risk. Initially the inflammatory symptoms predominate, so that arthritis, tendinitis, and bursitis may be mistaken for SHS. Laboratory studies, including tests for rheumatoid factor levels or the presence of uric acid crystals in a joint effusion, can help differentiate these from SHS. A myofascial pain syndrome should be assessed by careful palpation. Most commonly the scalene, deltoid, sternocleidomastoid, and suprascapular muscles are involved. Scalenus anterior or thoracic outlet syndromes may cause vasomotor changes and can be identified by palpation, checking pulses with the arms abducted, and radiography to identify a cervical rib. Evidence of cervical disk disease (extremity weakness, numbness, and paresthesias) can be evaluated by CT, MRI, or myelography as needed. The diagnosis of SHS can be confirmed by relief of pain with a diagnostic stellate ganglion block (p 242).

C. Initiate treatment immediately after diagnosis to avoid irreversible musculoskeletal changes. Recent treatment has concentrated on analgesics, physical therapy, and sympathetic blocks.

D. The early use of physical therapy (PT), including passive and active exercises of the shoulder and hand, has proved effective alone or in combination with stellate ganglion blocks or steroid therapy. There is one reported caveat: avoid orthopedic manipulation under anesthesia. Whether this includes PT after brachial plexus, suprascapular, or dorsal scapular nerve blocks has not been determined.

E. NSAIDs should be begun promptly because the early phase of this syndrome involves inflammation. Analgesia is also necessary to allow the patient to participate more fully in PT. If NSAIDs are not effective, narcotics can be added temporarily for adequate pain control.

F. Stellate ganglion blocks have been advocated for the treatment of SHS since its discovery. Early studies have shown good to excellent improvement in >80% of patients treated with PT and stellate ganglion blocks. Coordination of PT and the blocks is important. Performance of these blocks before PT will decrease pain during therapy and enhance progress. Usually a series of three to five blocks at 2- to 7-day intervals is necessary. The injections should be continued if deemed appropriate; a patient in one study needed a series of 14 blocks for effective pain relief. Brachial plexus continuous catheter techniques can provide prolonged sympathetic blockade, allowing aggressive PT in an inpatient setting (p 208).

G. Trigger point injections (TPIs) have been recommended to treat SHS itself or an associated myofascial pain syndrome. Anecdotal reports suggest that TPIs alone are not very effective. Combination of other therapy with adjunctive treatment of a myofascial pain syndrome has a higher success rate. The use of steroids in TPIs has been suggested, but their efficacy in comparison with local anesthetic injections has not been studied.

H. High-dose oral steroid therapy (prednisone, 40 to 60 mg/day) has been proposed for treatment of this syndrome since 1947. Two recent reports have confirmed the effectiveness of this treatment. One study in patients with SHS after cerebrovascular accidents described a 100% "cure" rate within 1 week of treatment; a 10% remission rate was also noted.

I. Prophylaxis should focus on PT and should be started early after the occurrence of a clinical entity associated with SHS (see Table 1). This may help prevent the latter stages of SHS. The use of prophylactic stellate ganglion blocks has not been evaluated and is not recommended at this time.

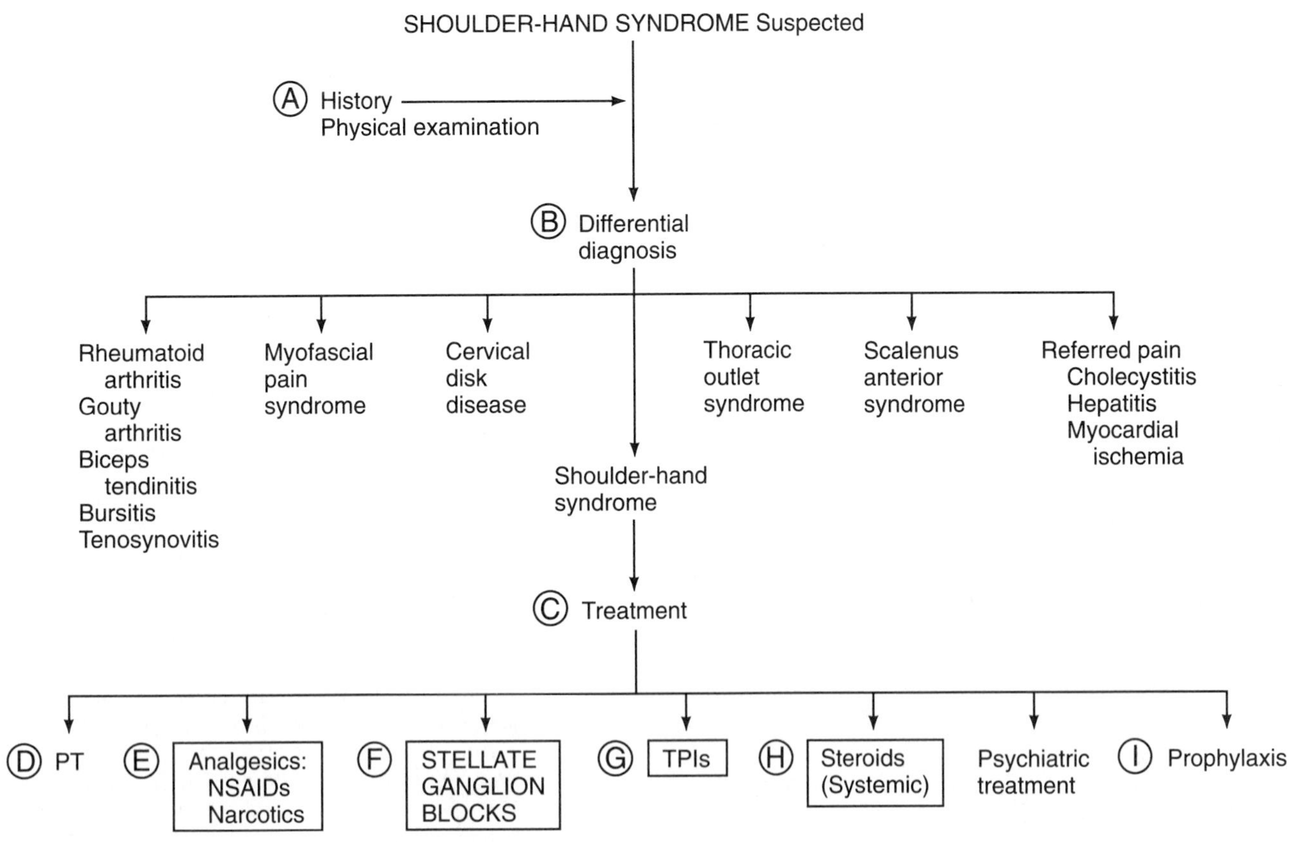

TABLE 1 Factors Associated with Shoulder-Hand Syndrome

Cardiovascular
  Post–myocardial infarction
Neurologic
  Post–cerebrovascular accident
  Intracranial/extracranial tumor
  Epilepsy
  Parkinson's disease
  Herpes zoster
Musculoskeletal
  Post-traumatic
  Arthritis
  Cervical disk degeneration
Idiopathic
Miscellaneous
  Barbiturate use
  Laparoscopic surgery
  Pulmonary tuberculosis
  Neoplasms
  Diabetes mellitus

References

Davis SW, Petrillo CR, Eichberg RD, Chu DS. Shoulder-hand syndrome in a hemiplegic population: A 5-year retrospective study. Arch Phys Med Rehabil 1977; 58:353.

Korst JK van der, Colenbrander H, Cats A. Phenobarbital and the shoulder-hand syndrome. Ann Rheum Dis 1966; 25:553.

Russek HI. Shoulder-hand syndrome following myocardial infarction. Med Clin North Am 1958; 42:1555.

Steinbrocker O. Painful homolateral disability of shoulder and hand with swelling and atrophy of hand. Ann Rheum Dis 1947; 6:80.

Steinbrocker O, Argyros TG. The shoulder-hand syndrome: Present status as a diagnostic and therapeutic entity. Med Clin North Am 1958; 42:1533.

Walker J, Belsole R, Germain B. Shoulder-hand syndrome in patients with intracranial neoplasms. Hand 1983; 347.

THORACIC OUTLET SYNDROME

Paul Dreyfuss, M.D.

Thoracic outlet syndrome (TOS), especially the disputed neurogenic type, is a highly controversial diagnosis. There is no general consensus on diagnostic criteria and whether tests such as provocative physical maneuvers and electrodiagnostic studies are helpful. The thoracic outlet is the opening bordered laterally by the first rib, medially by the vertebral column, and anteriorly by the claviculomanubrium complex. Symptoms result from mechanical compression of the neurovascular bundle through this outlet. Contributing causes include anomalies such as a cervical rib or an incomplete cervical rib with fibrous bands. Compression may occur anywhere along the three zones of the cervicoaxillary canal (the interscalene triangle, the costoclavicular triangle, and the subcoracoid space). Depending on the anatomy and compressive site, either vascular (arterial or venous) or neurogenic symptoms occur. Rarely does a combination occur. Subsets have been created to better define diagnostic and treatment strategies.

A. Numerous provocative physical examination maneuvers have been described to identify TOS or its subsets; examples include Adson's test, the exaggerated military maneuver, the hyperabduction test, and the elevated arm stress test. Because many of these tests are positive in a normal population, they must exactly reproduce the patient's symptoms to be truly positive.

B. Cervical films are needed to identify anomalies. Occasionally a lordotic view is needed to view a cervical rib. A chest radiograph can identify an apical mass or clavicular abnormalities. Electrodiagnostic tests include techniques such as nerve conduction studies and electromyography. Certain findings are characteristic but not pathognomonic for true neurogenic-type TOS. Electrodiagnostic studies are helpful in ruling out radiculopathies and peripheral nerve entrapments that may mimic TOS.

C. TOS is truly a rare entity. Other, more common entities, including brachial plexus neuritis, cervical radiculopathy, peripheral nerve entrapments, cervical cord lesions, and myofascial syndromes, must be excluded. Vasculitis, thromboangiitis obliterans, and secondary subclavian compression from metastasis also must be excluded.

D. The incidence of true neurogenic TOS is estimated to be as low as one case per million. It comprises <2% of all TOSs and usually affects young and middle-aged women. In true neurogenic TOS, a cervical rib or other anomaly compresses the lower trunk of the brachial plexus or the C8–T1 roots. Paresthesias and aches occur in the medial aspect of the upper extremity and hand. The small muscles of the hand become weak, especially the lateral thenar muscles. Electrodiagnostic testing shows chronic axonal loss in a lower trunk distribution: If there is continuing axonal loss or if conservative treatment fails, surgery is indicated.

E. Conservative treatment includes weight reduction and strengthening exercises to correct drooping shoulders and poor posture. Mobilization and scalene muscle stretching are sometimes needed. Positioning or postures that aggravate the pain should be avoided. Occupational modifications may be necessary.

F. Disputed neurogenic TOS is the most commonly diagnosed subset (>90%), for which the largest number of surgeries are performed, yet there are no objective criteria or clinical tests to confirm this disorder. Many feel it is not a true entity. No cervical ribs or other anomalies exist. There are subjective complaints, but no muscle wasting or electrodiagnostic abnormalities. Conservative treatment is usually effective in mild to moderate cases. Surgery is rarely indicated, surgical results have not been entirely successful, and complications such as brachial plexus injury are possible.

G. Droopy shoulder syndrome is a subset of disputed neurogenic TOS that typically occurs in young women with low-set shoulders and long necks. Symptoms are pain and paresthesias in the neck, chest, shoulders, and arms, usually bilateral and asymmetric. There are no objective abnormalities. Conservative treatment is usually effective.

H. Arterial vascular TOS comprises 5% of all TOSs. Symptoms are secondary to subclavian artery compression and may include coldness, diffuse pain, weakness, loss of radial pulse, and signs of peripheral embolization. The major arterial type requires arteriographic demonstration of compression, and surgery is indicated to prevent further arterial damage. The minor type occurs in 80% of young adults as a normal variant but may be problematic with shoulder elevation. Surgery, if indicated, is done not to treat arterial damage but for occupational reasons.

I. Venous vascular TOS comprises <2% of TOSs. Venography demonstrates compression. Symptoms are secondary to subclavian vein compression and may include edema, discoloration of the arm, and distention of superficial proximal veins.

J. Combined arterial vascular and true neurogenic TOS is most often due to a significant structural abnormality. Evaluation and treatment as described previously for each type of TOS are appropriate. Surgical consultation may be necessary.

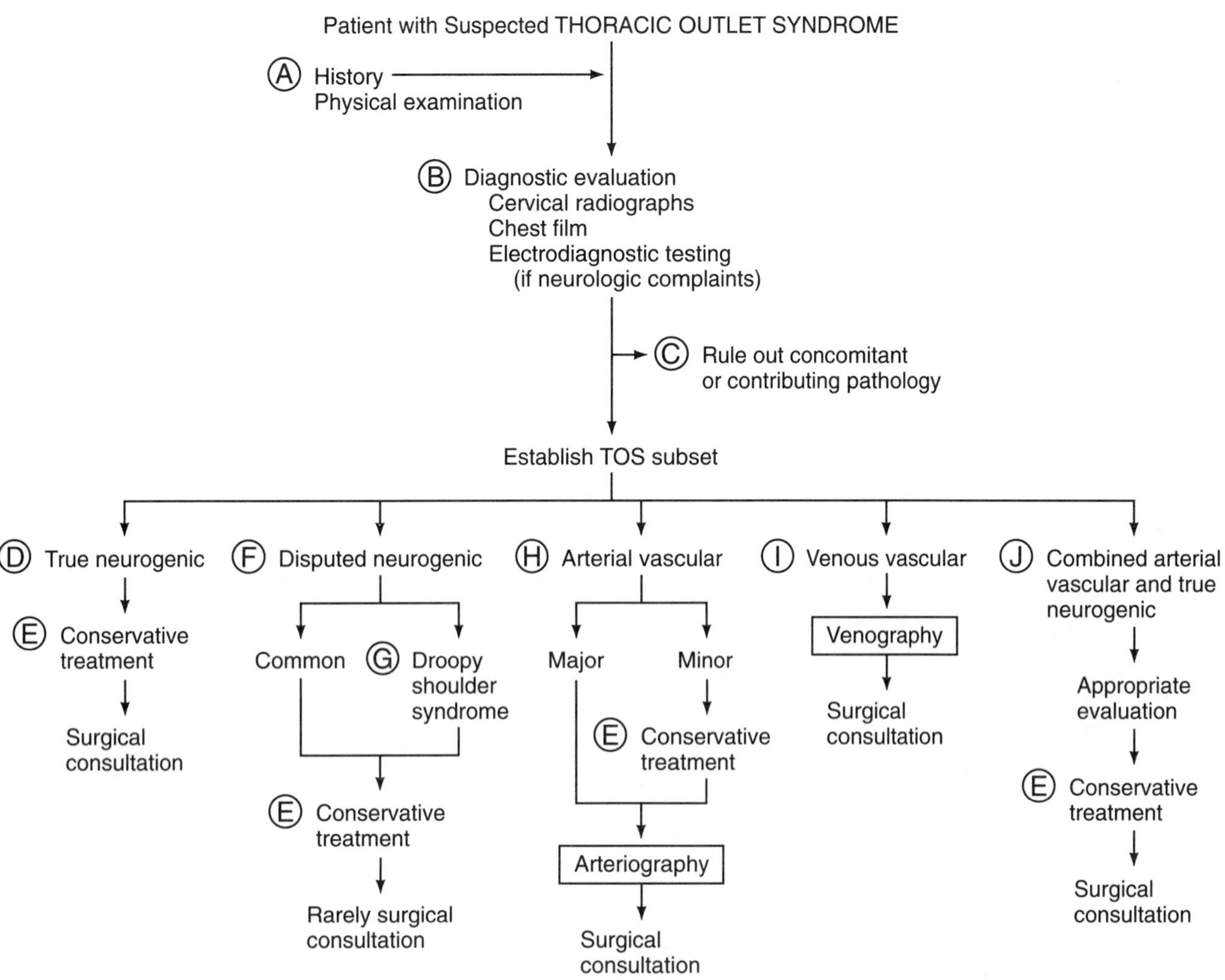

References

Cuetter AC, Bartoszek DM. The thoracic outlet syndrome: Controversies, overdiagnosis, overtreatment and recommendations for management. Muscle Nerve 1989; 12:410.

Pang D, Wessel HB. Thoracic outlet syndrome. Neurosurgery 1988; 22:105.

Wilbourn AJ, Porter JM. Thoracic outlet syndromes. In: Weiner MA, ed. Spine: State of the art reviews. Philadelphia: Hanley & Belfus, 1988.

CARPAL TUNNEL SYNDROME

Somayaji Ramamurthy, M.D.

Carpal tunnel syndrome (CTS) is the most common compression neuropathy in the upper extremity.

A. The usual symptoms are weakness or clumsiness of the hand, hyperesthesia or paresthesias in the distribution of the median nerve, increase of symptoms with the use of the hand, numbness of the fingers, and pain in the wrist and forearm, occasionally involving even the shoulder and neck. The pain is reproduced by wrist flexion (Phalen's test). Tinel's sign may be present on tapping the median nerve over the wrist. Sensory findings are limited to the distribution to the median nerve.

B. EMG nerve conduction velocity (NCV) studies are very useful in confirming the diagnosis.

C. The diagnosis of CTS may be associated with rheumatoid arthritis, myxedema, multiple myeloma, diabetes mellitus, trauma, or pregnancy.

D. Conservative measures such as splinting, injection of a local anesthetic with steroids usually provide significant pain relief. In temporary conditions such as CTS aggravated by pregnancy, these may produce long-term pain relief.

E. If conservative measures provide only temporary relief, carpal tunnel surgery is very successful in relieving the symptoms.

References

Eversman WW Jr. Entrapment and compression neuropathies. In: Green DP, ed. Operative hand surgery. New York: Churchill Livingstone, 1988:1430.

Green DP. Diagnostic and therapeutic value of carpal tunnel injection. J Hand Surg 1984; 9A:850.

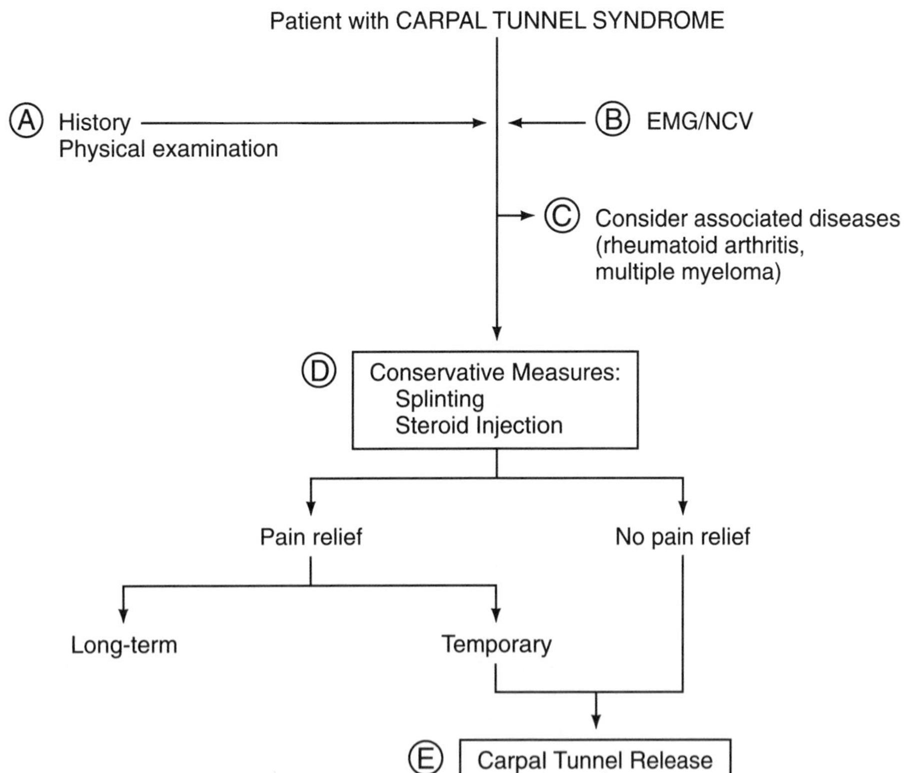
Patient with CARPAL TUNNEL SYNDROME
(A) History
Physical examination
(B) EMG/NCV
(C) Consider associated diseases
(rheumatoid arthritis,
multiple myeloma)
(D) Conservative Measures:
Splinting
Steroid Injection
Pain relief
No pain relief
Long-term
Temporary
(E) Carpal Tunnel Release

THORACIC PAIN

CHRONIC THORACIC PAIN

John D. Merwin, M.D.

Chronic thoracic pain may be the result of many different processes. The initiating disease or trauma may well have resolved but the pain persists. It is also possible that the patient may not be able to identify an initiating event. The diagnosis requires a thorough history and physical examination. A multidisciplinary pain management approach is often necessary to obtain significant relief in these patients.

A. Myofascial pain syndrome (MPS) is one of the most common causes of chest pain. Pain can vary from slight ache to severe, disabling discomfort. Muscles should be carefully evaluated for trigger points (TPs). Muscles should be examined in both the relaxed and stretched positions. TPs may be primary or secondary causes of pain. Spray and stretch or TP injection with a local anesthetic should be part of a comprehensive physical therapy program (p 190).

B. Cancer can cause visceral, chest wall, or neuropathic pain. After identifying the lesion, pain relief may be achieved by radiation, chemotherapy, hormone therapy, or surgery to relieve compression of nerves and other vital structures. Persistent pain may respond well to NSAIDs (bony pain), tricyclic antidepressants (neuropathic pain), and systemic and/or neuraxial narcotics (visceral pain). Neurolytic blockade may be appropriate in well-localized cancer pain in patients with a limited life expectancy (p 216).

C. Postsurgical pain such as in post-thoracotomy and postmastectomy syndromes (pp 114 and 117) usually is easily diagnosed, but the cause of the pain is not so easily identified. In many patients the pain may be the result of tumor recurrence. Again, a thorough evaluation is necessary. Often these pain syndromes are the result of injury or disruption of nerves causing neuropathic or sympathetically mediated pain. Diagnostic sympathetic and somatic intercostal blocks can confirm the diagnosis.

D. Postherpetic neuralgia has been discussed earlier (p 48). Herpes zoster occurs in the thoracic region approximately 50% of the time.

E. Disorders of the thoracic spine, although not as common as lumbar or cervical disorders, can be a significant source of pain. Thoracic facet joints can suffer excessive stress and strain from sudden, unguarded twisting movements, or from prolonged working with the hands above the head. Treatment consists of heat, physical therapy, and infiltration of the facet joint (p 266).

F. Intractable thoracic pain may require more invasive procedures such as neurolytic blocks, surgical ablation, dorsal column stimulation, or intracerebral stimulation.

G. As in any patient with chronic pain, the psychological and emotional factors must be evaluated and treated along with the organic causes of pain. Environmental, psychological, social, marital, and family problems may contribute to chronic depression and worsening of pain. Clues to depression such as persistent irritability, insomnia, chronic malaise, weight change, or suicidal ideation should be elicited.

References

Bonica JJ. Chest pain caused by other disorders. In: Bonica JJ, ed. The management of pain. 2nd ed. Philadelphia: Lea & Febiger, 1990:1114.

Levene DL, ed. Chest pain: An integrated diagnostic approach. Philadelphia: Lea & Febiger, 1977.

Portenoy RK, Lipton RB, Foley KM. Back pain in the cancer patient: An algorithm for evaluation and management. Neurology 1987; 37:134.

Swerdlow M. Role of nerve blocks and pain involving the chest and brachial plexus. In: Bonica JJ, Ventafridda V, eds. Advances in pain research and therapy. Vol. 2. New York: Raven Press, 1979:325.

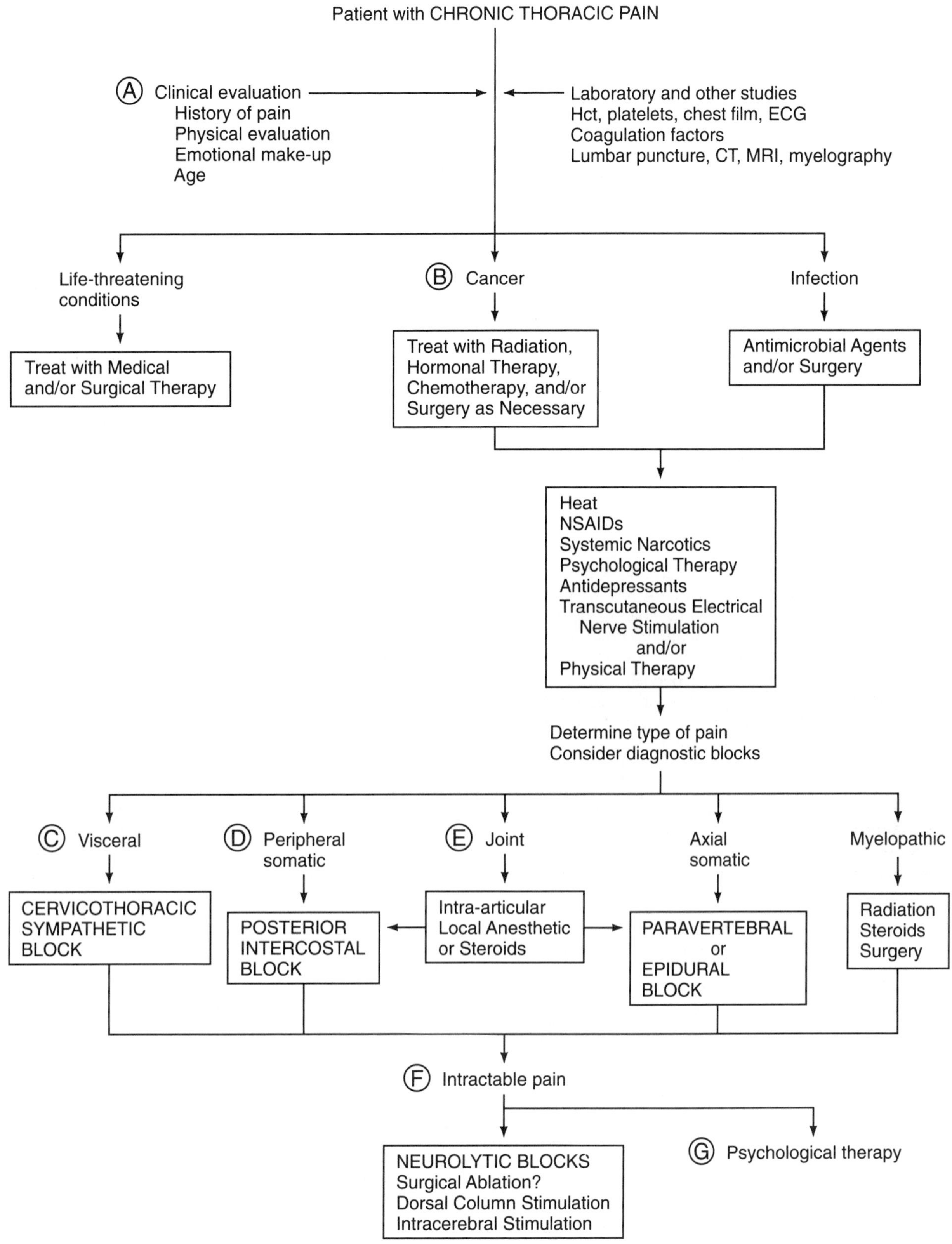

Patient with CHRONIC THORACIC PAIN
(A) Clinical evaluation
History of pain
Physical evaluation
Emotional make-up
Age
Laboratory and other studies
Hct, platelets, chest film, ECG
Coagulation factors
Lumbar puncture, CT, MRI, myelography
Life-threatening conditions
Treat with Medical and/or Surgical Therapy
(B) Cancer
Treat with Radiation, Hormonal Therapy, Chemotherapy, and/or Surgery as Necessary
Infection
Antimicrobial Agents and/or Surgery
Heat
NSAIDs
Systemic Narcotics
Psychological Therapy
Antidepressants
Transcutaneous Electrical Nerve Stimulation
and/or
Physical Therapy
Determine type of pain
Consider diagnostic blocks
(C) Visceral
CERVICOTHORACIC SYMPATHETIC BLOCK
(D) Peripheral somatic
POSTERIOR INTERCOSTAL BLOCK
(E) Joint
Intra-articular Local Anesthetic or Steroids
Axial somatic
PARAVERTEBRAL or EPIDURAL BLOCK
Myelopathic
Radiation
Steroids
Surgery
(F) Intractable pain
NEUROLYTIC BLOCKS
Surgical Ablation?
Dorsal Column Stimulation
Intracerebral Stimulation
(G) Psychological therapy

POSTMASTECTOMY PAIN

Scott D. Murtha, M.D.

Postmastectomy pain (PMP) is also referred to as intercostobrachial nerve entrapment or postmastectomy pain syndrome. PMP may occur from minor procedures such as a lumpectomy, but it is more common following radical mastectomy and axillary node dissection. This syndrome develops in approximately 4 to 6% of women who have had surgical procedures on the breast. Pain is thought to be due to traumatic neuroma formation of the intercostobrachial nerve (ICBN). The ICBN is the lateral cutaneous branch of T2, with minor contribution from other upper thoracic nerves. There is marked anatomic variation in size and distribution of the ICBN; consequently there are varying degrees of surgical injury to this nerve. As noted, only a small percentage of patients who suffer ICBN damage will have associated PMP.

A. The diagnosis of PMP syndrome is based primarily on a detailed description of the pain, history of breast surgery, and physical examination.

B. PMP is intractable pain characterized as tight, burning, and constricting. It involves the medial and posterior arm, the axilla, and the anterior chest wall. Symptoms can occur immediately or very shortly after surgery and are present for longer than one month. PMP often is associated with hyperesthesia, allodynia, and hyperalgesia, making the wearing of undergarments uncomfortable. The pain is exacerbated by arm movement and relieved by immobilization. Patients often posture the affected arm in a flexed position close to the chest wall; thus they are at risk for developing a "frozen shoulder." There are intermittent episodes of lancinating pain, paresthesia, and dysthesia. PMP is more common in patients with postoperative wound infections or fluid retention, presumably from local perineuronal fibrosis.

C. Physical examination reveals hyperesthesia of the anterior chest wall, axilla, and medial/posterior arm. Diffuse, light touch can aggravate the pain; palpation of a neuroma elicits lancinating pain.

D. The differential diagnosis includes brachial plexopathy due to carcinomatous infiltration or radiofibrosis. If the history and examination are not definitive, relief of symptoms by a posterior intercostal block (p 252) of the affected dermatomes helps to differentiate PMP from brachial plexopathy. Pain relief by a local trigger point injection of a neuroma can aid in the differential diagnosis.

E. Treatment consists of pain relief and aggressive physical therapy. This combination helps prevent frozen shoulder and disuse atrophy pain. Initial pain relief modalities include conservative measures, particularly the use of an NSAID with a tricyclic antidepressant. Topical capsaicin has been reported to be an effective noninvasive modality.

References

Foley KM. Pain syndromes in patients with cancer. Med Clin North Am 1987; 71:177.

Granek I, Ashikari RA, Foley K. The postmastectomy pain syndrome: Clinical and anatomical correlates. Proc ASCO 1984; 3:122.

Vecht CJ, Van de Brand HJ, Wajer OJM. Post-axillary dissection pain in the breast cancer due to a lesion of the intercostobrachial nerve. Pain 1989; 38:171.

Watson LPN, Evans RJ, Watt VR. The post-mastectomy pain syndrome and the effect of topical capsaicin. Pain 1989; 38:177.

Wood KM. Intercostobrachial nerve entrapment syndrome. South Med J 1978; 662.

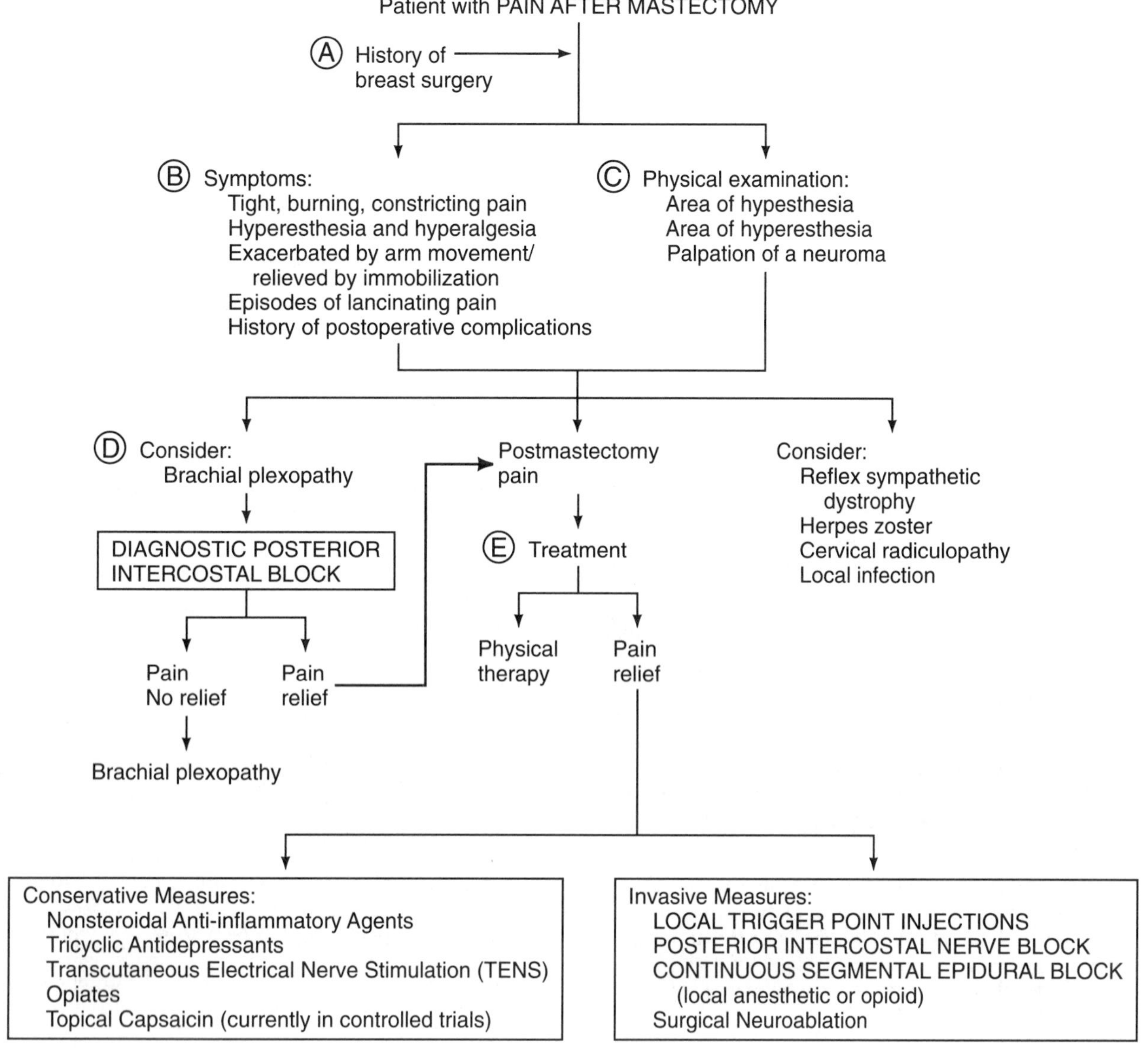
Patient with PAIN AFTER MASTECTOMY
(A) History of breast surgery
(B) Symptoms:
Tight, burning, constricting pain
Hyperesthesia and hyperalgesia
Exacerbated by arm movement/ relieved by immobilization
Episodes of lancinating pain
History of postoperative complications
(C) Physical examination:
Area of hypesthesia
Area of hyperesthesia
Palpation of a neuroma
(D) Consider:
Brachial plexopathy
DIAGNOSTIC POSTERIOR INTERCOSTAL BLOCK
Pain No relief
Pain relief
Brachial plexopathy
Postmastectomy pain
(E) Treatment
Physical therapy
Pain relief
Consider:
Reflex sympathetic dystrophy
Herpes zoster
Cervical radiculopathy
Local infection
Conservative Measures:
Nonsteroidal Anti-inflammatory Agents
Tricyclic Antidepressants
Transcutaneous Electrical Nerve Stimulation (TENS)
Opiates
Topical Capsaicin (currently in controlled trials)
Invasive Measures:
LOCAL TRIGGER POINT INJECTIONS
POSTERIOR INTERCOSTAL NERVE BLOCK
CONTINUOUS SEGMENTAL EPIDURAL BLOCK
(local anesthetic or opioid)
Surgical Neuroablation

POST-THORACOTOMY PAIN SYNDROME

John D. Merwin, M.D.

Post-thoracotomy syndrome consists of pain that recurs or persists along a thoracotomy scar in the distribution of one or more intercostal nerves. All patients undergoing thoracotomy experience pain, but it usually lasts 7 to 10 days. In a small percentage of patients, the pain continues or may recur weeks to months after the procedure. The pain is often moderate to severe and lasts at least 2 months after the surgical procedure. Perioperative treatment of the acute pain injury response may reduce the incidence of persistent pain syndromes.

A. The pain is often associated with paresthesia, dysesthesia, and other sensory changes. Allodynia and hyperesthesia may be noted on palpation of the scar. Reflex sympathetic dystrophy may develop in the ipsilateral arm and chest. Persistent or recurrent pain in a patient with cancer is most likely due to recurrent tumor. A few patients develop pain from a traumatic neuroma at the site of the surgical procedure. Diagnostic intercostal blocks with local anesthetic (LA) localize the source of the pain. A CT or bone scan helps localize recurrent tumor. A conservative attitude in which the patient receives psychological support in combination with nerve blockade, transcutaneous electrical nerve stimulation (TENS), and physical therapy has been advocated as a first-line form of treatment.

B. Cancer recurrence may require further surgical excision, radiation, chemotherapy, or hormonal therapy to reduce the painful symptoms. Once the tumor mass has been reduced, psychological, systemic, or regional anesthetic techniques should be more effective.

C. Antidepressants and psychological interventions are often helpful in patients with post-thoracotomy syndrome. Many of these patients exhibit signs and symptoms of clinical depression because of the nature of their disease process. Lancinating pain is often responsive to antidepressants.

D. Adequate pain relief with either segmental epidural, intercostal, or paravertebral blockade with LA, coupled with physical therapy, can provide relief in patients with a peripheral neuropathic or sympathetically mediated pain. Myofascial pain may be primary or secondary and should be treated accordingly. Some clinicians have advocated injection of the scar with LA and steroids. TENS may also prove helpful in selected patients.

E. Reflex sympathetic dystrophy should be suspected and diagnosed with a sympathetic blockade (p 244). Treatment should be aggressive. In patients with a terminal disease process who do not respond to more conservative measures, neurolytic or neuroablative techniques may be required.

References

Carlsson CA, Persson K, Pelletieri L. Painful scars after thoracic and abdominal surgery. Acta Chir Scand 1985; 151:309.

Cousins MJ. Acute pain and the injury response: Immediate and prolonged effects. Reg Anesth 1989; 14:170.

Tasker RR, Dostrovsky JO. In: Wall PS, Melzack R, eds. Textbook of pain. 2nd ed. New York: Churchill Livingstone, 1989:154.

Ventafridda V, Tamburini M, De Conno F. Comprehensive treatment in cancer pain. In: Fields HL, Dubner R, Cervero F, eds. Advances in pain research and therapy. Vol. 9. New York: Raven Press, 1985:617.

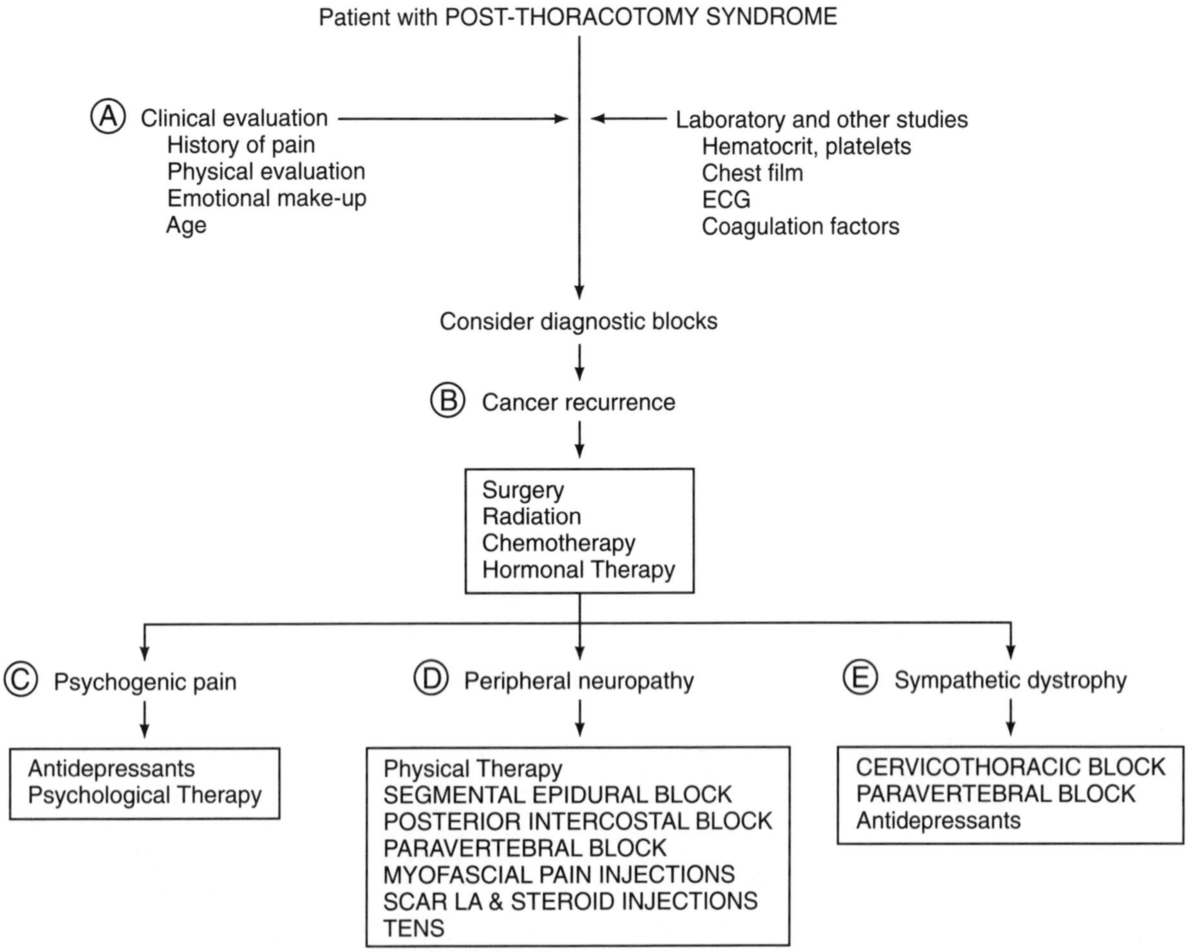

Patient with POST-THORACOTOMY SYNDROME

(A) Clinical evaluation
- History of pain
- Physical evaluation
- Emotional make-up
- Age

Laboratory and other studies
- Hematocrit, platelets
- Chest film
- ECG
- Coagulation factors

↓

Consider diagnostic blocks

↓

(B) Cancer recurrence

↓

Surgery
Radiation
Chemotherapy
Hormonal Therapy

↓

(C) Psychogenic pain
↓
Antidepressants
Psychological Therapy

(D) Peripheral neuropathy
↓
Physical Therapy
SEGMENTAL EPIDURAL BLOCK
POSTERIOR INTERCOSTAL BLOCK
PARAVERTEBRAL BLOCK
MYOFASCIAL PAIN INJECTIONS
SCAR LA & STEROID INJECTIONS
TENS

(E) Sympathetic dystrophy
↓
CERVICOTHORACIC BLOCK
PARAVERTEBRAL BLOCK
Antidepressants

COMPRESSION FRACTURE PAIN OF THE BACK

Diane Gilbert, M.D.

A. The history should include a thorough description of the pain, age at menopause, medications, and any evidence of endocrinopathy. Lower back pain is the presenting symptom in 90% of patients with senile or postmenopausal osteoporosis. Compression fractures often are associated with trivial trauma or with routine daily activities with sudden onset of pain, often excruciating, associated with paraspinal muscle spasms. Back pain often radiates anteriorly along the costal margin of the affected spinal nerve; worsens with standing, sitting, coughing, sneezing, or the Valsalva maneuver; and is relieved considerably with recumbent bed rest. There is tenderness with deep palpation and percussion over the vertebral body, but often not directly over the spinous process. On physical examination, note posture, the presence of thoracic kyphosis (dowager's hump), scoliosis, spinal range of motion, height (arm span and vertical height should be equal), and evidence of ileus (from reflex sympathetic hyperactivity). Careful neurologic examination for deficits, especially evidence of cauda equina syndrome, is mandatory.

B. The thoracolumbar spine is the primary target for osteoporotic fractures, the most common occurring between T8 and L2. If there is a history of trauma, look for noncontiguous fractures. A compression fracture is present if the height of the symptomatic vertebrae is one-third less than that of adjacent vertebrae. CT permits visualization of the status of the posterior wall of the vertebral body if there is a question of burst fracture.

C. A fracture is unstable if two of three columns are disrupted, as described by Dennis. A compression fracture is failure under pressure of the anterior column. If the vertebral body is >50% of the height of adjacent vertebrae, the fracture is usually stable; if <50%, the fracture is usually unstable because of associated traumatic kyphosis or posterior ligament disruption. The pain associated with an unstable compression fracture is often alleviated by proper surgical stabilization.

D. Osteoporosis is the most common skeletal disorder in the world and is one of the most frequent causes of pain and disability, especially in elderly women. The patient is usually a small, sedentary, nulliparous, postmenopausal white woman with a lifelong history of insufficient dietary calcium intake. Other risk factors include light-colored hair; freckles; scoliosis; strong family history of osteoporosis; early menopause; immobilization; hypogonadism; denervation of peripheral nerve or spinal cord injury; anorexia nervosa; chronic, heavy alcohol use; cigarette smoking; use of certain drugs (heparin, methotrexate, anticonvulsants, aluminum-containing phosphate binders, heavy metals). Decreased weight bearing can lead to profound and rapid loss of skeletal density activity, as seen with astronauts in a weightless environment.

E. Routine lab work-up should include CBC, erythrocyte sedimentation rate (ESR), and serum protein electrophoresis (SPEP) to rule out anemia of chronic disease, multiple myeloma, leukemia, and benign marrow disorders. An endocrine screen to determine parathormone (PTH) and thyroid levels should also be performed. Suspect osteomalacia when there is generalized myopathy, bone pain, tenderness, and symmetric long bone fractures. Measurement of levels of serum and urine calcium, phosphorus, alkaline phosphatase (may be transiently high after acute fracture or with metastasis), blood urea nitrogen (BUN), and 25(OH)$_2$ vitamin D can differentiate osteoporosis from osteomalacia. Chest radiography may reveal occult malignancy and rib fractures. A bone scan can be used to detect metastatic disease and determine the age of the fracture.

(Continued on page 120)

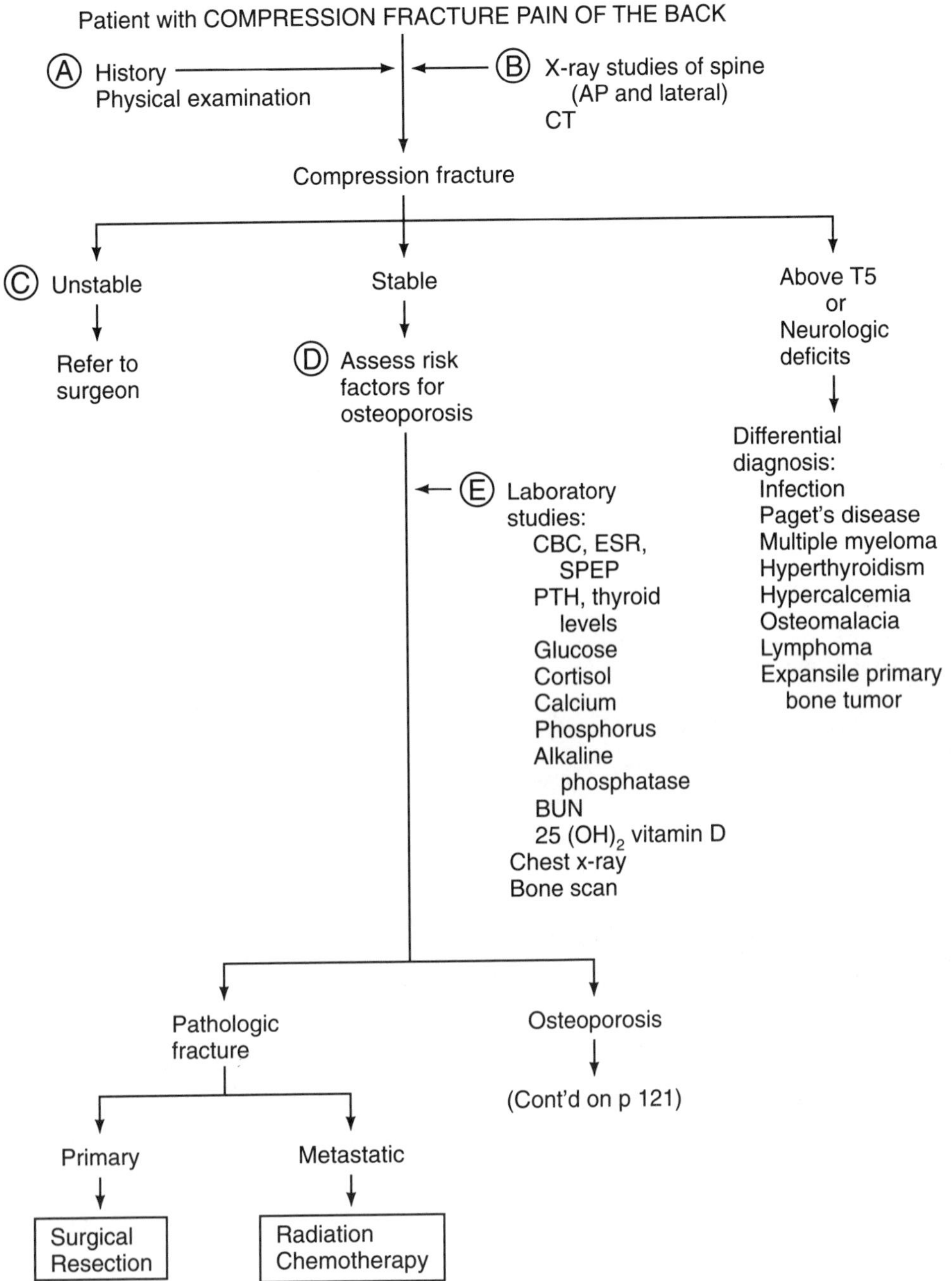

Patient with COMPRESSION FRACTURE PAIN OF THE BACK
Ⓐ History
Physical examination
Ⓑ X-ray studies of spine
(AP and lateral)
CT
Compression fracture
Ⓒ Unstable
Refer to surgeon
Stable
Ⓓ Assess risk factors for osteoporosis
Above T5
or
Neurologic deficits
Differential diagnosis:
Infection
Paget's disease
Multiple myeloma
Hyperthyroidism
Hypercalcemia
Osteomalacia
Lymphoma
Expansile primary bone tumor
Ⓔ Laboratory studies:
CBC, ESR, SPEP
PTH, thyroid levels
Glucose
Cortisol
Calcium
Phosphorus
Alkaline phosphatase
BUN
25 (OH)$_2$ vitamin D
Chest x-ray
Bone scan
Pathologic fracture
Osteoporosis
(Cont'd on p 121)
Primary
Metastatic
Surgical Resection
Radiation Chemotherapy

F. Spinal pain and loss of height occur in 25% of the 60-year-old population; however, 70% of that population shows radiologic changes of osteoporosis. Vertebral fractures are seen in 40% of women over the age of 70. These are often found during routine studies of asymptomatic patients. These women are at an increased risk for hip fracture and distal radius fracture. Therefore, every effort should be made to ensure adequate nutrition, weight-bearing activity, and proper back care.

G. Even in severely osteopenic patients, compression fractures heal quickly regardless of treatment. Limit bed rest, as immobilization can lead to further bone resorption. Adequate pain relief decreases muscle spasm and allows mobility.

H. Regional analgesia, such as epidural blockade, is recommended for those patients with severe pain and muscle spasms not responding to systemic analgesics and patients with cardiac and/or respiratory disorders. Duration of immobilization and the risk of ileus are decreased (p 238).

I. Extension or isometric back and abdominal strengthening exercises with pectoral stretching and deep breathing are recommended. Avoid flexion exercises, which can cause further compression fractures. Encourage short, intermittent bed rest. Proper back mechanics in lifting and bending are taught to avoid unnecessary spinal compressive forces. Swimming or exercises performed in water are good for cardiovascular fitness but are not weight bearing. The etiology of falls should be investigated.

J. Bracing may be necessary to immobilize painful joints and should be used when the patient is erect. The goal is pain relief with the least cumbersome, lightest, and easiest-to-wear orthosis. A rigid, thoracolumbar hyperextension orthosis provides external support, alleviates flexion forces, discourages kyphotic posture, and allows for more comfortable mobilization. These braces allow increased mobilization and do not contribute to osteopenia. Plastizote inserts in shoes cushion concussive forces.

K. Chronic pain may develop after fracture healing. It has been suggested that the lordotic curve is accentuated to compensate for increased thoracic kyphosis, leading to stress and strain of the paraspinal muscles. A lumbosacral corset may add support while the patient develops tolerance to the new posture. Patients with chronic vertebral instability with persistent midline back pain and a positive instability test should have a comprehensive program of paraspinous muscle strengthening.

L. Osteoporosis is more effectively prevented than treated. Estrogen is the single most effective measure for prevention of postmenopausal osteoporosis, but there are contraindications and side effects. Calcitonin might be best reserved for women who are unable to take estrogen and who have documented osteoporosis and vertebral fractures. Fluoride is still considered experimental, but in cases with significant morbidity from vertebral fractures its use may be justified.

References

Barth R, Lane J. Osteoporosis. Orthop Clin North Am 1988; 19:845.

Bonica JJ, ed. The management of pain. 2nd ed. Philadelphia: Lea and Febiger, 1990.

Cohen I. Fractures of the osteoporotic spine. Orthop Clin North Am 1990; 21:143.

Denis F. Spinal instability as defined by the three-column spine concept in acute spinal trauma. Clin Orthop Rel Res 1984: 189:65.

Kaplan F. Osteoporosis: Pathophysiology and prevention. Clin Symp 1987.

Sinaki M. Exercise and osteoporosis. Arch Phys Med Rehabil 1989; 70:220–29.

Weinerman S, Bockman R. Medical therapy of osteoporosis. Orthop Clin North Am. 1990; 21:109–24.

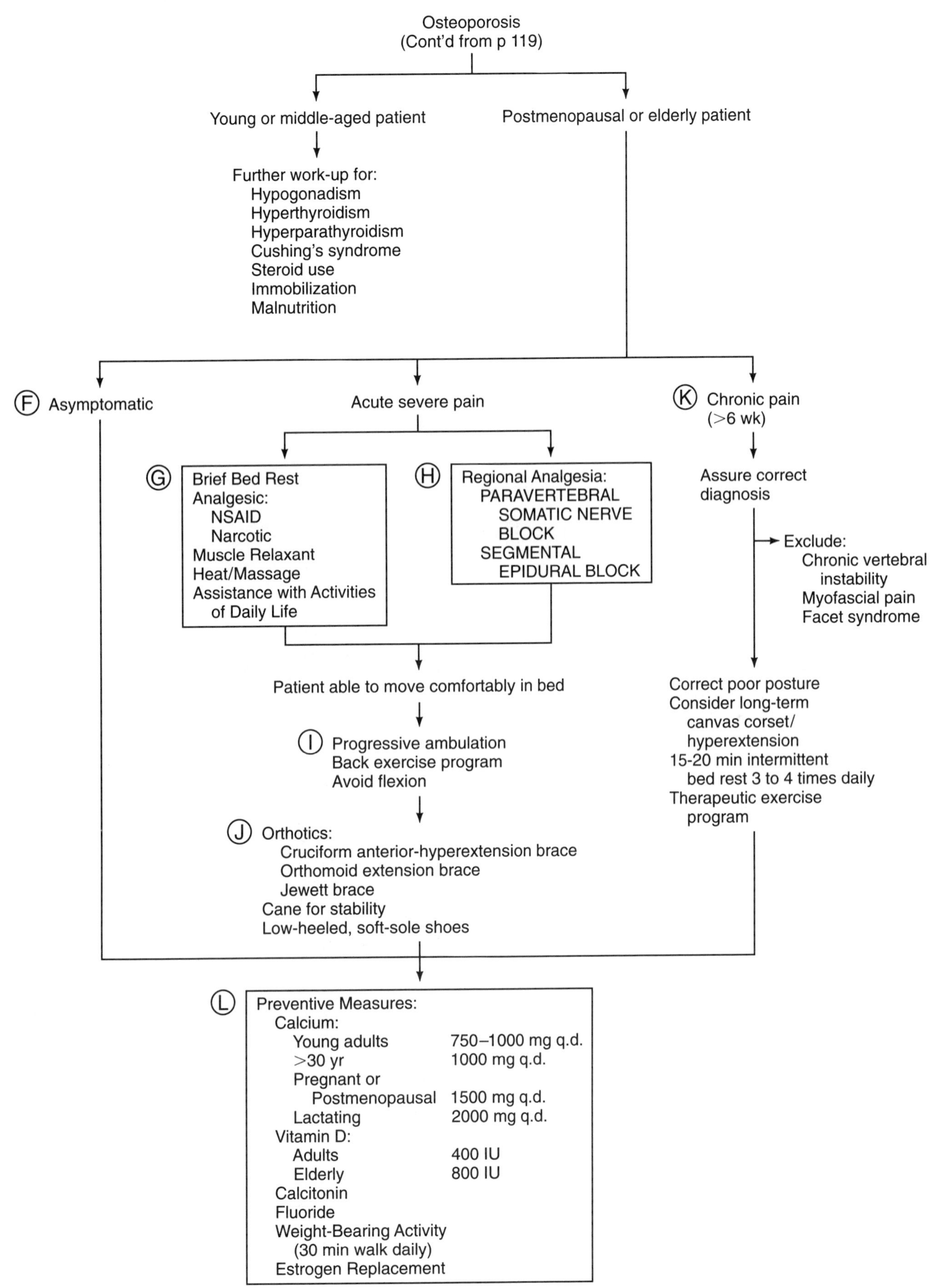

Osteoporosis
(Cont'd from p 119)
Young or middle-aged patient
Postmenopausal or elderly patient
Further work-up for:
Hypogonadism
Hyperthyroidism
Hyperparathyroidism
Cushing's syndrome
Steroid use
Immobilization
Malnutrition
(F) Asymptomatic
Acute severe pain
(K) Chronic pain (>6 wk)
(G) Brief Bed Rest
Analgesic:
NSAID
Narcotic
Muscle Relaxant
Heat/Massage
Assistance with Activities of Daily Life
(H) Regional Analgesia:
PARAVERTEBRAL SOMATIC NERVE BLOCK
SEGMENTAL EPIDURAL BLOCK
Assure correct diagnosis
Exclude:
Chronic vertebral instability
Myofascial pain
Facet syndrome
Patient able to move comfortably in bed
(I) Progressive ambulation
Back exercise program
Avoid flexion
Correct poor posture
Consider long-term canvas corset/ hyperextension
15-20 min intermittent bed rest 3 to 4 times daily
Therapeutic exercise program
(J) Orthotics:
Cruciform anterior-hyperextension brace
Orthomoid extension brace
Jewett brace
Cane for stability
Low-heeled, soft-sole shoes
(L) Preventive Measures:
Calcium:
Young adults 750–1000 mg q.d.
>30 yr 1000 mg q.d.
Pregnant or Postmenopausal 1500 mg q.d.
Lactating 2000 mg q.d.
Vitamin D:
Adults 400 IU
Elderly 800 IU
Calcitonin
Fluoride
Weight-Bearing Activity (30 min walk daily)
Estrogen Replacement

BACK PAIN

Acute Low Back Pain
Chronic Low Back Pain
Lumbosacral Radiculopathy
Spinal Stenosis
Ankylosing Spondylitis
Failed Laminectomy Syndrome
Facet Joint Syndrome
Sacroiliac Joint Pain

ACUTE LOW BACK PAIN

Jonathan P. Lester, M.D.

Acute low back pain is a common medical disorder in industrialized societies. Most cases are self-limited and may be treated successfully with conservative care. Accurate diagnosis may be made from the history and physical examination. Laboratory studies, radiologic imaging, and electrophysiologic studies are used to confirm the diagnosis or clarify the pathology in difficult cases. Treatment strategies utilize patient education, pain control measures, and physical rehabilitation. Early return to functional activities and prevention of chronic back pain are the goals of treatment.

A. Traumatic injury raises the question of spinal fracture. Flexion and rotation injuries may cause injury to the intervertebral disc, while repetitive stress or sudden overload in the extended position may injure the posterior elements including the facet joints and pars interarticularis. Back pain radiating into the lower extremity with or without neurologic loss may indicate lumbosacral (LS) radiculopathy secondary to a herniated nucleus pulposus (HNP). Back pain associated with systemic complaints including fever, weight loss, a change in bowel or bladder habits, night pain, or morning stiffness suggest the possibility of malignancy, infection, or spondyloarthropathy and should be thoroughly evaluated with the appropriate laboratory studies. Acute bowel or bladder dysfunction with or without saddle anesthesia or radicular pain suggests cauda equina syndrome and should be referred immediately for surgical evaluation.

B. A history of radicular pain associated with dural tension signs (straight leg raise, bowstring, Laségue's sign) suggests acute LS radiculopathy secondary to an HNP. Conservative care consisting of NSAIDs, epidural steroid injections (ESIs), and specialized physical therapy programs will resolve symptoms in most cases. Imaging studies (CT and MRI) and electrophysiologic studies (EMG and dermatomal somatosensory evoked potentials [DSEPs]) can define the pathology in those patients unresponsive to conservative care and in those with neurologic deficits. Refer patients with progressive neurologic loss or intractable pain for surgical management.

C. Acute low back pain not associated with traumatic etiology, systemic symptoms, radicular complaints, or dural tension signs suggests an isolated soft tissue or articular etiology. Myofascial pain syndrome, piriformis syndrome, annular tear, facet syndrome, and sacroiliac (SI) joint syndrome are easily recognized by their specific historical aspects, their response to provocative stress on physical examination, and their response to diagnostic injection. Conservative therapy is successful in resolving symptoms in most cases. In some patients no specific diagnosis will be reached. For lack of a better term, these individuals are "diagnosed" as having nonspecific low back strain and are treated conservatively.

D. A positive bone scan can differentiate acute pars interarticularis fracture from isthmic spondylolisthesis. Acute pars injuries require immobilization and are referred to an orthopedic surgeon for definitive management. Back pain associated with low grades of spondylolisthesis (<50% slippage) may be treated conservatively. Those with high grades of listhesis (>50%) or neurologic loss should be referred for surgical evaluation.

References

Berhard T, Kirkaldy-Willis W. Recognizing specific characteristics of nonspecific low back pain. Clin Orthop 1987; 217:266.

Derby R. Diagnostic block procedures: Use in pain localization. Spine: State of the Art Reviews 1986; 1:47.

Hadler N. The patient with low back pain. Hosp Pract 1987; 22:17.

Saal J. Rehabilitation of sports-related lumbar spine injuries. Physical Medicine and Rehabilitation: State of the Art Reviews 1987; 1:42.

Saal J. Diagnostic studies of industrial low back injuries. Top Acute Care Trauma Rehabil 1988; 2:31.

Warfield C. Facet syndrome and the relief of low back pain. Hosp Pract 23(10A):41–42. 1988.

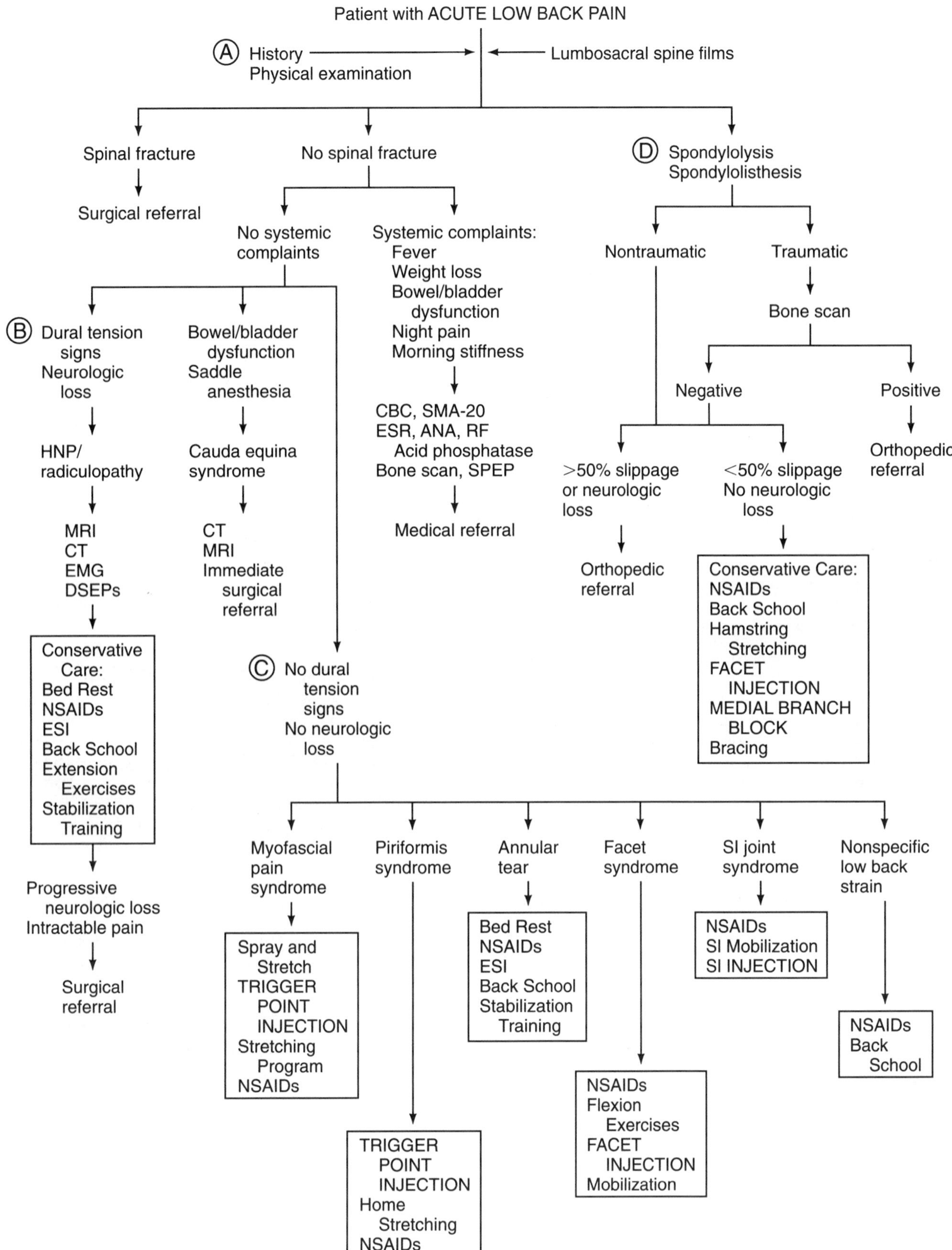

Patient with ACUTE LOW BACK PAIN
(A) History
Physical examination
Lumbosacral spine films
Spinal fracture
Surgical referral
No spinal fracture
(D) Spondylolysis
Spondylolisthesis
No systemic complaints
Systemic complaints:
Fever
Weight loss
Bowel/bladder dysfunction
Night pain
Morning stiffness
CBC, SMA-20
ESR, ANA, RF
Acid phosphatase
Bone scan, SPEP
Medical referral
Nontraumatic
Traumatic
Bone scan
Negative
Positive
Orthopedic referral
>50% slippage or neurologic loss
Orthopedic referral
<50% slippage
No neurologic loss
Conservative Care:
NSAIDs
Back School
Hamstring Stretching
FACET INJECTION
MEDIAL BRANCH BLOCK
Bracing
(B) Dural tension signs
Neurologic loss
HNP/ radiculopathy
MRI
CT
EMG
DSEPs
Conservative Care:
Bed Rest
NSAIDs
ESI
Back School
Extension Exercises
Stabilization Training
Progressive neurologic loss
Intractable pain
Surgical referral
Bowel/bladder dysfunction
Saddle anesthesia
Cauda equina syndrome
CT
MRI
Immediate surgical referral
(C) No dural tension signs
No neurologic loss
Myofascial pain syndrome
Spray and Stretch
TRIGGER POINT INJECTION
Stretching Program
NSAIDs
Piriformis syndrome
TRIGGER POINT INJECTION
Home Stretching
NSAIDs
Annular tear
Bed Rest
NSAIDs
ESI
Back School
Stabilization Training
Facet syndrome
NSAIDs
Flexion Exercises
FACET INJECTION
Mobilization
SI joint syndrome
NSAIDs
SI Mobilization
SI INJECTION
Nonspecific low back strain
NSAIDs
Back School

CHRONIC LOW BACK PAIN

John King, M.D.

Evaluation of the chronic low back pain patient must be thorough to rule out reversible causes, even though most of these patients do not have disease amenable to pharmacologic or surgical interventions alone. The chronicity of the pain leads to physical, social, and psychologic adaptations that may manifest in illness behavior, which is reinforced. Such learned behavior can be "unlearned" with appropriate reinforcers for improved function and healthy living. Frequently a team approach is required to deal with the physical, psychologic, and social factors that both impede performance and add to the suffering of these patients.

A. Narcotics and tranquilizing muscle relaxants offer effective short-term benefits but are not useful adjuncts to chronic pain management because of their (1) limited effectiveness, secondary to tolerance; (2) creation of medical dependency; and (3) adverse effects on mood and cognition. These unnecessary and unhelpful medications are easily eliminated, usually without any increase in the pain pattern or intensity during inpatient programs, over a 2- to 3-week period. Outpatient deceleration is more difficult and typically requires 6 to 8 weeks in motivated, cooperative patients.

B. In chronic pain syndrome, the patient experiences pain for >6 months (occasionally less), and the pain has led to disability and problems in physical, psychologic, social, and vocational areas. This is a learned and dysfunctional adjustment pattern that requires behavioral intervention to restore optimal functioning in all spheres.

C. Tricyclic antidepressants, anticonvulsants, and occasionally phenothiazines, with or without NSAIDs, may be useful chronic pain medications, but all require some monitoring. If benefit is uncertain, the trial should be stopped (usually by tapering off over 2 weeks) every 6 months. If pain exacerbates, medication is likely to be of benefit; if it does not and the trial was adequate, the medication should be discontinued and its failure documented. Other medications that have less clear chronic effects but occasionally are found beneficial include mexilitine (oral lidocaine-like medication) and alprazolam (difficult to wean off, even if not helpful for pain).

D. Treatment should consist no longer of passive modalities such as hot packs, massage, or ultrasonography, but should involve active therapies that increase self-reliance and self-management: exercises; stretching; self-pacing; and planning of workload, rest, and recreation. If no actively or progressively destructive processes (e.g., cancer) are found, pain should not be interpreted as a signal to stop activities and withdraw from life. The functional perspective, or rehabilitation model in which the impairments caused by the pain are treated, becomes the most beneficial approach toward decreasing suffering. The goals are increased activity, decreased medication, and no increased pain. The ability to do more, without necessarily hurting more, helps to decrease suffering. Suffering aspects can also be minimized by concurrent cognitive therapy.

E. Reassuring patients with a chronically painful condition requires significant time for exhaustive evaluation and review of records and patient education. Many pain patients think "no one has ever really listened to me." Treat both the mind and the body.

F. Pure psychogenic pain is rarely encountered. Absence of clinical signs along with normal laboratory and imaging studies do not rule out all causes of physical pain (e.g., chronic bursitis, early osteoarthritis, fibromyalgia). When, in addition, no conformance or consistency of the pain pattern to activities, surreptitious testing, or observation exists, purely psychogenic causes or motivational issues should be pursued. Most chronic pain patients have both a physical problem and secondary psychosocial changes with variable premorbid psychologic strengths.

G. If no psychogenic causes are found and there are no apparent possible physical causes, malingering and secondary gain issues may be related to the decreased function. Unless there is a severe antisocial personality, dementia, or uncontrolled schizophrenia, behavior modification inpatient programs may still be effective in improving function.

(Continued on page 128)

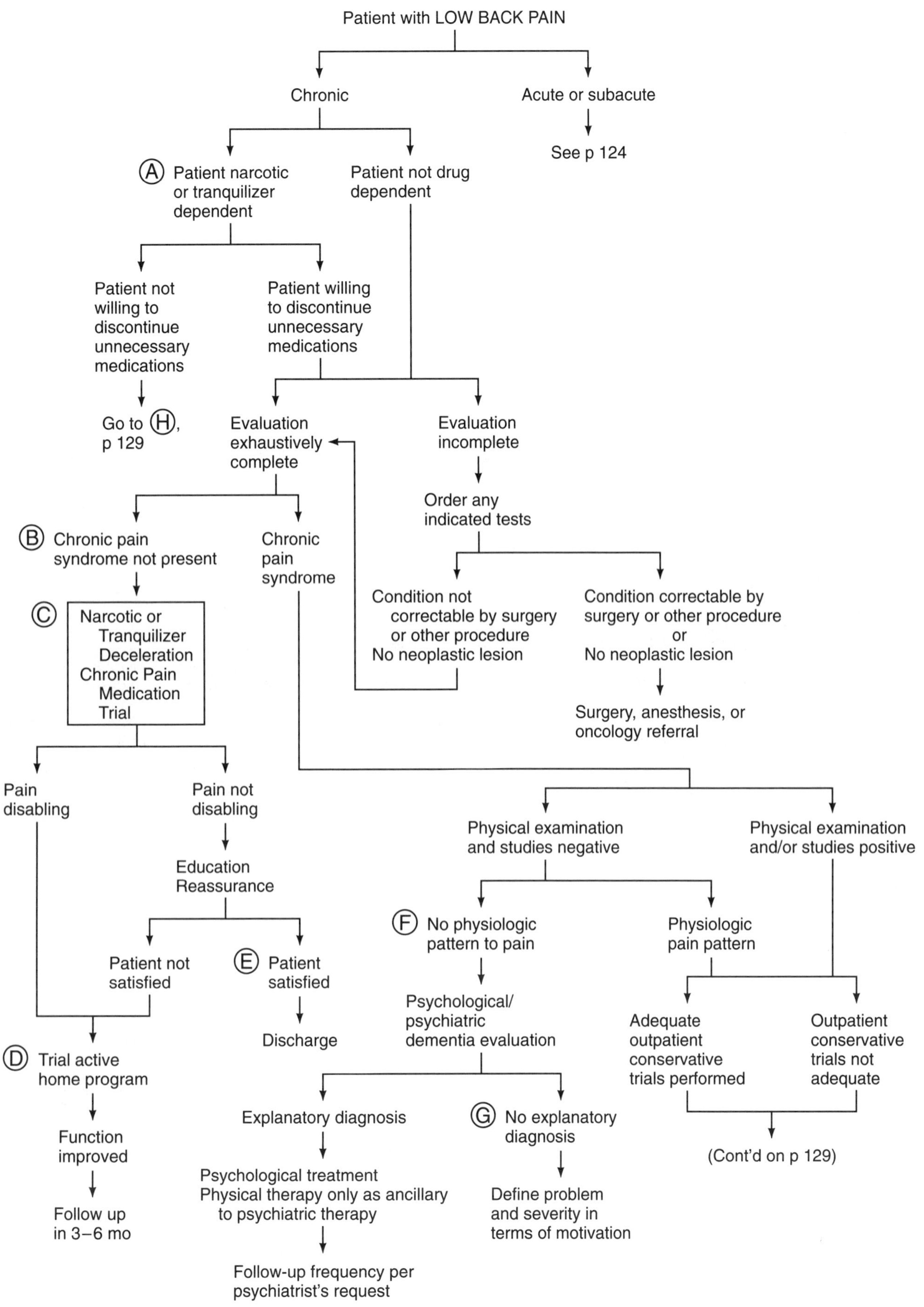
Patient with LOW BACK PAIN
Chronic
Acute or subacute
See p 124
Ⓐ Patient narcotic or tranquilizer dependent
Patient not drug dependent
Patient not willing to discontinue unnecessary medications
Patient willing to discontinue unnecessary medications
Go to Ⓗ, p 129
Evaluation exhaustively complete
Evaluation incomplete
Order any indicated tests
Ⓑ Chronic pain syndrome not present
Chronic pain syndrome
Condition not correctable by surgery or other procedure
No neoplastic lesion
Condition correctable by surgery or other procedure
or
No neoplastic lesion
Surgery, anesthesia, or oncology referral
Ⓒ Narcotic or Tranquilizer Deceleration
Chronic Pain Medication Trial
Pain disabling
Pain not disabling
Education
Reassurance
Physical examination and studies negative
Physical examination and/or studies positive
Patient not satisfied
Ⓔ Patient satisfied
Discharge
Ⓕ No physiologic pattern to pain
Physiologic pain pattern
Psychological/ psychiatric dementia evaluation
Adequate outpatient conservative trials performed
Outpatient conservative trials not adequate
Ⓓ Trial active home program
Function improved
Follow up in 3–6 mo
Explanatory diagnosis
Psychological treatment
Physical therapy only as ancillary to psychiatric therapy
Follow-up frequency per psychiatrist's request
Ⓖ No explanatory diagnosis
Define problem and severity in terms of motivation
(Cont'd on p 129)

H. Inpatient programs should not be dualistic: "It's all in your mind" or "It's all in your body." They should deal with the physical, psychological, social, family, vocational, and avocational aspects of the disabling pain.

I. If patients are reasonably screened, it is rare for medical problems to absolutely preclude progression to the patient's premorbid capabilities. An unchanging pattern of pain is not a reason to end a rehabilitation program that is increasing physical abilities.

J. A home program is best done daily and consists of fewer than seven exercises that require less than 45 minutes to complete.

K. Follow up every 3 to 12 months if necessary to evaluate long-term effectiveness of the interventions and to minimize "doctor shopping," which increases the risk of unnecessary invasive procedures. Initially, PRN follow up is allowed to alleviate any anxiety associated with the initial transition back to a full active lifestyle, but this should become progressively less frequent. Having comprehensively evaluated and followed the patient, you are in the best position to evaluate any new pain. For routine follow-ups, Fordyce's "Ten Steps to Help Chronic Pain Patients" offers practical suggestions:

1. Accept patients' pain as real. Find out *why* they hurt, not whether they hurt.
2. Protect the patient from unnecessary invasive procedures.
3. Set realistic goals. Expect to manage rather than cure.
4. Evaluate chronic pain in terms of what patients do, not what they say.
5. Let the patient know that *you* are the expert on medications and procedures.
6. Shift patients to oral, time-contingent medications (not PRN).
7. Prescribe exercises to start at easily achieved levels, but increase at a preset rate.
8. Educate patients' families to encourage increased activity.
9. Focus your attention on patients' activity rather on the pain. Ask not how patients feel, but what they have done.
10. Help patients get involved in pleasurable activities. Remember, people who have something better to do don't hurt as much.

References

Abramowicz M, ed. Alprazolam for panic disorder. Med Letter 1991; 33:3.

Bowsher D. Assessment of the chronic pain sufferer. Surg Rounds Orthop 1989; 3:70.

Fordyce WE, Fowler RS, Lehman JF, De Lateur BJ: Ten steps to help patients with chronic pain. Patient Care 12:263, 1978.

King JC, Kelleher WJ. The chronic pain syndrome. In: Walsh NE, ed. Rehabilitation of chronic pain. Phys Med Rehabil 1991; 5:168.

Linton SJ. Behavioral remediation of chronic pain: A status report. Pain 1986; 24:125.

Lipman RS. Pharmacotherapy of anxiety and depression. Psychopharmacol Bull 1981; 171:91.

Loeser JO, Eyar KJ, eds. Managing the chronic pain patient. New York: Raven Press, 1989.

Mayer TG, Gatchel RJ, Mayer H, et al: A prospective two-year study of functional restoration in industrial low-back injury. JAMA 1987; 258:1763.

Vlok GJ, Hendrix MRG. The lumbar disc: Evaluating the causes of pain. Orthopedics 1991; 14:419.

(Cont'd from p 127)

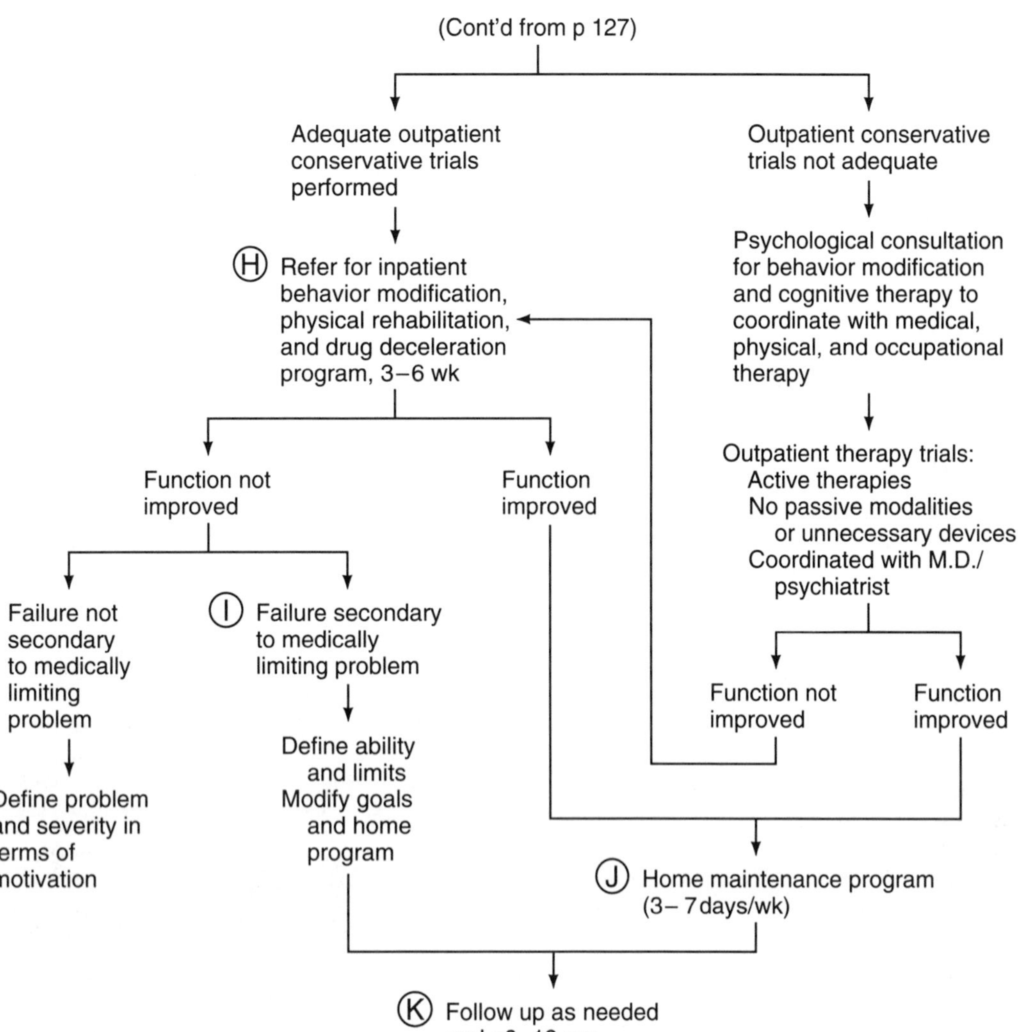

LUMBOSACRAL RADICULOPATHY

Jonathan P. Lester, M.D.

Suspected lumbosacral (LS) radiculopathy is one of the most common diagnoses assigned to patients with low back pain. The disorder is suggested by complaints of pain, sensory disturbance, weakness, and reflex changes in a radicular pattern. Most LS radiculopathies involve the L5 or S1 roots. Radiologic imaging techniques can define the structural etiology, and electrophysiologic studies are used to evaluate the severity and specificity of root compromise. Many causes of LS radiculopathy can be treated successfully with conservative measures.

A. The evaluation of LS radiculopathy should begin with a complete history, physical examination, and in most cases a complete set of LS spine radiographs.

B. A history of acute onset of symptoms following spinal trauma suggests the possibility of spinal fracture with radicular, cauda equina, or spinal cord injury. If the index of suspicion for one of these problems is high or if plain films reveal a fracture, refer the patient to a spine surgeon immediately for further evaluation.

C. Acute LS radiculopathy associated with a flexion-rotation injury is most often due to a herniated nucleus pulposus (HNP). Most cases can be managed with a program of conservative measures. Refer patients with intractable pain or progressive neurologic loss for surgical evaluation.

D. Peripheral entrapment neuropathies of the lower extremity may closely mimic LS radiculopathy (pseudoradiculopathy). Electrodiagnostic studies in combination with peripheral nerve blocks and selective root blocks are used to make the diagnosis. Most cases are successfully resolved with peripheral nerve blocks or neurolysis.

E. Spinal stenosis is a common cause of monoradicular and polyradicular disease. Stenosis may compromise either the central portion of the spinal canal with polyradicular or cauda equina symptoms, or the lateral portion of the canal with isolated monoradicular symptoms. Symptoms are usually exacerbated by activity in an extended position. LS spine x-rays often reveal sclerotic hypertrophy and subluxation of the facet joints, and narrowing of the interlaminar space. Definitive diagnosis is made by CT scanning. EMG and dermatomal somatosensory evoked potential (DSEP) studies can define the extent of neurologic compromise. A variety of conservative measures are available to reduce the severity of symptoms, but surgical management is often required to address the fixed bony lesion (p 132).

F. Isthmic or degenerative spondylolisthesis may cause lateral spinal stenosis with resultant radiculopathy. LS spine films readily reveal the anatomic defect. EMG and DSEP are utilized to determine the severity of neurologic compromise. Conservative care may be attempted, but surgical management is often necessary.

G. Herpes zoster infection may result in localized radiculitis. In most cases, patients present with pain, weakness, and sensory loss in the same radicular distribution as the skin lesions. Treatment goals are to reduce the duration of the viral infection, to minimize the severity of the clinical symptoms, and, in patients over age 50, to prevent postherpetic neuralgia (p 48).

H. Diabetic polyneuropathy (DPN) is a common finding in association with chronic LS radiculopathy. Toxicity from abnormal glucose metabolism may predispose peripheral nerves to injury at common sites of entrapment such as the neuroforamina. In addition, DPN may also cause a localized mononeuritis (most often involving the femoral nerve) that may mimic radiculopathy. The diagnosis of LS radiculopathy in association with DPN is made by medical evaluation of serum glucose metabolism in concert with EMG and nerve conduction studies (NCS). Some improvement may be realized with improved glucose control (p 56).

I. A spinal cord or bony tumor may first present as LS radiculopathy. Night pain, pain unrelieved by rest, or pain worse in the supine position should alert the physician and prompt a thorough evaluation for such a lesion.

J. Metabolic bone disease such as Paget's disease may cause radicular pain if the extensive bony remodeling causes stenosis of the spinal canal. LS spine x-rays will reveal hyperostotic vertebrae, and a skeletal survey will reveal tibial bowing and an increase in skull size. Refer these patients to the medical specialist for further evaluation and treatment.

References

Amundson G, Wenger D. Spondylolisthesis: Natural history and treatment. Spine: State of the Art Reviews 1987; 1:323.

Couldwell W, Weiss M. Leg radicular pain and sensory disturbance: The differential diagnosis. Spine: State of the Art Reviews 1988; 2:669.

Kimura J. Electrodiagnosis in diseases of nerve and muscle: Principles and practice. 2nd ed. Philadelphia: FA Davis, 1989.

McNab I. The pathogenesis of spinal stenosis. Spine: State of the Art Reviews 1987; 1:369.

Saal J. Diagnostic studies of industrial low back injuries. Top Acute Care Trauma Rehabil 1988; 2:31.

Saal J, Dillingham M, Gamburd R, Fanton G. The pseudoradicular syndrome: Lower extremity peripheral entrapment masquerading as lumbar radiculopathy. Spine 1988; 13:926.

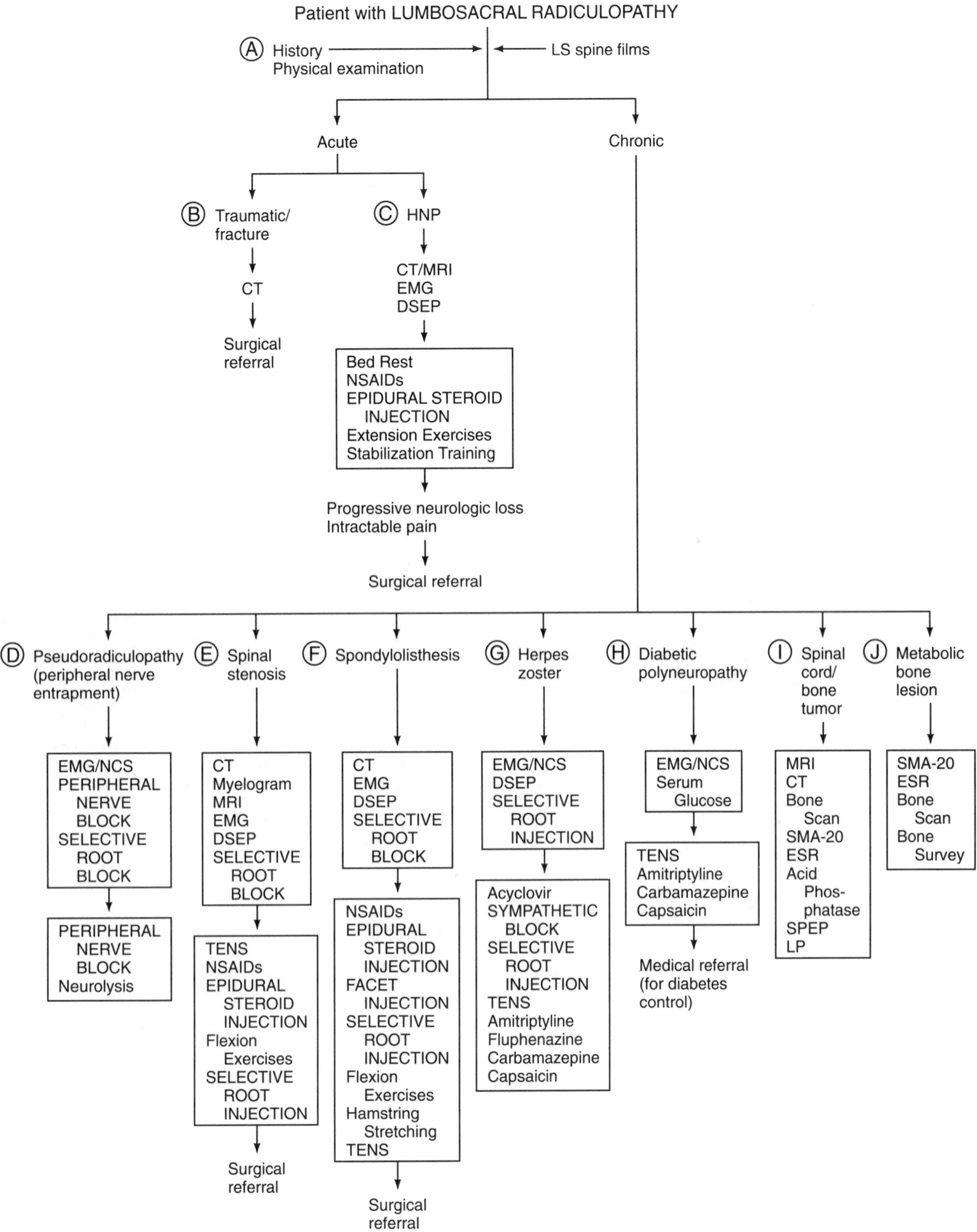

Patient with LUMBOSACRAL RADICULOPATHY
(A) History
Physical examination
LS spine films
Acute
Chronic
(B) Traumatic/fracture
CT
Surgical referral
(C) HNP
CT/MRI
EMG
DSEP
Bed Rest
NSAIDs
EPIDURAL STEROID INJECTION
Extension Exercises
Stabilization Training
Progressive neurologic loss
Intractable pain
Surgical referral
(D) Pseudoradiculopathy (peripheral nerve entrapment)
EMG/NCS
PERIPHERAL NERVE BLOCK
SELECTIVE ROOT BLOCK
PERIPHERAL NERVE BLOCK
Neurolysis
(E) Spinal stenosis
CT
Myelogram
MRI
EMG
DSEP
SELECTIVE ROOT BLOCK
TENS
NSAIDs
EPIDURAL STEROID INJECTION
Flexion Exercises
SELECTIVE ROOT INJECTION
Surgical referral
(F) Spondylolisthesis
CT
EMG
DSEP
SELECTIVE ROOT BLOCK
NSAIDs
EPIDURAL STEROID INJECTION
FACET INJECTION
SELECTIVE ROOT INJECTION
Flexion Exercises
Hamstring Stretching
TENS
Surgical referral
(G) Herpes zoster
EMG/NCS
DSEP
SELECTIVE ROOT INJECTION
Acyclovir
SYMPATHETIC BLOCK
SELECTIVE ROOT INJECTION
TENS
Amitriptyline
Fluphenazine
Carbamazepine
Capsaicin
(H) Diabetic polyneuropathy
EMG/NCS
Serum Glucose
TENS
Amitriptyline
Carbamazepine
Capsaicin
Medical referral (for diabetes control)
(I) Spinal cord/bone tumor
MRI
CT
Bone Scan
SMA-20
ESR
Acid Phos-phatase
SPEP
LP
(J) Metabolic bone lesion
SMA-20
ESR
Bone Scan
Bone Survey

SPINAL STENOSIS

Susan J. Dreyer, M.D.

Spinal stenosis is the narrowing of the spinal canal in either the lateral (apophyseal) or anterior-posterior (laminar) direction, resulting in nerve compression laterally of the spinal roots and anteroposteriorly of the cauda equina. This narrowing can occur anywhere along the spinal column from occiput to sacrum, for which there may be asymptomatic radiographic evidence. The origin of the stenosis can be congenital or acquired; however, most cases are caused by degenerative arthritis. Typical onset is in the fifth decade, although those persons with absolute stenosis (AP diameter of the spinal canal <10 mm) may show spinal stenosis as early as the third decade. Much controversy still exists regarding treatment, especially surgical timing and technique. Current literature indicates that degenerative lumbar stenosis is not as ubiquitous as had been originally thought.

A. Classic symptoms include low back and leg pain, especially when standing, walking, or hyperextending. The lower extremity pain and paresthesias are relieved by flexing the spine. Unlike vascular claudication, this pseudoclaudication is less predictable in onset, slower to subside, and not relieved by standing alone. Physical examinations show strong peripheral pulses (unless concomitant vascular disease exists) and minimal sciatic tension signs such as straight leg raises. Presenting symptoms of cervical stenosis may be those of myelopathy with weakness, atrophy, hyperreflexia, and spasticity.

B. Plain radiographs usually demonstrate spondylosis with loss of disc height, osteophytes, and sclerosis of the facet joints. CT, myelography, and MRI can all further delineate the lesion, although far lateral stenosis is often missed with myelography. Degenerative lumbar stenosis most frequently involves the L4-5 facet joint. In the neck, the C5-6 level is most commonly involved. Clinical decisions cannot be based on isolated radiographic findings. Each radiographic examination has its limitations; for example, false-negative rates of 10% to 25% are reported with myelography. Electrodiagnostic studies such as electromyography and somatosensory-evoked potentials (SEPs) also aid in localization.

C. Much of the discomfort is believed to stem from concomitant soft tissue disorders, which should be treated aggressively.

D. Identify the cause of the spinal stenosis as well as the region involved to better dictate treatment. Spinal stenosis secondary to Paget's disease responds to calcitonin; other types of spinal stenoses do not. Surgical procedures are dictated by the underlying disorder.

E. Most patients deserve a trial of aggressive conservative therapy, including modalities such as stretching, back school, and the use of NSAIDs. Best results are achieved with a multidisciplinary team focused on returning the patient to productivity.

F. Epidural blocks with or without steroids help delay the need for surgery, especially in older patients with sciatica.

G. Selective nerve root blocks aid in diagnosing the symptomatic levels, as multilevel stenosis is commonly seen on radiographs. Limiting surgical decompression to symptomatic levels minimizes iatrogenic instability.

H. Surgery is indicated in those patients who have significant neurologic involvement, such as marked or progressive muscle weakness. A neurogenic bowel or bladder requires emergent decompression of the cauda equina to prevent irreversible damage. Consider surgery in those patients who have failed to achieve pain relief through conservative treatment. The basic goals of surgery for spinal stenosis are to achieve adequate decompression and adequate stability.

References

Hopp E, ed. Spine: State of the Art Reviews, spinal stenosis. Vol. 2, no. 3. Philadelphia: Hanley & Belfus, 1987.

Lispon SJ, Branch WT: Low back pain. In: Branch W. Office practice of medicine, 2nd ed. Philadelphia: WB Saunders, 1987:875.

Loeser JD, Bigos SJ, Fordyce WE, Volinn EP. Low back pain. In: Bonica JJ, ed. The management of pain. 2nd ed. Philadelphia: Lea & Febiger, 1990:1468.

Wood GW. Other disorders of the spine. In: Creshaw AH, ed. Campbell's operative orthopaedics. St. Louis: CV Mosby, 1987:3347.

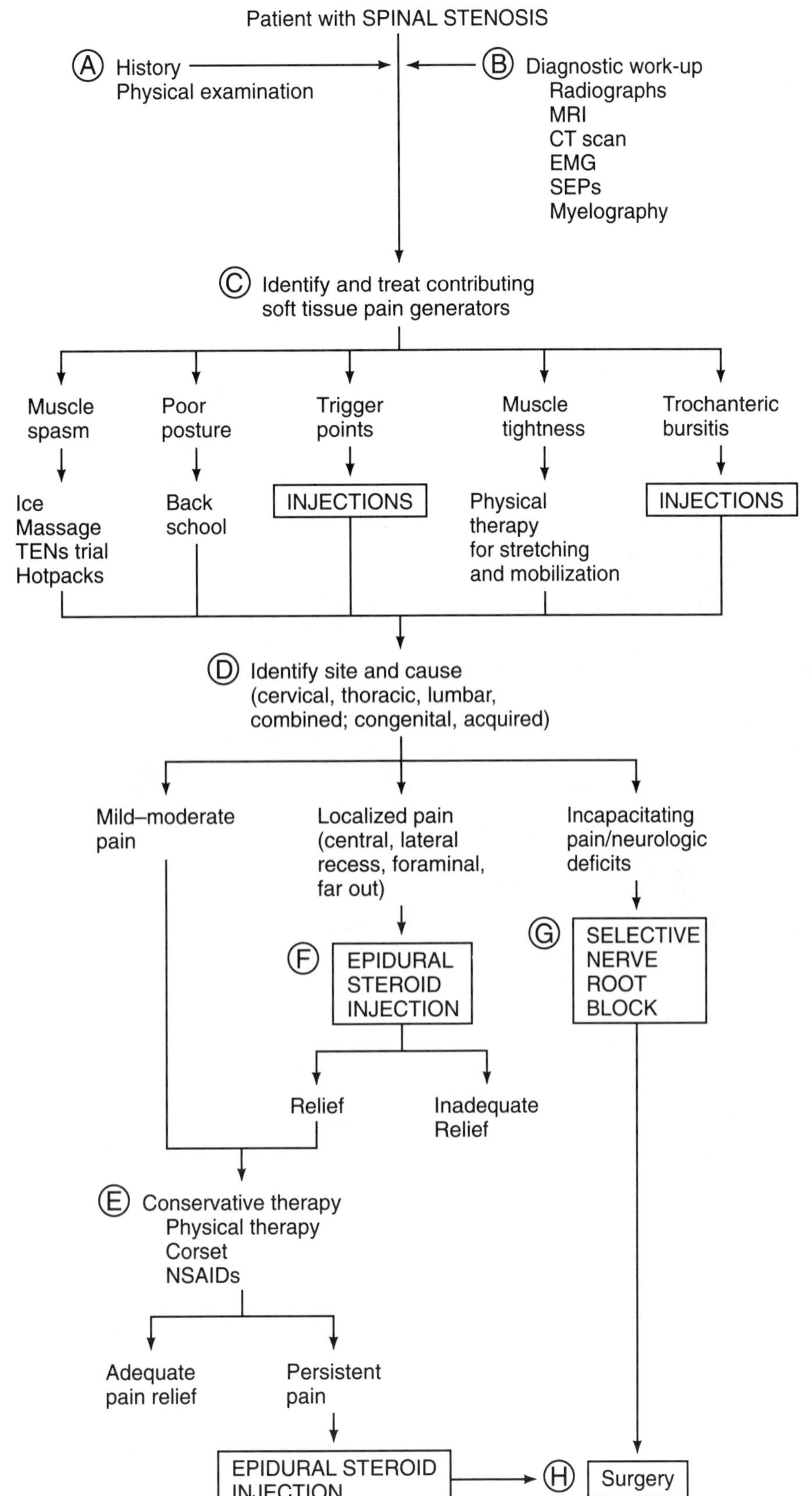
Patient with SPINAL STENOSIS
(A) History
Physical examination
(B) Diagnostic work-up
Radiographs
MRI
CT scan
EMG
SEPs
Myelography
(C) Identify and treat contributing soft tissue pain generators
Muscle spasm
Poor posture
Trigger points
Muscle tightness
Trochanteric bursitis
Ice
Massage
TENs trial
Hotpacks
Back school
INJECTIONS
Physical therapy for stretching and mobilization
INJECTIONS
(D) Identify site and cause (cervical, thoracic, lumbar, combined; congenital, acquired)
Mild–moderate pain
Localized pain (central, lateral recess, foraminal, far out)
Incapacitating pain/neurologic deficits
(F) EPIDURAL STEROID INJECTION
(G) SELECTIVE NERVE ROOT BLOCK
Relief
Inadequate Relief
(E) Conservative therapy
Physical therapy
Corset
NSAIDs
Adequate pain relief
Persistent pain
EPIDURAL STEROID INJECTION
(H) Surgery

ANKYLOSING SPONDYLITIS

Ellen Leonard, M.D.

Ninety percent of persons with ankylosing spondylitis (Marie-Strumpell disease), a seronegative spondyloarthropathy that predominantly affects young men, are found to be positive for the HLA-B27 antigen.

A. Patients <40 years of age who complain of back pain of insidious onset, which is worse in the morning, should be considered for a diagnosis of spondyloarthropathy. A careful history should be taken, with particular attention paid to family history of psoriasis; past medical history of uveitis and prostatitis; and symptoms of weight loss, fatigue, malaise, morning stiffness, and anterior chest pain. Complete a detailed physical examination, paying special attention to flexibility of the spine (Schober's test), pain in sacroiliac joints, and chest expansion.

B. Laboratory data should include sedimentation rate and presence or absence of HLA-B27. The sedimentation rate may or may not be increased, but HLA-B27 is found in 90% of patients with this disease. Radiography is essential. Findings can range from "blurring" of the sacroiliac joints to "bamboo" spine. The New York criteria grade radiographs from 0 to IV.

C. Three stages of pain occur in progression of the disease:
Stage I. Early sacroiliac inflammation is described as hip pain and is often mislabeled as sciatica. The pain awakens the patient at night and abates after he or she gets up and moves around.
Stage II. The chronic middle phase of the disease is characterized by morning stiffness that improves by afternoon. Many patients also experience anterior chest pain of mechanical origin.
Stage III. Late in the disease, patients have no morning stiffness and pain at rest but continue to have nagging interscapular neck and low back pain. By this stage, patients have rigid spines and dorsal kyphosis. If these patients have severe focal pain, a pseudoarthrosis should be suspected.

D. The treatment of ankylosing spondylitis pain is twofold: decrease the pain, and decrease deformity and maintain function. Radiotherapy is no longer used because of the risk of leukemia. Pharmacologic treatment consists of the administration of NSAIDs. The first choice is indomethacin, 25 to 50 mg, 3 to 4 times per day. The other traditional choice, phenylbutazone, carries the risk of marrow aplasia. Other NSAIDs such as sulindac, 150 to 200 mg twice a day, may be used. The second prong of treatment is physical therapy and education. Instruct patients to sleep on a firm mattress with no pillow. Exercises are aimed at preventing kyphosis and maintaining flexibility, range of motion, and pulmonary function. Instruct patients in extension exercises, morning warm-up exercises, and flexibility exercises. Have patients perform chest expansion exercises to prevent restrictive lung disease, and encourage general endurance activities.

E. In the late stages of the disease, patients may develop painful pseudoarthroses, which should be treated with immobilization. Instruct patients in rest and positioning to decrease the strain on neck muscles. Surgery for vertebral wedge osteotomy may be indicated in some patients.

References

Calliet R. Low back pain syndrome. Philadelphia: FA Davis, 1986:197.

Delisa J, ed. Rehabilitation medicine: Principles and practices. Philadelphia: JB Lippincott, 1988:726.

Good A. The pain of ankylosing spondylitis. Am J Med 1986; 80:118.

Kottke F, Lehmann JF. Krusen's handbook of physical medicine and rehabilitation. 4th ed. Philadelphia: WB Saunders, 1990:631.

Rodnan G. Primer on the rheumatic diseases. Atlanta: Arthritis Foundation, 1983:85.

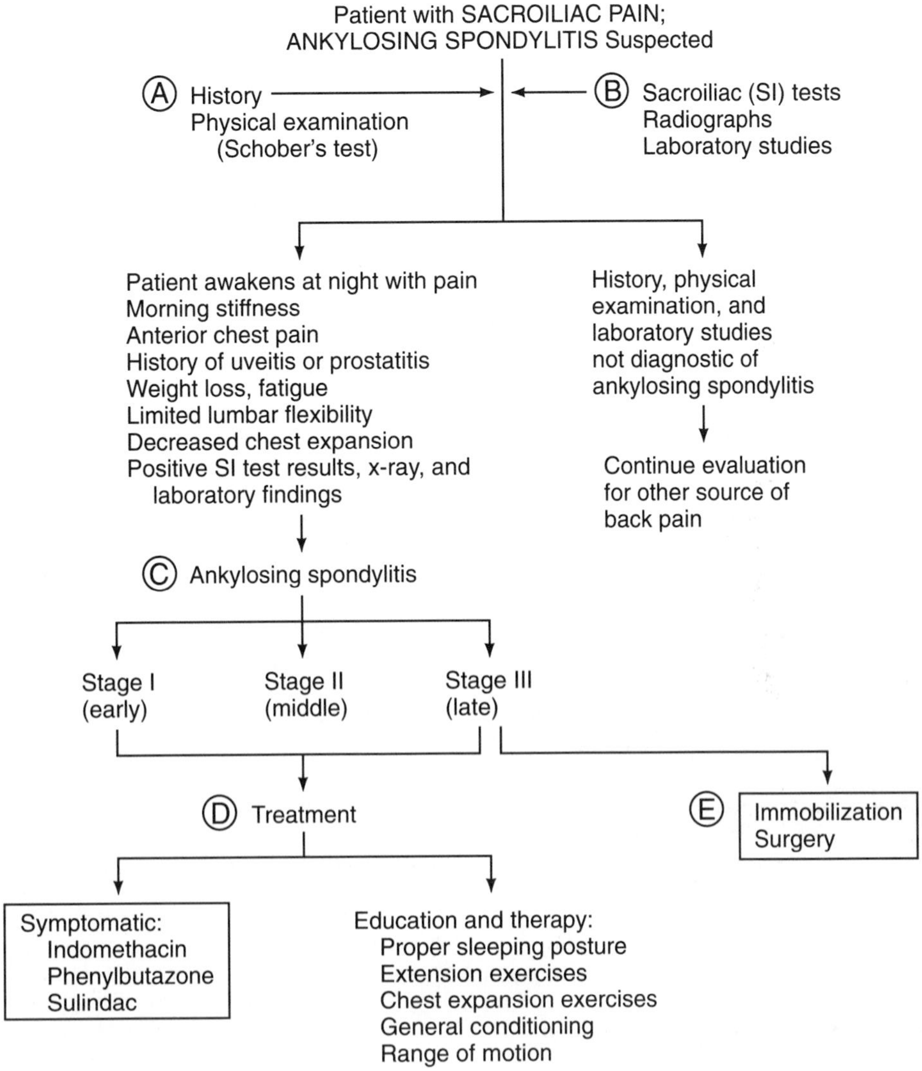

Patient with SACROILIAC PAIN;
ANKYLOSING SPONDYLITIS Suspected

(A) History
Physical examination
(Schober's test)

(B) Sacroiliac (SI) tests
Radiographs
Laboratory studies

Patient awakens at night with pain
Morning stiffness
Anterior chest pain
History of uveitis or prostatitis
Weight loss, fatigue
Limited lumbar flexibility
Decreased chest expansion
Positive SI test results, x-ray, and laboratory findings

(C) Ankylosing spondylitis

Stage I (early)

Stage II (middle)

Stage III (late)

(D) Treatment

Symptomatic:
- Indomethacin
- Phenylbutazone
- Sulindac

Education and therapy:
- Proper sleeping posture
- Extension exercises
- Chest expansion exercises
- General conditioning
- Range of motion

(E) Immobilization
Surgery

History, physical examination, and laboratory studies not diagnostic of ankylosing spondylitis

Continue evaluation for other source of back pain

FAILED LAMINECTOMY SYNDROME

Mark E. Romanoff, M.D.

The failed laminectomy syndrome (FLS) is not a single entity. Bony abnormalities (spondylolisthesis, pseudarthrosis), joint problems (facet arthropathy, degenerative joint disease), muscular changes (myofascial pain syndrome, atrophy), neural disorders (nerve root impingement, arachnoiditis, deafferentation), and psychological difficulties (depression, compensation/litigation), may all play roles in this difficult-to-treat syndrome. Signs and symptoms vary, depending on which factor is prominent. A 40% failure rate for laminectomy surgery has been quoted when the preoperative diagnosis is in doubt. A failure rate of 10% to 15% with resultant pain and compromised mobility is more commonly observed.

Treatment for FLS must be individualized and creative. Success rates are poor and in most studies do not approach 50%. FLS is produced by inappropriate surgery, surgical complications, and patient factors. Strict guidelines concerning the indications for back surgery have been approved by the American Academy of Orthopedic Surgeons and the Association of Neurological Surgeons to help prevent inappropriate surgery.

A. A complete history, including previous surgical diagnosis, the number and types of previous surgery, medication use, and the extent of disability, is necessary. The work and home environment should be evaluated. Psychological screening should be performed. A comprehensive treatment plan taking into account all these factors is required for a good outcome. A thorough physical examination, including a detailed neurologic examination, should help confirm or refute preliminary diagnostic suspicions and may be used to follow progress. Provocative tests to elicit discomfort (straight leg raise; sitting root test; lasegue; palpation of muscles, ligaments, and joints) are important aspects of the physical examination. It can reveal valuable information, and also reassure patients that you are actively looking for the cause of their problem. An extensive search should be made for a myofascial pain syndrome (MFPS) (p 46), which usually coexists with almost all FLS diagnoses. Early treatment may alleviate many symptoms and allow therapy to progress more rapidly. A differential spinal block and/or thiopental testing can help determine the source of pain.

B. Diagnostic studies focus on mechanical causes for pain in these patients, but other pathologic conditions should not be overlooked. The history, physical examination, laboratory studies, and radiographic procedures should be used to rule out important diagnoses such as osteomyelitis, spinal cord neoplasm, Paget's disease, hemachromatosis, and referred pain from the kidney, pancreas, or abdominal aorta.

C. Conservative treatment should begin soon after the initial history taking and physical examination. Most patients have tried or are taking NSAIDs at the time of evaluation. NSAIDs should be given an adequate trial of at least 8 weeks before changing or discontinuing medications. If one class of NSAIDs fails, one from another class should be substituted. Antidepressant medications can lessen depressive symptoms and sleep disturbances and affect pain thresholds. The choice of antidepressant should be made with the drug's side effects and the patient's medical profile, and psychological state in mind (see p 182). Narcotic medications usually are not helpful and should be discontinued. Physical and/or occupational therapy (PT/OT) should be begun. Increasing activity levels may help reverse learned patient behavior as well as improve muscular tone and flexibility. Transcutaneous electrical nerve stimulation (TENS) is often effective in decreasing pain in MFPS, degenerative joint disease, and nerve root irritation. TENS has often been tried in the past and deemed ineffective by the patient. A TENS trial should be repeated (p 194). Psychological interventions may also help manage the pain.

D. Imaging techniques during the initial phase of therapy should be limited to patients with suspected surgical disease (radicular symptoms on physical examination), those with new symptoms, or those whose response to conservative treatment has not been optimal. An enhanced MRI or CT scan can aid in the diagnosis of epidural fibrosis versus retained disk material. MRI produces sharper images of soft tissues, but CT is more effective in imaging bony abnormalities. Patients with metal appliances should not undergo MRI.

E. Repeat operations should be performed only if there is overwhelming evidence of a surgically correctable lesion. Examples include retained disk material or a recurrent disk at the site of previous surgery; a new herniated nucleus pulposus; or instability or a pseudarthrosis at the site of a previous fusion (this may be diagnosed by CT/MRI but requires confirmation by lateral flexion-extension radiography—motion may be found but is not always the cause of pain); or spinal stenosis. One study that evaluated repeat operations in patients with FLS found that >80% of 67 patients had some pain relief and 43% discontinued narcotic use. However, only 12% of these patients experienced good relief of pain, and a 13% complication rate was also noted. Approximately 50% of patients with epidural fibrosis showed a poor result after repeat surgery. The best outcomes after repeat surgery were associated with four factors: (1) a pain-free interval of >1 year after the initial surgery, (2) a complete myelographic block, (3) a true disk herniation, and (4) evidence of instability.

(Continued on page 138)

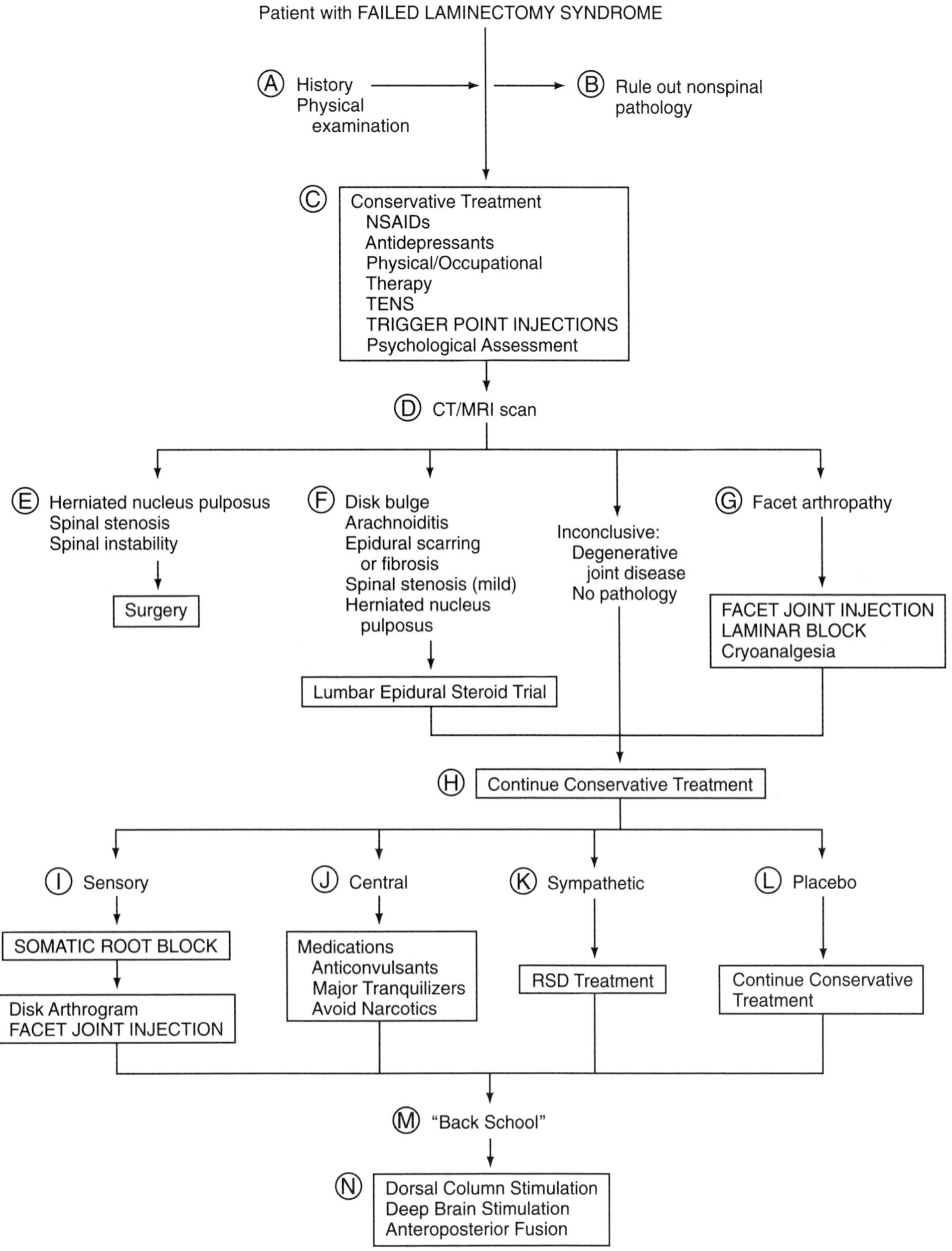

Patient with FAILED LAMINECTOMY SYNDROME
(A) History
Physical examination
(B) Rule out nonspinal pathology
(C) Conservative Treatment
NSAIDs
Antidepressants
Physical/Occupational Therapy
TENS
TRIGGER POINT INJECTIONS
Psychological Assessment
(D) CT/MRI scan
(E) Herniated nucleus pulposus
Spinal stenosis
Spinal instability
Surgery
(F) Disk bulge
Arachnoiditis
Epidural scarring or fibrosis
Spinal stenosis (mild)
Herniated nucleus pulposus
Lumbar Epidural Steroid Trial
Inconclusive:
Degenerative joint disease
No pathology
(G) Facet arthropathy
FACET JOINT INJECTION
LAMINAR BLOCK
Cryoanalgesia
(H) Continue Conservative Treatment
(I) Sensory
SOMATIC ROOT BLOCK
Disk Arthrogram
FACET JOINT INJECTION
(J) Central
Medications
Anticonvulsants
Major Tranquilizers
Avoid Narcotics
(K) Sympathetic
RSD Treatment
(L) Placebo
Continue Conservative Treatment
(M) "Back School"
(N) Dorsal Column Stimulation
Deep Brain Stimulation
Anteroposterior Fusion

F. Lumbar epidural steroid injections (ESIs) appear to have the highest efficacy in patients with low back pain and radicular symptoms. Patients with arachnoiditis or epidural scarring may respond to lumbar ESI, but if fibrosis is present the anti-inflammatory effect of the steroids will be of little benefit.

G. Facet syndrome may mimic the signs and symptoms of nerve root compression (p 140). It tends to be forgotten as an entity in the differential diagnosis of FLS. Facet joint injections with a local anesthetic and steroid can be performed, or the nerve supply to the joint can be interrupted (p 266). If these are effective but demonstrate short-lived pain relief, cryoanalgesia (p 226), radiofrequency lesion, or neurolytic block can be attempted for long-term pain control.

H. Other conservative methods may be added to the regimen at this time. Biofeedback, relaxation techniques, and hypnosis may be useful. Dosages of NSAIDs and antidepressants may be increased or the medications changed as appropriate.

I. Lumbar or transsacral nerve root blocks can be effective forms of treatment in these patients. Temporary relief of pain after a series of blocks may indicate nerve root compression. Causes of this compression should be actively sought. Failure of these blocks may indicate disk pain or facet pain. A disk arthrogram that reproduces the patient's pain is justification for surgical intervention. If a facet joint injection has not been attempted recently, it should be performed at this time.

J. Patients with a central pain syndrome may benefit from a trial of anticonvulsant medications. Narcotics are unlikely to be useful.

K. Sympathetically mediated pain should be managed as reflex sympathetic dystrophy (p 50).

L. Some patients respond to placebo or show evidence of psychologically mediated pain are best treated conservatively.

M. "Back school" should be started in patients when no further interventional therapy is planned. This should involve operant conditioning, behavior modification, PT/OT, and often drug detoxification. Success rates of >70% have been achieved in these intensive programs. Opponents cite the high relapse rates as one problem with this approach.

N. Dorsal column stimulation (p 224) or spinal cord stimulation has proved effective in some patients. In one study of 89 patients with arachnoiditis and FLS, an excellent response was seen in 85% after 3 months of implantation, but this decreased to only 35% after 4 to 8 years of follow-up. A 24% complication rate was also noted, electrode migration and infection being the most common. For patients not responding to spinal cord stimulation, deep brain stimulation has been attempted. Medial thalamus stimulation appears to be more effective for deep, crushing pain. Burning, sharp, and searing pain is controlled with lateral thalamus stimulation. Some studies using periventricular gray stimulation have produced 80% success rates. Complications cited include intraventricular hemorrhage, infection, and electrode movement.

Simultaneous combined anterior and posterior fusion has been recommended for patients with disabling low back pain. With this technique, 61% of patients showed good results and 14% had fair pain relief; a complication rate of 23% was experienced. Patients with combined multilevel pathology, single-level or multilevel annular tears, and herniated nucleus pulposus responded best, whereas those with multilevel degenerative disk disease fared poorly.

References

Bogduk N. Back pain: Zygapophyseal blocks and epidural steroids. In: Cousins MJ, Bridenbaugh PO, eds. Neural blockade in clinical anesthesia and management of pain. 2nd ed. Philadelphia: JB Lippincott, 1988:935.

Burton CV, Kirkaldy-Willis WH, Yong-Hing K, et al. Causes of failure of surgery on the lumbar spine. Clin Orthop 1981; 157:191.

Finnegan WJ, Fenlin JM, Marvel JP, et al. Results of surgical intervention in the symptomatic multiply-operated back patient. J Bone Joint Surg 1979; 61A:1077.

Kozak JA, O'Brien JP. Simultaneous combined anterior and posterior fusion. An independent analysis of a treatment of the disabled low-back pain patient. Spine 1990; 15:322.

Long DM, Filtzer DL, BenDebba M, Hendler NH. Clinical features of the failed-back syndrome. J Neurosurg 1988; 69:61.

Plotkin R. Results in 60 cases of deep brain stimulation for chronic intractable pain. Proc. 8th Meeting World Soc. Stereotactic and Functional Neurosurgery, Part I, Zurich, 1981. Appl Neurophysiol 1982; 45:201.

Siegfried J, Lazorthes J. Long-term follow-up of dorsal cord stimulation for chronic pain syndrome after multiple lumbar operations. Proc. 8th Meeting World Soc. Stereotactic and Functional Neurosurgery, Part I, Zurich, 1981. Appl Neurophysiol 1982; 45:201.

Spangfort E. Disc surgery. In: Wall P, Melzack R, eds. Textbook of pain. New York: Churchill Livingstone, 1984:795.

Turk DC, Meichenbaum D. A cognitive-behavioural approach to pain management. In: Wall P, Melzack R, eds. Textbook of pain. New York: Churchill Livingstone, 1984:1001.

Wilkinson HA. Failed-back syndrome. J Neurosurg 1989; 70:659.

FACET JOINT SYNDROME

Emil J. Menk, M.D.

The differential diagnosis of back pain remains a major diagnostic dilemma. Although facet joint syndrome was first described more than 50 years ago, it remains a vague but significant clinical problem, and, although an alert clinician can make a tentative diagnosis based on a combination of symptoms, signs, and investigative test results, definitive determinations depend on results of diagnostic nerve blocks.

A basic understanding of the pathogenesis of this syndrome has gradually developed. One explanation involves the gradual degeneration of the articular cartilages. These synovial joints, like others, are subject to progressive degenerative changes. The overall process has been described as a steady progression from synovitis to capsule laxity to subluxation of the joint surfaces, with eventual facet enlargement and loss of articular cartilage. This process produces irritation and inflammation of the involved nerves. The imprecise and varying pain pattern that arises from a diseased facet joint becomes more understandable when one considers the complex innervation.

A. The patient may give a history of an aching low back pain at the lower lumbar or lumbosacral levels. The pain may present unilaterally if only one side of facets is involved. The patient may relate a history of referred pain to the ipsilateral buttocks and posterolateral thigh, but rarely below the level of the knee—this pain is worse with sustained posture and may be somewhat relieved in a slightly flexed neutral position. The patient may or may not have a history of trauma.

B. A physical examination may reveal pain on extension (especially with hip extension in the prone position), lateral flexion, and rotation of the spine. The patient's posture may be rigid, with loss of lordosis. The patient may have reduced spinal mobility at the affected level, and mild to moderate discomfort along the paraspinal muscles of the affected side. Deep palpation may elicit significant discomfort over the involved facet joint. Patients with a pars defect may exhibit all the above signs; however, this defect should be readily diagnosed with radiography.

C. None of the listed tests are diagnostically specific for facet joint syndrome; however, they may have been done in the general work-up for low back pain. EMG and myelographic studies should be normal. A radiograph of the facet joints may show degenerative changes, disc narrowing, and joint asymmetries. CT and MRI may show the same and subchondral sclerosis, erosions, and facet hypertrophy; however, no studies have shown these disorders to be pathognomonic of facet joint disease or to cause pain. The role of radionuclide scanning is controversial. Although one study indicated that radionuclide scanning was not helpful, I have found high resolution scans to be very useful when evaluated in conjunction with a history and physical examination.

D. Ultimately, the diagnosis of facet joint syndrome relies exclusively on fluoroscopically directed intra-articular injections. The diagnosis is confirmed when pain is relieved during extension, lateral flexion, and rotation maneuvers after the injection (p 266).

E. The treatment of facet joint syndrome routinely involves several modalities. Unless contraindicated, all patients should receive an NSAID. Although rest is beneficial during acute phases, exercises should be recommended once adequate pain relief has been obtained. Maintenance of strength, function, and mobility is essential for effective long-term management. Both transcutaneous electrical nerve stimulation (TENS) and manipulation of the spine may help in the acute phases. Applications of heat and cold also may relieve painful muscle spasms. Facet joint injections often produce immediate relief and, when performed with steroids, can lead to long-term improvement. In refractory cases, denervation techniques such as cryoanalgesia, radiofrequency, or chemical neurolysis can be useful.

References

Boas RA. Facet joint injections. In: Stanton-Hicks M, Boas R, eds. Chronic low back pain. New York: Raven Press, 1982:199.

Bogdak N. Back pain: zygapophysial blocks and epidural steroids. In: Cousins MJ, Bridenbaugh PO, eds. Neural blockade in clinical anesthesia and management of pain. 2nd ed. Philadelphia: JB Lippincott, 1988:935.

Raymond JR, Dumas JM, Lisbona R. Nuclear imaging as a screening test for patients referred for intra-articular facet block. J Can Assoc Radiol 1984; 35:291.

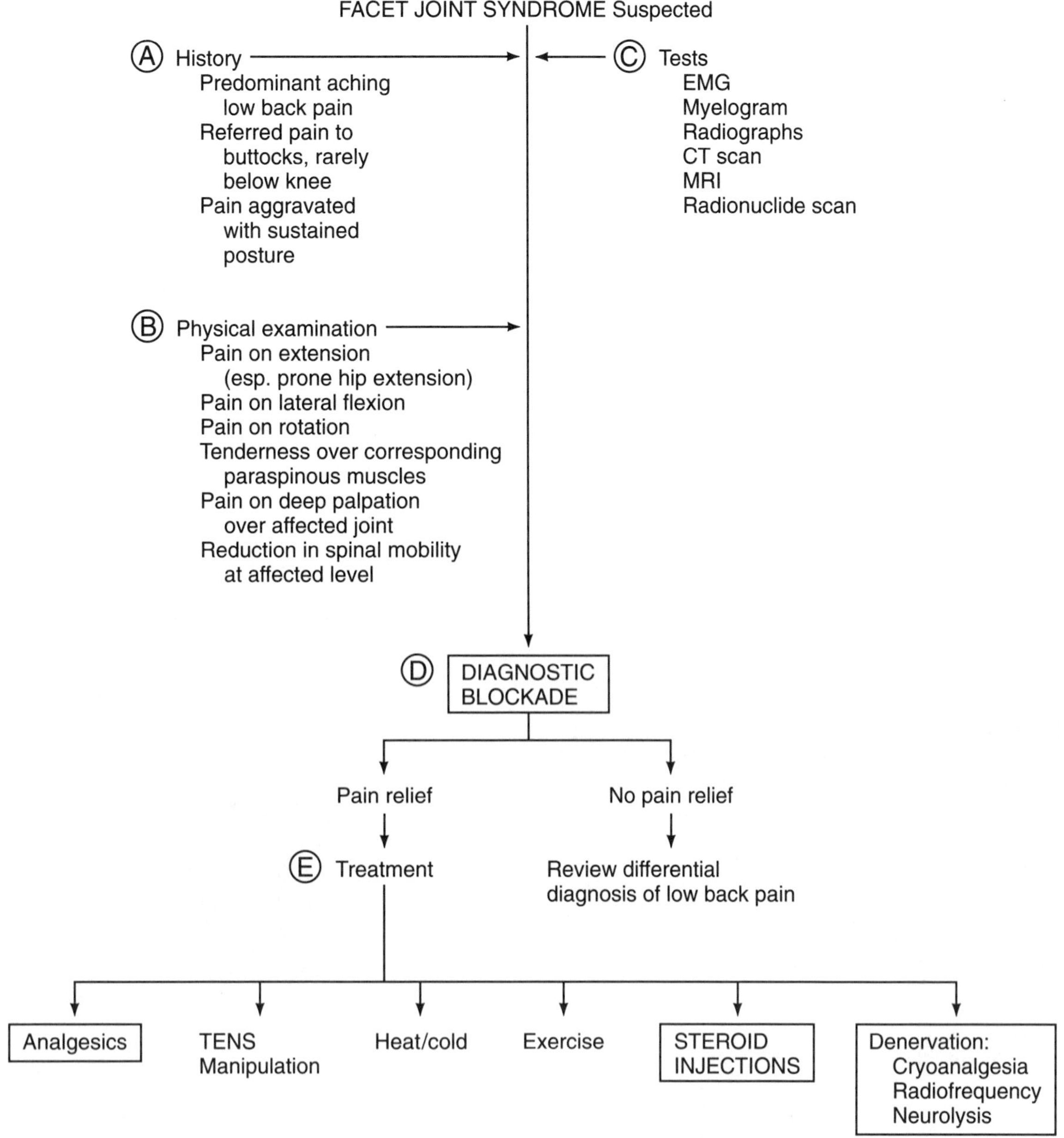

FACET JOINT SYNDROME Suspected
A History
Predominant aching low back pain
Referred pain to buttocks, rarely below knee
Pain aggravated with sustained posture
C Tests
EMG
Myelogram
Radiographs
CT scan
MRI
Radionuclide scan
B Physical examination
Pain on extension (esp. prone hip extension)
Pain on lateral flexion
Pain on rotation
Tenderness over corresponding paraspinous muscles
Pain on deep palpation over affected joint
Reduction in spinal mobility at affected level
D DIAGNOSTIC BLOCKADE
Pain relief
No pain relief
E Treatment
Review differential diagnosis of low back pain
Analgesics
TENS
Manipulation
Heat/cold
Exercise
STEROID INJECTIONS
Denervation:
Cryoanalgesia
Radiofrequency
Neurolysis

SACROILIAC JOINT PAIN

James Griffin, P.T., A.T.C.

The sacroiliac (SI) joint can be a primary source of pain. Pain may be referred to the SI joint or from the SI joint to the lumbar facets, iliolumbar ligament, and gluteal, piriformis, iliopsoas, and adductor muscles. Visceral referral may occur from the reproductive organs in women and from the large intestine. Systemic conditions such as ankylosing spondylitis, regional ileitis, and gout can also produce pain in the SI joint. If the treatment of these sources of pain decreases but does not eliminate SI joint pain, then SI joint involvement must also be considered. Conversely, SI pain unresponsive to treatment may be a symptom of another problem.

A. Primary SI problems frequently result from an accident or injury, but can result from an unguarded or unexpected movement, chronic strain in the workplace, or with repetitive activity, such as swinging a golf club. SI joint pain is not uncommon during or after pregnancy.

B. Persons with an anatomically short leg or increased unilateral pronation can have SI joint pain as a result. The removal or correction of these stresses may easily relieve the problem. SI joint problems frequently exist in conjunction with other musculoskeletal disorders, which must be treated to ensure complete relief. Tightness and trigger points commonly exist in the musculature surrounding the SI joint and pelvis. These points respond to the methods devised by Travell, which use vapocoolant spray while the muscle is being stretched; trigger point injections may be necessary for adequate relief, however.

C. SI joint problems that require direct attention may be treated by injection (p 268) or manipulation. Treatment by manipulation requires the practitioner to have a knowledge of pelvic mechanics for evaluation and the skill to perform the appropriate manipulative technique to restore normal mechanics. Techniques used may involve high-velocity, low-amplitude thrust techniques, or muscle energy techniques, which are a form of precise contract-relax muscle stretches that mobilize the joint. By itself, manipulation may be sufficient to resolve many SI problems. An SI belt worn tightly around the pelvis just below the level of the iliac crest and above the pubic symphysis while weight bearing can provide stability in hypermobile patients by compressing the SI joint.

D. If manual skills are unavailable, if manipulation fails, or in patients who are too irritable to tolerate manual treatment, injection of the joint under fluoroscopic observation is effective. An injection of 0.25% bupivacaine distributed 1 ml to the joint and 3 ml to the posterior ligament and muscle can restore normal pelvic mechanics as well as relieve pain in some patients. In some cases a combination of injection and manipulation may be required to restore normal mechanics and relieve irritation in the joint. Dysfunction in the lower lumbar spine must be recognized and treated. Also, compensatory changes in the vertebral column secondary to SI dysfunction may occur even as far proximal as the cervical spine and should be evaluated in nonresponsive patients. Patients with chronic SI pain suffer some degree of deconditioning and must be placed on a program to regain strength, flexibility, and endurance. Encourage the use of proper back hygiene.

E. The use of a neurolytic injection may be required in persistent cases of SI joint pain that are resistant to other therapy, and an injection of sclerosing agents may stabilize the joint.

References

Aitken GS. Syndromes of lumbo-pelvic dysfunction. In: Grieve GP, ed. Modern manual therapy of the vertebral column. New York: Churchill Livingstone, 1986.

Bernard TN, Kirkaldy-Willis WH. Making a specific diagnosis. In: Kirkaldy-Willis WH, ed. Managing low back pain. 2nd ed. New York: Churchill Livingstone, 1988.

Bourdillon JF, Day EA. Spinal manipulation. 4th ed. Norwalk, CT: Appleton & Lange, 1987.

Cassidy JD, Kirkaldy-Willis WH. Manipulation. In: Kirkaldy-Willis WH, ed. Managing low back pain. 2nd ed. New York: Churchill Livingstone, 1988.

Greenman PE. Principles of manual medicine. Baltimore: Williams & Wilkins, 1989.

Grieve GP. Referred pain and other clinical features. In: Grieve GP, ed. Modern manual therapy of the vertebral column. New York: Churchill Livingstone, 1986.

Kirkaldy-Willis WH. A comprehensive outline of treatment. In: Kirkaldy-Willis WH, ed. Managing low back pain. 2nd ed. New York: Churchill Livingstone, 1988.

Kirkaldy-Willis WH. The site and nature of the lesion. In: Kirkaldy-Willis WH, ed. Managing low back pain. 2nd ed. New York: Churchill Livingstone, 1988.

Travell JG, Simmons DG. Myofascial pain and dysfunction. Baltimore: Williams & Wilkins, 1983.

Wallace LA. Limb length difference and back pain. In: Grieve GP, ed. Modern manual therapy of the vertebral column. New York: Churchill Livingstone, 1986.

Wells PE. The examination of the pelvic joints. In: Grieve GP, ed. Modern manual therapy of the vertebral column. New York: Churchill Livingstone, 1986.

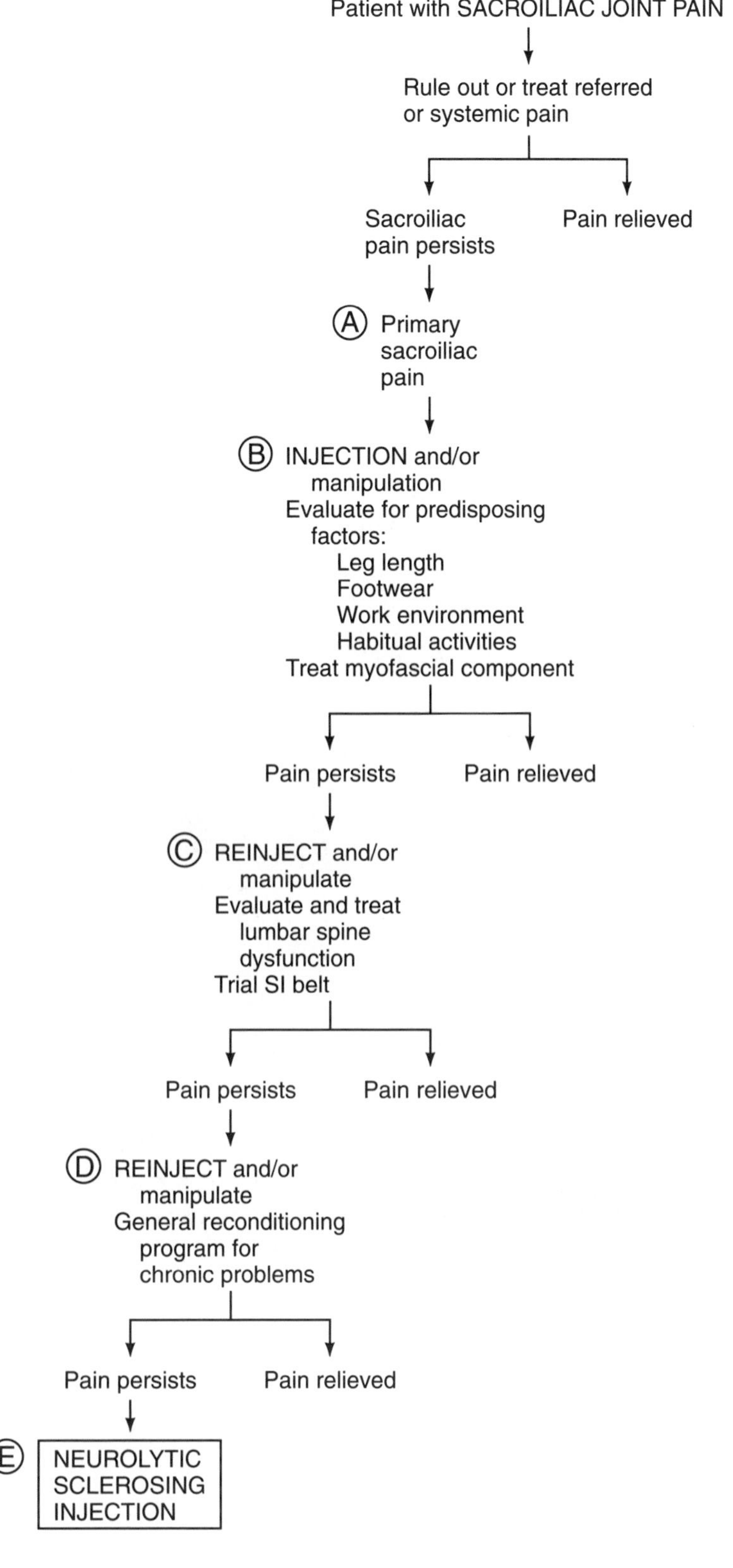

Patient with SACROILIAC JOINT PAIN
Rule out or treat referred or systemic pain
Sacroiliac pain persists
Pain relieved
(A) Primary sacroiliac pain
(B) INJECTION and/or manipulation
Evaluate for predisposing factors:
Leg length
Footwear
Work environment
Habitual activities
Treat myofascial component
Pain persists
Pain relieved
(C) REINJECT and/or manipulate
Evaluate and treat lumbar spine dysfunction
Trial SI belt
Pain persists
Pain relieved
(D) REINJECT and/or manipulate
General reconditioning program for chronic problems
Pain persists
Pain relieved
(E) NEUROLYTIC SCLEROSING INJECTION

LOWER EXTREMITY PAIN

SCIATICA

Jonathan P. Lester, M.D.

Pain radiating down the posterior thigh and leg in the distribution of the sciatic nerve may be caused by various disorders of the bony elements and overlying soft tissues of the lumbosacral spine. The cause is often suggested by the duration of symptoms. Most cases can be diagnosed with the aid of a thorough history and physical examination. Difficult cases or those with multiple causes may require additional evaluation with imaging studies, electrodiagnostic examination, and diagnostic blocks. Most causes of sciatica can be managed successfully with conservative therapy.

A. The acute onset of sciatica is often secondary to a herniated nucleus pulposus (HNP) that causes a lumbosacral radiculopathy. A history of a precipitating flexion-rotation injury and associated radicular complaints are highly suggestive of an HNP. Conservative treatment often relieves pain. Educate patients on appropriate back care to prevent recurrences, and refer persons with progressive neurologic loss or intractable pain unresponsive to conservative therapy for surgical evaluation.

B. Complaints of bowel or bladder disturbance in association with saddle anesthesia or radicular pain indicate a possible cauda equina syndrome. Refer the patient immediately for surgical evaluation.

C. Myofascial pain syndrome is readily recognized by the finding of specific trigger points that produce local and referred pain patterns. Aim treatment at abolishing the hyperirritable focus of contracted muscle fibers that form the trigger point. Many techniques have been found to be effective including spray-and-stretch, trigger point injection (TPI), soft tissue mobilization, and aggressive stretching programs (p 46).

D. Piriformis syndrome is a myofascial pain disorder that involves a trigger point in the belly of the piriformis muscle and should be treated similarly (p 148).

E. Facet syndrome is produced by painful inflammation or dysfunction of the facet joint (p 140). Use conservative treatment to reduce any chemical irritation of the joint and to restore normal joint biomechanics. Patients with a temporary response to serial facet injections or medial branch nerve blocks may be candidates for chemical, radiofrequency, or cryodorsal rhizotomies.

F. Spinal stenosis can be readily diagnosed by CT scan. Patients may complain of claudication of the lower extremities in association with monoradicular or polyradicular symptoms. Conservative therapy is often beneficial, although many patients may eventually require surgery (p 132).

G. Spondylolisthesis can be readily identified on oblique lumbosacral radiographs. Whether this disorder is an incidental finding in a patient with sciatica or the cause of the pain is often unclear. Patients with low grades of listhesis (<50%) often benefit from conservative therapy. Refer those with high grades of listhesis (>50%) or those with signs of radicular compromise for surgical evaluation.

H. Repeated flexion-rotation injuries of the annular fibers of the intervertebral disc may lead to a chaotic, painful disturbance of disc architecture known as internal disc disruption (IDD). IDD is best diagnosed by provocative CT and discography, but grossly degenerated disc levels may also be identified by MRI. Conservative therapy is limited, and those patients with isolated one- or two-level disc disease may be candidates for surgical fusion.

I. Chronic sciatica following previous lumbar spine surgery is not uncommon and is often referred to as failed back surgery syndrome. Common causes of sciatica for these patients include recurrent HNP, spinal stenosis, segmental instability, and arachnoiditis. Aggressive evaluation of these patients requires both imaging and electrophysiologic studies. Conservative treatment is based on the appropriate diagnosis (p 136).

References

Frymoyer J. Back pain and sciatica. N Engl J Med 1988; 318:291.

Saal J. Diagnostic studies of industrialized low back injuries. Top Acute Care Trauma Rehabil 1988; 2:31.

Saal J. Rehabilitation of sports-related lumbar spine injuries. Phys Med Rehabil: State of the Art Reviews 1987; 1.

Zucherman J, Schofferman J. Pathology of failed back surgery syndrome: background and diagnostic alternatives. Spine: State of the Art Reviews 1986; 1:1.

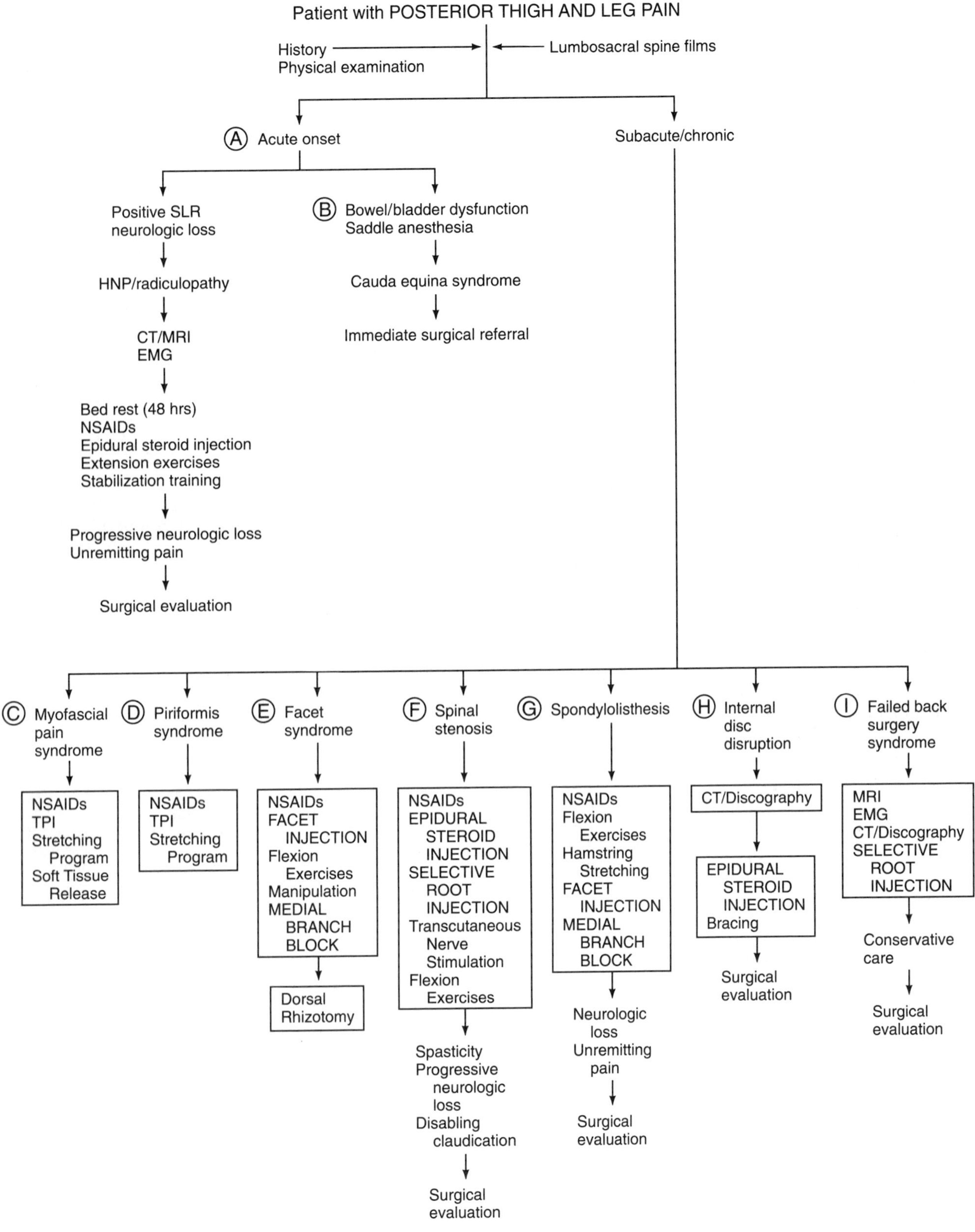

Patient with POSTERIOR THIGH AND LEG PAIN
History
Physical examination
Lumbosacral spine films
(A) Acute onset
Subacute/chronic
Positive SLR
neurologic loss
HNP/radiculopathy
CT/MRI
EMG
Bed rest (48 hrs)
NSAIDs
Epidural steroid injection
Extension exercises
Stabilization training
Progressive neurologic loss
Unremitting pain
Surgical evaluation
(B) Bowel/bladder dysfunction
Saddle anesthesia
Cauda equina syndrome
Immediate surgical referral
(C) Myofascial pain syndrome
NSAIDs
TPI
Stretching Program
Soft Tissue Release
(D) Piriformis syndrome
NSAIDs
TPI
Stretching Program
(E) Facet syndrome
NSAIDs
FACET INJECTION
Flexion Exercises
Manipulation
MEDIAL BRANCH BLOCK
Dorsal Rhizotomy
(F) Spinal stenosis
NSAIDs
EPIDURAL STEROID INJECTION
SELECTIVE ROOT INJECTION
Transcutaneous Nerve Stimulation
Flexion Exercises
Spasticity
Progressive neurologic loss
Disabling claudication
Surgical evaluation
(G) Spondylolisthesis
NSAIDs
Flexion Exercises
Hamstring Stretching
FACET INJECTION
MEDIAL BRANCH BLOCK
Neurologic loss
Unremitting pain
Surgical evaluation
(H) Internal disc disruption
CT/Discography
EPIDURAL STEROID INJECTION
Bracing
Surgical evaluation
(I) Failed back surgery syndrome
MRI
EMG
CT/Discography
SELECTIVE ROOT INJECTION
Conservative care
Surgical evaluation

PIRIFORMIS SYNDROME

Jonathan P. Lester, M.D.
Kevin L. Kenworthy, M.D., C.P.T., M.C.

Piriformis syndrome is a benign, myofascial pain disorder that may closely mimic other causes of low back pain and disability. The piriformis muscle arises from the inner aspect of the sacrum, runs laterally through the sciatic notch, passes over the sciatic nerve, and inserts onto the greater trochanter. In some cases a portion of the sciatic nerve may pass through the piriformis. Contraction of the piriformis muscle assists in external rotation of the hip.

A. Mild trauma to the buttocks or hips, postural overuse, or disturbance of the pelvic musculature may initiate the formation of a painful trigger point in the piriformis muscle belly. Secondary spasm of the piriformis muscle may irritate the sciatic nerve and produce radicular pain complaints. Accurate diagnosis is made by appropriate historical information and physical examination. Treatment is conservative, and complete resolution of symptoms is achieved in most cases.

B. Patients with piriformis syndrome may complain of deep aching pain radiating to the hip, groin, buttock, or posterior thigh. The pain is often described as aching or cramping and is made worse with stooping, sitting, squatting, or lifting. Patients may also describe radicular symptoms in the distribution of the sciatic nerve. The onset of symptoms is often related to pelvic trauma or overuse. Women may complain of dyspareunia. Physical examination is remarkable for tenderness over the piriformis muscle belly and is exacerbated by passive internal rotation of the hip (Freiberg's sign) or resisted external rotation of the hip (Pace's sign). Rectal examination is very helpful in confirming the diagnosis. Other causes of low back and posterior thigh pain are excluded by additional physical examination techniques.

C. Conservative care consists of local trigger point injection (TPI), aggressive stretching protocols, and NSAIDs. Narcotics and muscle relaxants are not indicated. In our pain clinic, TPI is performed by injecting 20 ml of 0.5% lidocaine through a 22-gauge 3 1/2 inch spinal needle into the piriformis muscle belly. Steroids have also been added to the injection and are thought by some to improve success. Some patients may experience partial block of the sciatic nerve and require observation in the clinic for the duration of the anesthesia. For this reason, we avoid the use of a long-acting local anesthetic such as bupivacaine. After the TPI, patients are taught an aggressive stretching program for the piriformis and gluteal muscles. Most cases are resolved with a few visits to the clinic, and recurrences are prevented by a maintenance stretching program. Severe cases unresponsive to conservative therapy may benefit from surgical resection of the piriformis muscle.

References

Bernard T, Kirkaldy-Willis W. Recognizing specific causes of nonspecific low back pain. Clin Orthop Rel Res 1987; 217:266.

Durrani Z, Winnie AP. Piriformis muscle syndrome: An underdiagnosed cause of sciatica. J Pain Sympt Manag 1991; 6:374.

Ludvig F, Siewer P, Bernhard P. The piriformis muscle syndrome: Sciatic nerve entrapment treated with section of the piriformis muscle. Acta Orthop Scand 1981; 52:73.

Pace J, Nagle D. Piriform syndrome. West J Med 1976; 124:435.

Steiner C, Staubs C, Buhlinger C. Piriformis syndrome: Pathogenesis, diagnosis, and treatment. JAOA 1987; 87:318.

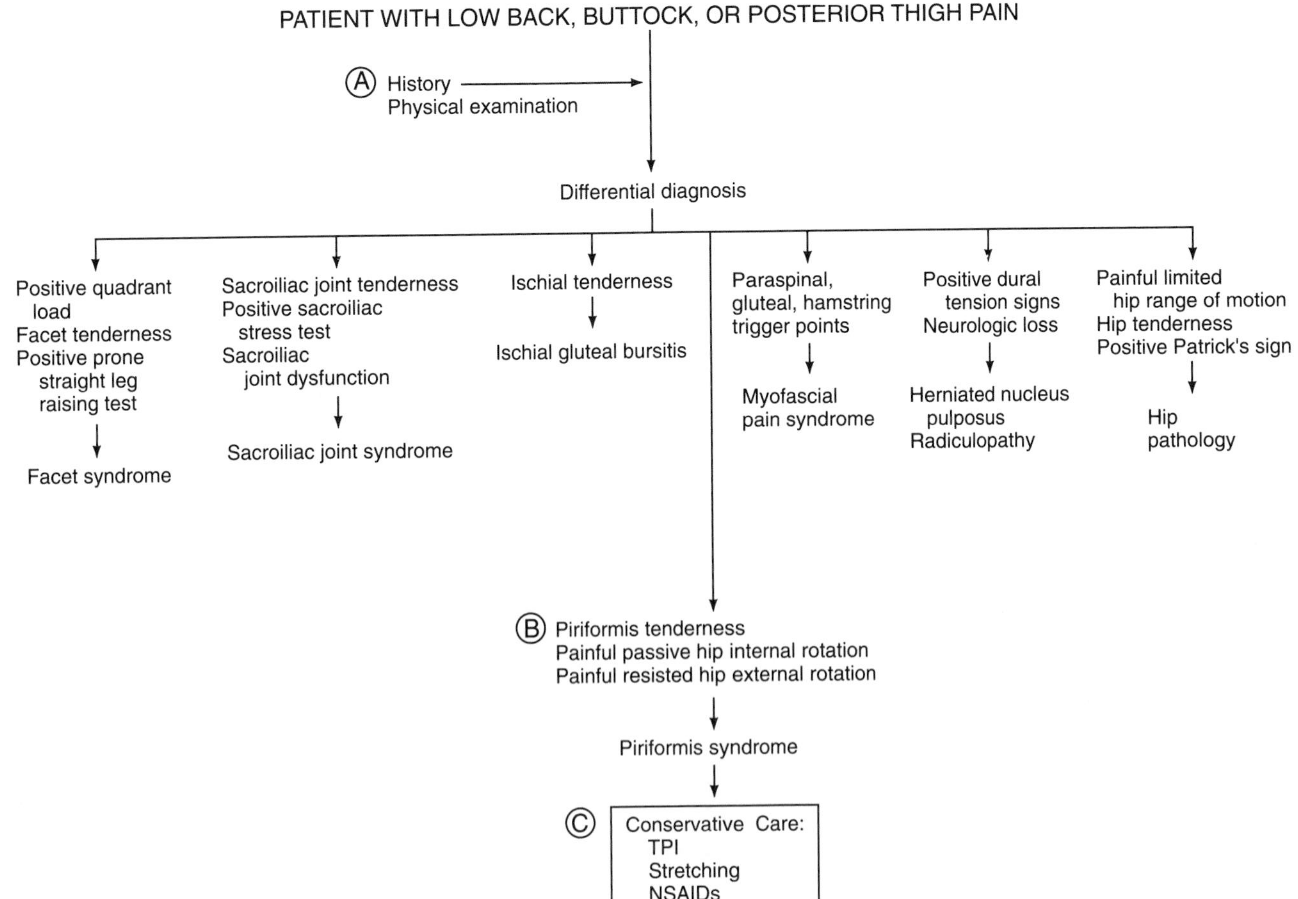

PATIENT WITH LOW BACK, BUTTOCK, OR POSTERIOR THIGH PAIN
(A) History
Physical examination
Differential diagnosis
Positive quadrant load
Facet tenderness
Positive prone straight leg raising test
Facet syndrome
Sacroiliac joint tenderness
Positive sacroiliac stress test
Sacroiliac joint dysfunction
Sacroiliac joint syndrome
Ischial tenderness
Ischial gluteal bursitis
Paraspinal, gluteal, hamstring trigger points
Myofascial pain syndrome
Positive dural tension signs
Neurologic loss
Herniated nucleus pulposus
Radiculopathy
Painful limited hip range of motion
Hip tenderness
Positive Patrick's sign
Hip pathology
(B) Piriformis tenderness
Painful passive hip internal rotation
Painful resisted hip external rotation
Piriformis syndrome
(C) Conservative Care:
TPI
Stretching
NSAIDs

REFLEX SYMPATHETIC DYSTROPHY OF THE LOWER EXTREMITIES

David Vanos, M.D.

Successful treatment of reflex sympathetic dystrophy (RSD) (sometimes now referred to as sympathetically maintained pain [SMP]) requires proper diagnosis of the condition through the recognition of its clinical features and confirmation of the diagnosis through the use of selective sympathetic blocks. After confirmation of the diagnosis, serial sympathetic blocks usually are required for definitive treatment along with physical therapy, medication, and psychological support and treatment. In addition, any concomitant pain entities (e.g., myofascial pain, bursitis, arthritis) that may be producing RSD secondarily must be addressed.

A. The clinical presentation of RSD is one of continuous burning pain in an extremity (or a portion of the extremity) after some form of trauma or microtrauma that does not involve major nerve injury and is associated with sympathetic overactivity. Symptoms include an early phase with vasodilation, swelling, stiffness, hyperhidrosis, allodynia, hyperalgesia, hyperpathia, and temperature increase. The late phase consists of vasoconstriction, coolness, atrophy of skin appendages, and atrophy of bone (Sudeck's atrophy). The evaluation may include radiography and bone scans to document bony atrophy and blood flow changes, respectively, consistent with RSD. Thermography may also aid diagnosis. The differential diagnosis should include fracture, sprain, strain, thrombosis, post-traumatic vasospasm, and causalgia.

B. The confirmation of lower extremity RSD by ablation of the pain using sympathetic blocks may be accomplished by lumbar sympathetic block (LSB), IV regional sympathetic block (with guanethidine), and with IV phentolamine.

C. Rule out placebo response to such blocks by carefully noting when pain relief occurs, correlation with signs of sympathetic block in the affected extremity, and duration of relief.

D. Once RSD is confirmed by diagnostic sympathetic blockade, serial blocks may be necessary to accomplish permanent ablation or near-ablation of the syndrome. Other variants of IV regional blocks that have been used to treat RSD pain include steroids, methyldopa, reserpine, prazocin, prostaglandins, hydralazine, diazoxide, and calcium channel blockers. I have used the recently released parenteral NSAID, ketorolac, in IV regional block for RSD pain.

E. Include physical therapy early to increase the range of motion of affected joints, decrease swelling, and desensitize the extremity to physical stimuli.

F. Medications including tricyclic antidepressants, NSAIDS, and oral calcium channel blockers may have some utility and should be used when indicated.

G. A psychological evaluation consisting of administration of the Minnesota Multiphasic Personality Inventory (MMPI) and an interview with a clinical psychologist may reveal evidence of depression and/or anxiety amenable to treatment (p 6). This evaluation may be a key element in the treatment of many RSD patients.

H. Consistent success in ablating RSD pain, but without long-term relief, may be an indication to consider permanent chemical, or even surgical, sympathectomy.

References

Löfström JB, Cousins MJ. Sympathetic neural blockade of the upper and lower extremity. In: Cousins MJ, Bridenbaugh PO, eds. Neural blockade in clinical anesthesia and management of pain. 2nd ed. Philadelphia: JB Lippincott, 1988:461.

Poplawski ZJ, et al. Post-traumatic dystrophy of the extremities: a clinical review and trial of treatment. J Bone Joint Surg 1983; 65A:642.

Raja SN, et al. Systemic alpha-adrenergic blockade with phentolamine: a diagnostic test for sympathetically maintained pain. Anesthesiology 1991; 74:691.

Vanos D, Ramamurthy S, et al. Intravenous regional block using ketorolac: preliminary results in the treatment of reflex sympathetic dystrophy. Anesth Analg 1992; 74:139.

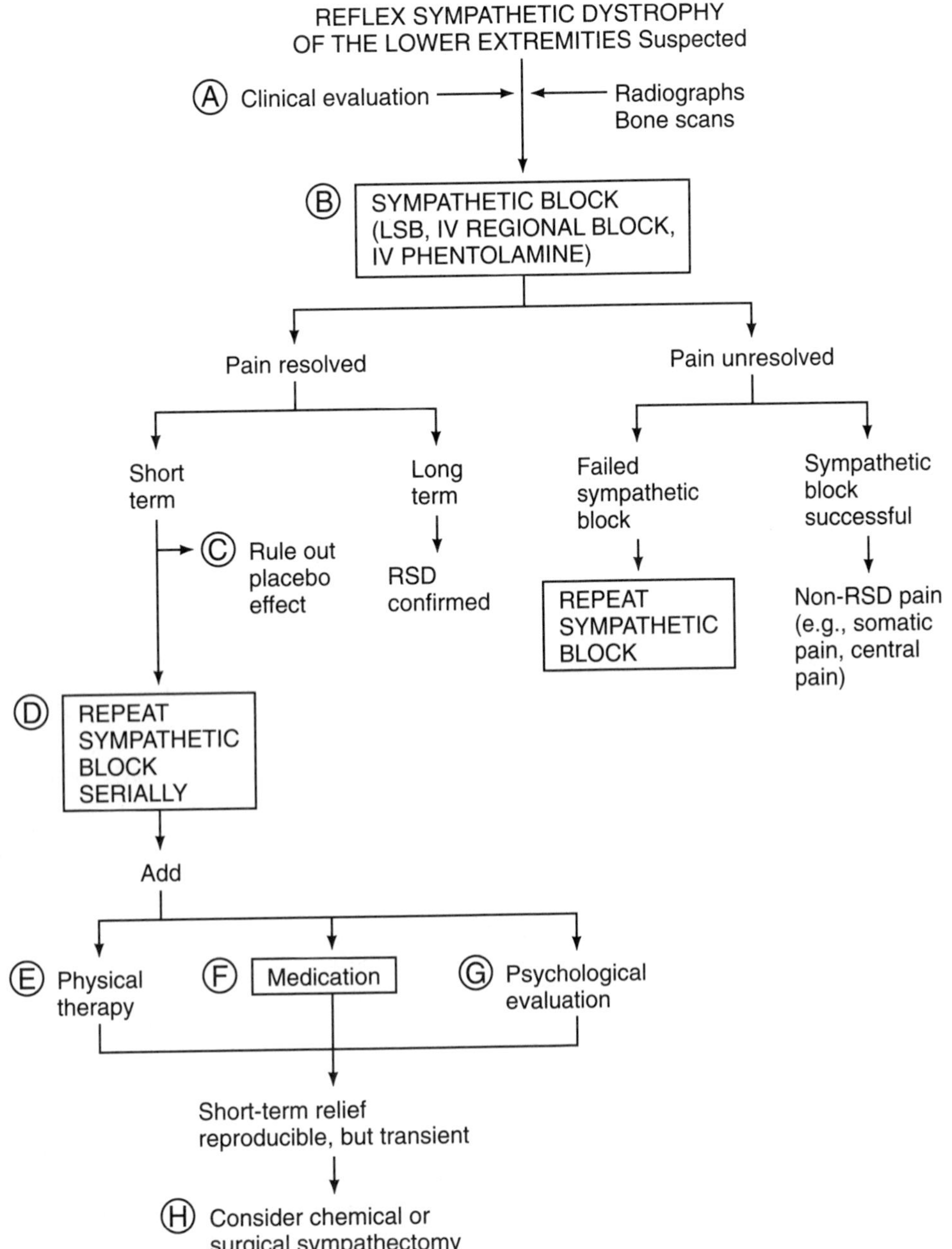
REFLEX SYMPATHETIC DYSTROPHY
OF THE LOWER EXTREMITIES Suspected
(A) Clinical evaluation
Radiographs
Bone scans
(B) SYMPATHETIC BLOCK
(LSB, IV REGIONAL BLOCK,
IV PHENTOLAMINE)
Pain resolved
Pain unresolved
Short
term
Long
term
Failed
sympathetic
block
Sympathetic
block
successful
(C) Rule out
placebo
effect
RSD
confirmed
REPEAT
SYMPATHETIC
BLOCK
Non-RSD pain
(e.g., somatic
pain, central
pain)
(D) REPEAT
SYMPATHETIC
BLOCK
SERIALLY
Add
(E) Physical
therapy
(F) Medication
(G) Psychological
evaluation
Short-term relief
reproducible, but transient
(H) Consider chemical or
surgical sympathectomy

FOOT PAIN

James Griffin, P.T., A.T.C.

Take a careful history to determine the location of pain, type of onset, intensity and quality of pain, pain profile over time, and factors that aggravate or relieve the patient's pain. The physical examination should include inspection, palpation, and evaluation of neurologic status and both active and passive range of motion. A biomechanical assessment should be made with the patient sitting, standing, and walking.

A. An evaluation of footwear must be a part of any treatment of foot pain. Poorly fitting or worn footwear can cause or contribute to pain in the lower extremity. Advise changing to well-fitting shoes or repairing or replacing worn shoes to relieve discomfort.

B. The radiographic examination should include anteroposterior, lateral, and oblique views, obtained while weight bearing if possible. Special views are required to visualize the sesamoids, talocalcaneal, and talonavicular coalitions. Stress views that compare the normal with the affected side can show instability. Bone scans reveal areas of increased uptake and are diagnostic for stress reactions. Soft tissue tumors may be evaluated with CT scan or MRI to determine size and composition.

C. Nerve conduction velocity tests and EMG may show peripheral neuropathies and tarsal tunnel entrapment. Other studies may be necessary to identify various disease processes.

D. Reflex sympathetic dystrophy (RSD) can occur as a result of even a trivial injury to the foot. Early RSD is commonly overlooked and must be suspected when pain is greatly out of proportion to expectation. Prompt recognition and treatment can prevent progression to an irreversible and debilitating condition (p 150).

E. Soft tissue pain from corns and calluses often results from ill-fitting footwear. Verrucae pedis (plantar warts) are differentiated from calluses by extreme sensitivity to lateral compression. Dorsal ganglia are caused by constant irritation from shoes. Myofascial pain can produce discomfort after injury or immobilization of the foot or lower extremity—a common problem, but not often considered as a primary cause of pain (p 46).

F. The great toe, the most common site of ingrown toenails, is subject to disorders of hypermobility, hypomobility, and deformation. The hypermobile first ray can shift weight to other areas, causing pain. Treat with padding or orthotics to normalize weight distribution. Hallux rigidus produces pain and dorsal exostosis in the first metacarpophalangeal (MP) joint, and may respond to NSAIDs and a stiff rocker sole shoe. Hallux valgus may be treated conservatively with accommodative footwear and orthotic control of excess pronation. Surgery may repair deformity and restore normal biomechanics. The sesamoids can become irritated and locally swollen; they respond to NSAIDs and decreased weight bearing until the inflammation resolves. Gout can be well localized to the first MP joint, but may affect the entire medial column of the foot. Medication can control the condition, but surgery may be needed for advanced degeneration.

G. Deformation of the small toes can result in corns and callouses. A long second ray with a hypermobile first ray can produce a painful maldistribution of weight across the metatarsal heads. Padding or orthotic support may be required and surgery may be indicated.

H. Forefoot pain under the metatarsal heads may occur with a splayed or pronated foot, resulting in disproportionate weight bearing. Treatment with a metatarsal bar or selective padding may be sufficient. Morton's neuroma to the space between the third and fourth toe is common and may respond to steroid injection. Suspect stress fractures with forefoot pain. Because radiographs and bone scans are normal in the acute setting, pain with activity and relief with rest may be the only findings.

I. Midfoot discomfort from arch strain may occur as an interaction of foot mechanics, usually excessive pronation, activity, poor footwear, and insufficiency of the musculature supporting the medial arch. Treatment may include supportive footwear, activity modification, and orthotic devices to control pronation of the foot. Severe injury may result in instability of the metatarsocuneiform joints, requiring casting or surgical stabilization. The cuboid may sublux with an inversion injury and be mistaken for a "chronic ankle sprain." The injury responds to manipulation and supportive padding or orthotics. Tarsal coalition produces pain with activity and may result in arthritis of the subtalar or other joints. Pain, lack of subtalar motion, and radiographic studies confirm the diagnosis. Conservative treatment with supportive shoes and biomechanical support precede surgical intervention.

J. Rear foot pain may be produced by a talar subluxation secondary to inversion stress. Like the cuboid subluxation, this pain is often treated as a "chronic sprain." This entity may require injection of the sinus tarsi followed by manipulation of the talus and ankle rehabilitation. Orthotic support may be required. Tarsal tunnel syndrome produces burning pain or numbness in the distribution of the posterior tibial nerve. The nerve is tender and a Tinel's sign may be present. Treat conservatively with NSAIDs, injection of local anesthetic and steroids, or TENS to correct hyperpronation. Persistent symptoms require surgical decompression. Plantar fasciitis is an irritation of the

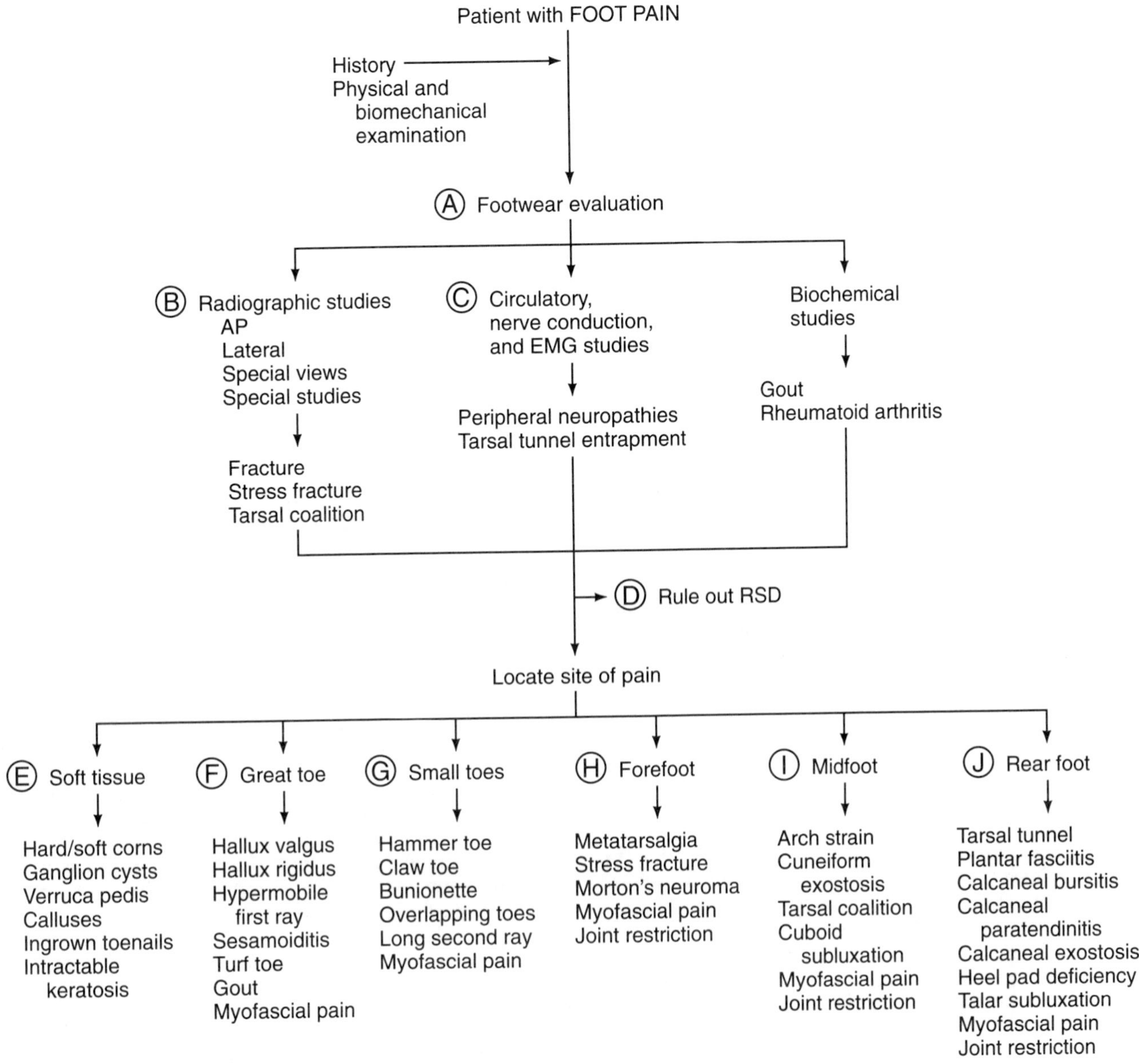

proximal insertion of the plantar fascia in which tenderness is found on the anteriomedial aspect of the heel. Treatment consists of NSAIDs and well-made shoes with medial arch support. Injection, a walking cast, or rarely, surgical release, is required in resistant cases. Posterior heel pain can originate with irritation of the insertion of the Achilles tendon, the bursa, or the loose tissue immediately around the Achilles insertion. Generally, treat conservatively. NSAIDs, use of a heel lift, moderation of activity, ice massage, and stretching of a tight Achilles tendon may all be beneficial. If simple measures fail, a short leg cast and immobilization may be required, but surgical removal of inflamed tissues is rarely required.

The goal of orthotic control of foot mechanics is to maintain the foot in a biomechanically neutral position and equally distribute stress. Well-made orthotics compensate for biomechanical disparities in the foot, ankle, and the lower extremity to achieve optimal results.

References

Beirane DR, Burckhardt JG, Peters VJ. Subtalar joint subluxation. J Am Podiatr Med Assoc 1984; 74:523.

Bonica JJ, Lippert FG. Pain in the leg, ankle, and foot. In: Bonica JJ, ed. The management of pain. 2nd ed. Vol 2. Philadelphia: Lea & Febiger, 1990.

McRae R. Clinical orthopedic examination. 3rd ed. New York: Churchill Livingstone, 1990.

Newell SG, Woodle A. Cuboid syndrome. Phys Sports Med 1981; 1:71.

Travell JG, Simmons DG. Myofascial pain and dysfunction. Baltimore: Williams & Wilkins, 1983.

Wooden MJ. Biomechanical evaluation for functional orthotics. In: Donatelli R, ed. The biomechanics of the foot and ankle. Philadelphia: FA Davis, 1990.

EVALUATION OF INTERMITTENT CLAUDICATION

Susan J. Dreyer, M.D.

Intermittent claudication is the most common presenting symptom of chronic obstructive peripheral arterial disease. Patients complain of buttock and leg pain with ambulation which is quickly relieved with rest. Pain in the buttocks and legs, extreme fatigue, and muscle cramping all occur more quickly if the speed of ambulation increases or the patient walks uphill. Atherosclerotic occlusive disease has a slow, insidious onset. The prevalence of claudication ranges from 1.3% to 5.8% of persons >60 years of age. The site of pain correlates well with the site of obstruction, occupation, and lifestyle.

A. Intermittent claudication is diagnosed by characteristic history and physical signs of decreased lower extremity perfusion.

B. Pain while walking, which is relieved promptly with rest, is characteristic. Unlike pseudoclaudication, the patient need not sit, squat, or recline to achieve relief. Dependent rubor is common, as is pallor with elevation. In severe cases, the pain diminishes with placement of the limb in a dependent position.

C. A differential diagnosis includes spinal stenosis, arthritis, degenerative disc disease, myofascial pain, thromboangiitis obliterans, acute arterial occlusion, compartment syndrome, muscle cramps, and McArdle's disease.

D. A comparison of systolic pressures between the arm and thigh, calf, and ankle provides noninvasive confirmation of the area of occlusion. Normal ankle–arm indices are >1. Sphygmomanometer determinations in diabetics are often not obtainable because of noncompressible, calcified vessels. Other flow studies such as directional Doppler flow velocity detection and pulse volume recording provide noninvasive means to study the blood flow to an extremity both before and after exercise. Postexercise values correlate better with the extent of disease.

E. In mild to moderate disease, pain occurs with activity and does not interfere with vocation or lifestyle.

F. Cessation of smoking is imperative. Exercise (e.g., walking, bicycling) is beneficial when done daily for 30 to 60 minutes at an unpainful level. Blood pressure should be controlled, maintaining diastolic pressure near 90 mm Hg to ensure adequate collateral perfusion. Foot care is essential, including trimming toenails straight; avoiding cold exposure; keeping the skin warm, dry, and supple; and inspecting the feet daily. Underlying systemic disease such as congestive heart failure, chronic obstructive pulmonary disease, and diabetes must be rigorously controlled. Treat polycythemia to keep the hematocrit <55%. Weight loss and control of hyperlipidemia are also recommended. Give NSAIDs for pain; more severe pain may require aspirin or acetaminophen with codeine. Vasodilators and anticoagulants are no longer considered effective treatment. Pentoxifylline's efficacy is still undetermined, and fibrinolytic therapy has negligible benefit in chronic occlusion.

G. Severe chronic obstructive peripheral arterial disease is characterized by pain at rest, ulcers, ischemic neuropathy causing numbness, and dysesthesias, or an ankle arm index <0.6 in addition to intermittent claudication.

H. Incapacitating symptoms that interfere with lifestyle or livelihood require surgical evaluation. Gangrene, nonhealing ulcers, ankle systolic pressure <45 mm Hg, or ischemic pain at rest are other surgical indications.

I. Patients with substantial surgical risk or nongraftable lesions are not candidates for surgery.

J. Surgical revascularization procedures include femoropopliteal bypass graft, aortoiliac endarterectomy or graft, femorotibial graft, femoroperoneal vein graft, infrapopliteal bypass graft, and percutaneous transluminal angioplasty for aortoiliac disease. Use of an adequate caliber vein (4 mm) is preferable to an artificial graft. When possible, use regional anesthesia for these procedures. Amputation is the alternative for life-threatening, nongraftable disease.

K. Chemical sympathectomy can bring significant relief to most nonsurgical candidates, with more relief being obtained from rest pain than from claudication pain. Percutaneous sympathetic blockade can be done as an outpatient procedure.

References

Bonica JJ. Pain due to vascular disease. In: Bonica JJ, ed. The management of pain. 2nd ed. Philadelphia: Lea & Febiger, 1990:506.

Radack K, Wyderski R. Conservative management of intermittent claudication. Ann Intern Med 1990; 113:135.

Whittemore AD, Mannick JA. Intermittent claudication. In: Branch WT Jr., ed. Office practice of medicine. 2nd ed. Philadelphia: WB Saunders, 1987:182.

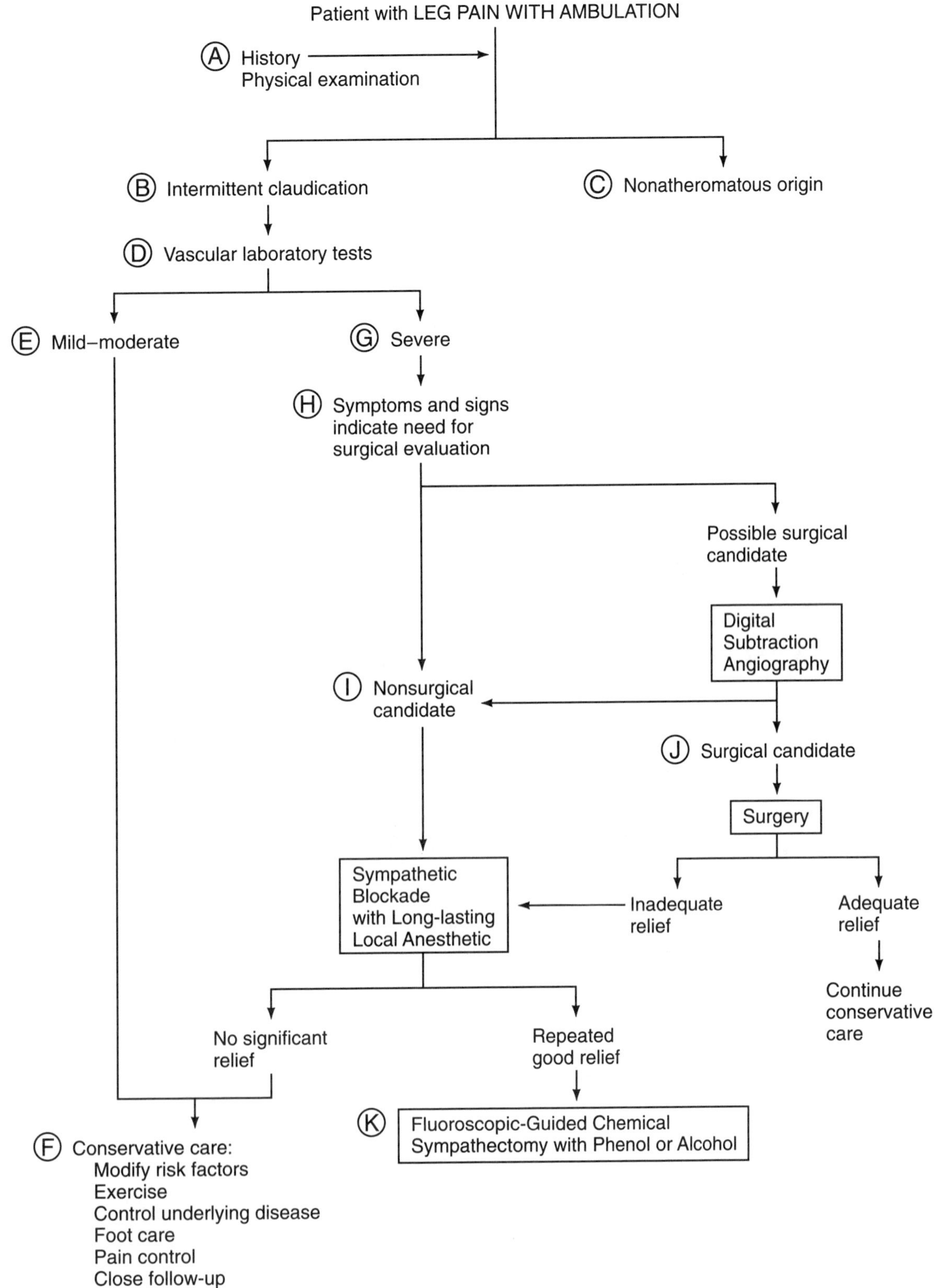

Patient with LEG PAIN WITH AMBULATION
(A) History
Physical examination
(B) Intermittent claudication
(C) Nonatheromatous origin
(D) Vascular laboratory tests
(E) Mild–moderate
(G) Severe
(H) Symptoms and signs indicate need for surgical evaluation
Possible surgical candidate
Digital Subtraction Angiography
(I) Nonsurgical candidate
(J) Surgical candidate
Surgery
Sympathetic Blockade with Long-lasting Local Anesthetic
Inadequate relief
Adequate relief
Continue conservative care
No significant relief
Repeated good relief
(K) Fluoroscopic-Guided Chemical Sympathectomy with Phenol or Alcohol
(F) Conservative care:
Modify risk factors
Exercise
Control underlying disease
Foot care
Pain control
Close follow-up

PEDIATRIC PAIN

ACUTE PAIN IN THE PEDIATRIC PATIENT

Dawn E. Webster, M.D.

Children experience pain as severely as if not more so than adults. The treatment of acute pain in children has been complicated, however, by difficulty in evaluating the child in pain, misconceptions concerning the use of narcotic analgesics in children, and the lack of experience with regional anesthetic techniques in children. Two areas of acute pain—postoperative pain and burn pain—are discussed here and may provide a basis for the treatment of acute pain of other types.

A. Postoperative pain varies for a given procedure and a given patient. There is no "right" amount of pain for a procedure, and children who complain of pain should be believed. Because some children do not complain of pain either because of fear or the lack of necessary communication skills, medical personnel should maintain a high index of suspicion. The use of developmentally appropriate pain measures, and the careful observation of behavioral and, to a lesser extent, physiologic, parameters may help in the evaluation. Parents' observations are also useful.

B. Regional anesthetic techniques are particularly valued in the postoperative setting, but their use may be extrapolated to other types of pain (trauma, burns, cancer pain). Toxic doses of local anesthetics are considered to be the same as for adults, because no evidence exists to the contrary. The most popular of techniques, the caudal block, is relatively easy to perform and has minimal complications. Other blocks that have been used with success in children include the ilioinguinal, iliohypogastric, penile, intercostal, interpleural, brachial plexus, femoral, and epidural. Perform regional techniques with general anesthetic or heavy sedation, because children are frightened of the needles and there may be some pain involved in placement of the block. Fentanyl and preservative-free morphine in the intrathecal and epidural space is useful in pediatric patients. Side effects are similar to those in adults and include respiratory depression, pruritus, and nausea and vomiting. Contraindications to this technique include infection at the site of block, parental refusal, and coagulopathy.

C. The mainstay of postoperative pain relief is pharmacologic (Table 1). For mild pain, acetaminophen, 10 mg per kilogram, in oral or suppository form, along with the comfort of a parent's presence may be all that is needed. For more severe pain, oral or IV narcotics titrated to effect and given on a routine basis will usually provide relief. Side effects should be actively monitored and treated. Children sometimes deny pain to avoid the nausea or somnolence associated with medication. Avoid intramuscular injections whenever possible, because children are notoriously fearful of needles. Children >3 months of age have no more predilection to respiratory depression from narcotics than do adults; do not withhold analgesics because of overexaggerated fear of this complication. Fear of addiction is also not a valid reason for withholding treatment for acute pain—addiction in the acute setting rarely, if ever, occurs in pediatric patients. Infants <3 months of age must also have relief from acute pain, but more intensive monitoring for respiratory depression and even more careful titration of the narcotic dose is needed. Use patient-controlled analgesia (PCA) in adolescents, for whom a sense of control is important. Postoperative patients as young as 5 years of age can also benefit from PCA. Topically administered anesthetic agents are useful in certain types of postoperative pain. Two percent lidocaine is effective in postcircumcision patients. Infiltration of the incision with 0.5% bupivacaine at the end of a hernia repair can prevent or ameliorate post-herniorrhaphy pain. These simple techniques have minimal complications when performed correctly and eliminate the systemic side effects incurred with narcotics.

TABLE 1 Recommended Starting Doses for Analgesia

Acetaminophen	10–15 mg/kg PO q4h
Codeine	0.5–1 mg/kg PO q4h
Fentanyl	0.5–2 μg/kg IV q1–2h
Morphine	0.08–0.1 mg/kg IV q2h
	0.2–0.4 mg/kg PO q4h
Meperidine	0.8–1 mg/kg IV q2h
	0.8–1.3 mg/kg IM/SC q3–4h

D. Burn pain originates not only from the injury itself, but also from the pain at graft donor sites, the anxiety-provoking pain of dressing changes and debridement, and the discomfort of physical therapy. The extent and depth of the burn directly relate to the intensity of the pain. Pain often is poorly controlled in these patients, and children with burns are even less likely to receive anesthetics and analgesics than are adults. The pharmacologic management of burn pain includes acetaminophen or choline magnesium trisalicylate for mild or background pain. These patients, already at risk for stress ulcers, are not given aspirin. The mainstay of management is with narcotics, preferably via oral or IV routes. IV narcotics may be given as infusions or regularly scheduled injections. Fentanyl may be useful for dressing changes, but may be limited as an infusion because of its association with chest wall rigidity, and with high-dose requirements, because of the development of tolerance. The pharmokinetics of morphine may be altered in burn patients, so titration to effect is required. The fear of addiction is unfounded in these patients. Physical dependence may be treated by slow, careful weaning from narcotics, once the pain is gone. Treat side effects of narcotics aggressively.

E. Management of the pain of dressing changes is of utmost importance in burn patients. Research indi-

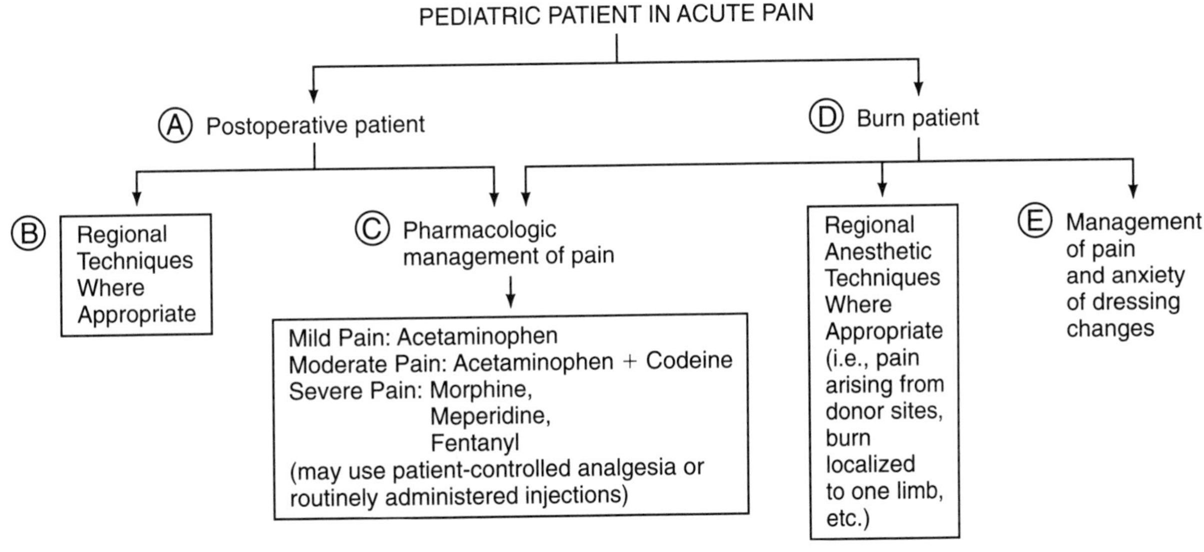

cates that one successful approach is to allow the patient some control during the dressing change: e.g., in some institutions the child is allowed to select the time of dressing change so that he or she knows other times are "safe." The patient can also be encouraged to help with the removal of bandages and application of creams. Helpfulness and cooperation should be positively reinforced with praise. Children who are not prepared for this approach may benefit from alternate techniques, such as keeping the injury from sight and distracting the child during the procedure. Medication with fentanyl or morphine 5 minutes prior to painful dressing changes and education of the patient about the importance of the dressing changes in the healing process are also important in improving tolerance to the procedure.

References

Mcgrath PJ, Unruh AM. Pain in children and adolescents. New York: Elsevier, 1987.

Rice LJ. Management of acute pain in the pediatric patient. Dannemiller Refresher Courses, 1991.

Rice LJ. Regional anesthesia. Dannemiller Refresher Courses, 1991.

Ross DM, Ross SA. Childhood pain: current issues, research and management. Baltimore: Urban & Schwarzenberg, 1988.

Shannon M, Berde CB. Pharmacologic management of pain in children and adolescents. Pediatr Clin North Am 1989; 36:855.

MANAGEMENT OF PAINFUL PROCEDURES IN PEDIATRIC PATIENTS

Dawn E. Webster, M.D.

Children experience many painful diagnostic and therapeutic procedures during treatment for various medical illnesses. For many children the pain associated with bone marrow aspiration and lumbar puncture is considered among the "worst imaginable" of pains, often more severe than that caused by the disease process. Also, it is thought that patients who undergo repeated painful procedures actually become sensitized, rather than desensitized, to these procedures. In spite of this, this pain is frequently ignored, partly because it is difficult for physicians, intent on patients' well-being, to accept that they may be causing a child distress, and partly because of a lack of established guidelines for management. Very few institutions have established protocols specifically addressing the issue of pain management during procedures. We must address this problem if we are to give conscientious, compassionate care to our pediatric patients.

A. The discomfort caused by a planned procedure should be anticipated and a careful, developmentally appropriate plan made. Since the first experience with a procedure sets the stage for future procedures, attention to the problem of painful procedures must be given early in the disease process, particularly for a child who is likely to require multiple procedures. Psychological preparation, including information and a chance to "rehearse" events, should begin as soon as a procedure is planned. Parents often give reliable information concerning how their child will respond to a situation, which can be helpful in the planning process. Therapy should be given in a treatment room, never in the patient's bed. Parents should be allowed as much contact as possible with their infant or child throughout the procedure. Adolescents should be allowed some control in the development of a pain management plan and a decision about the extent of parental involvement. Finally, when possible, the best qualified individual should perform the procedure, particularly in a child who will require multiple procedures.

B. Psychological methods that may help in preparation for procedures include hypnosis, behavior therapy, and cognitive-behavioral intervention. Hypnosis has proved effective in ameliorating the pain of lumbar punctures and bone marrow aspirations in some children and adolescents. Cognitive-behavioral intervention (a combination of "thought-stopping" positive reinforcement, emotive imagery, and behavior rehearsal) has been used effectively in children with cancer. In "thought stopping," a child learns to cope with fear about a procedure by thinking of positive things about the procedure, condensing them, and repeating them anytime fearfulness or anxiety prevails. Emotive imagery calls for including the child's fantasy heroes (e.g., Superman or Batman) into the scheme. Behavior rehearsal, encouraging the child to play "doctor" to a doll or teddy, is done under the care of a child life specialist or under nursing supervision.

C. Sedation is an useful adjunct in preparing children for procedures (Table 1). The American Academy of Pediatrics has issued safety guidelines for sedation. The practitioner should have equipment readily available to assist ventilation and to resuscitate the child. Sedated patients must have heart rate, respiratory rate, the color of mucous membranes, and airway patency monitored by a second person. The patient must never be left unattended. Conscious sedation, that which allows the patient to make appropriate responses to verbal or physical stimulation, requires the use of an agent with a large margin of safety, e.g., chloral hydrate. Deep sedation requires BP monitoring in addition to other monitors and a third person to assist the operator. Adherence to an NPO schedule is necessary to help prevent aspiration (Table 2).

D. Painful "sticks" (venipuncture) should be consolidated, intramuscular injections avoided, and local anesthetics used to place IV catheters. If a central or arterial line is in place, consider whether some samples could be drawn from them to avoid venipuncture. Any child >2 years of age should be informed about the procedure that is to take place. Distraction of the child during the procedure may be

TABLE 1 Dosages of Sedatives and Opioids for Painful Procedures*

	Oral	*Intravenous (give 3–5 min before procedure)*
Midazolam	0.5 mg/kg up to 15 mg max 15 min before procedure	0.05 mg/kg
Diazepam	0.2–0.3 mg/kg max	
Morphine		0.05–0.1 mg/kg over 2 min
Fentanyl†		1–2 μg/kg‡

*These doses are guidelines only; titrate to effect.
†Fentanyl has been noted to cause chest wall rigidity, bradycardia, and respiratory depression, particularly when administered with midazolam.
‡Naxolone must be readily available if narcotics are used.

TABLE 2 NPO Schedule for Procedures

	No solids or milk after midnight
0–3 years	Clear liquids up to 4 hours before procedure
3–6 years	Clear liquids up to 6 hours before procedure
>7 years	Clear liquids up to 8 hours before procedure

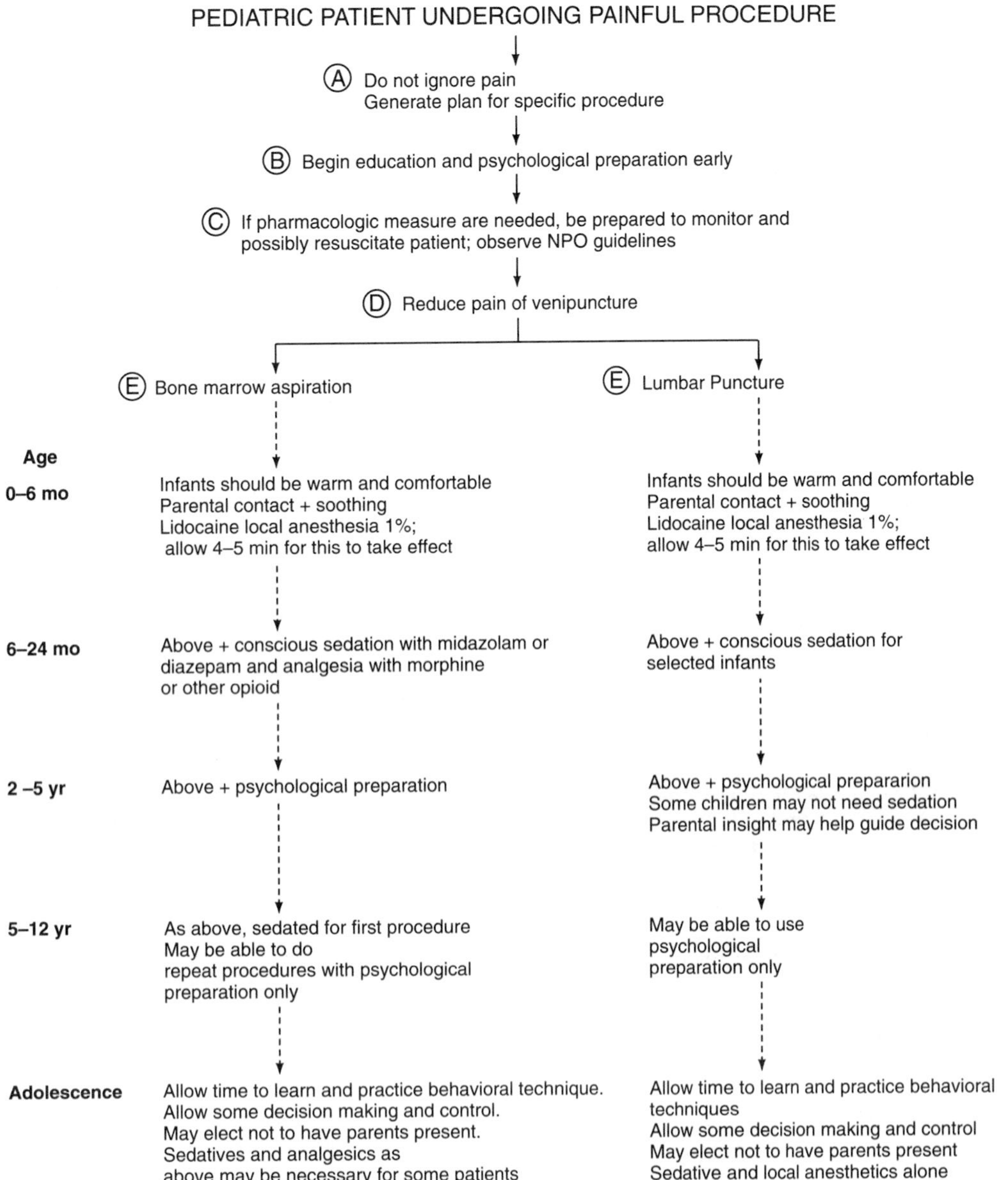

helpful. Skin patches have been developed that may be applied to the skin before venipuncture, but these must remain in place for a prolonged period before analgesia is adequate. Sedation is recommended for central line placement in children. Development of techniques and equipment that reduce the pain of these other "sticks" (e.g., heel and finger lances) is needed.

E. Bone marrow aspirations and lumbar punctures are among the most painful of procedures and must be performed repeatedly in some children. The use of a developmentally appropriate approach to preparation, sedation, and analgesia for these procedures is recommended. They should be performed by the most skilled practitioner available, using as painless a technique as possible.

References

American Academy of Pediatrics, Committee on Drugs, Section on Anesthesiology. Guidelines for the elective use of conscious sedation, deep sedation, and general anesthesia in pediatric patients. Pediatrics 1985; 76:317.

McGrath PJ, Unruh AM. Medically caused pain. In: Pain in children and adolescents. New York: Elsevier, 1987.

Report of the Consensus Conference on the Management of Pain in Childhood Cancer. Part 2. Pediatrics (Suppl) 1990; 86:5.

Schecter NL. The undertreatment of pain in children: An overview. Pediatr Clin North Am 1989; 36:781.

Zeltzer L, Jay S, Fisher DM. The management of pain associated with pediatric procedures. Pediatr Clin North Am 1989; 36:941.

CHRONIC AND RECURRENT PAIN DURING CHILDHOOD

Dawn E. Webster, M.D.

Chronic pain, pain that lasts for a long time and serves no useful function, exists in children and must be treated. To fail to treat a child's pain is inhumane and may lead to long-term physical, cognitive, and developmental problems. The evaluation of pain in infants and children is difficult, not only because young children cannot report pain, but also because they may be afraid to report it or may not realize that they should be able to have relief. In addition, children who try to complain of pain are sometimes ignored, misunderstood, or simply not believed.

A. Classic recurrent abdominal pain includes, by definition, at least three attacks of pain severe enough to affect activities, with no known organic cause, occurring over 3 months. It is relatively common in school-aged children. No one cause has been established but many factors have been implicated, including stress, parental role models, and depression. Guidelines for evaluation and treatment include a history and physical examination and appropriate laboratory tests (CBC, sedimentation rate, urinalysis, and others as indicated) to rule out organic causes. Therapy begins by defining all possible organic and psychological factors. Reassure the patient and parents of the benign nature of the pain. A trial of fiber in the diet (10 g supplementary fiber per day for 6 weeks) brings relief to 50% of patients. Techniques that may be beneficial include stress management, behavior modification for parents who unintentionally reward pain behavior, treatment of depression, and dietary changes in the case of constipation or lactose intolerance. Children who do not improve should be considered for further investigation only if the pain is severe enough to warrant the cost and possible iatrogenic effects of such a work-up.

B. Colic is defined as inconsolable crying with no physical cause for more than 3 hours a day, 3 days a week, and which continues for at least 3 weeks. It usually resolves by 9 months of age. The cause is undetermined and may be multifactorial. Many therapies have been tried, including rocking, swaddling (extreme swaddling results in hip dislocation and inhibited development), use of a pacifier, auditory stimuli, warmth, change of feedings, response to crying, visual distraction, and carrying. Colic is associated with severe stress to the family and an increased incidence of child abuse. It may also alter long-term child-parent interaction. Management includes empathetic listening, reassurance, and assistance to the mother in obtaining help from spouses, friends, family, or social agencies. Teach the systematic use of soothing methods but discourage frequent changes in feedings.

C. As with adults, headaches in children require that underlying disease be determined by history, physical examination, and indicated laboratory tests. Children's headaches differ from those of adults in that muscular and migrainous types are less distinct and the headaches often seem to be a blend of both components. Also, nausea, vomiting, and abdominal pain are more often present in the child. There are contradictory reports on the effects of migraines on school performance and coexistence with learning disabilities. If migraine is suspected, the child should be evaluated by someone experienced with childhood migraines. Migraine headaches in children are usually palliated with aspirin or acetaminophen as opposed to treatment with ergotamine preparations. Propranolol appears to have some prophylactic value as do psychological techniques such as relaxation, biofeedback, and cognitive interventions. Muscle-contraction headaches are also palliated with acetaminophen or aspirin and biofeedback or relaxation techniques. Most children cope with headaches well, without missing school. If a child misses school because of headaches, the syndrome of chronic intractable pain must be considered.

(Continued on page 164)

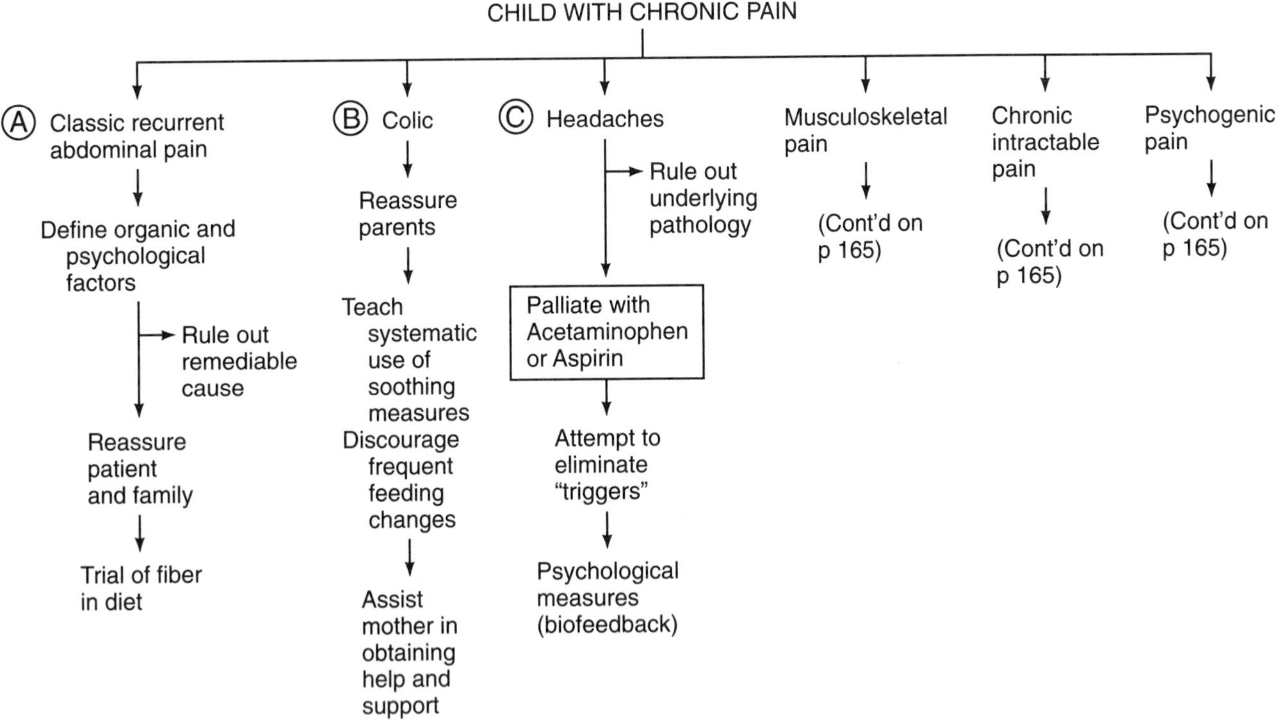
CHILD WITH CHRONIC PAIN
A Classic recurrent abdominal pain
Define organic and psychological factors
Rule out remediable cause
Reassure patient and family
Trial of fiber in diet
B Colic
Reassure parents
Teach systematic use of soothing measures
Discourage frequent feeding changes
Assist mother in obtaining help and support
C Headaches
Rule out underlying pathology
Palliate with Acetaminophen or Aspirin
Attempt to eliminate "triggers"
Psychological measures (biofeedback)
Musculoskeletal pain
(Cont'd on p 165)
Chronic intractable pain
(Cont'd on p 165)
Psychogenic pain
(Cont'd on p 165)

D. Musculoskeletal pain is a common childhood problem, present in 15.5% of school-aged children, with 4.5% of children experiencing reduction in activity for more than 3 months. Included in this category is the acute recurrent pain of juvenile rheumatoid arthritis (JRA). Children with JRA frequently complain of increasing pain as they become older, possibly because they learn to associate the pain with joint disintegration. Counseling these patients may be helpful. Medical treatment includes aspirin and NSAIDs. Fibromyalgia—aches, pains, and stiffness at many sites—which is exaggerated by fatigue, stress, inactivity, and cold damp weather occurs in children (the incidence is unknown). It is treated with NSAIDs and warmth. Reflex sympathetic dystrophy is being recognized with increasing frequency in children after sprains, fractures, or surgery. Again, the incidence is unknown. As with adults, early therapy is needed to prevent dystrophic changes. Treatment includes aggressive physical therapy, sympathetic blockade, and possible high-dose steroids. "Growing" pains—intermittent, incapacitating pain felt deep in the arms or legs, frequently experienced at night—are treated with heat, massage, palliation with aspirin or acetaminophen, stretching exercises, and reassurance. Back pain is rare in children. It usually represents a pathologic condition and warrants a thorough search for underlying disease.

E. Any type of pain syndrome can eventually become a syndrome of chronic intractable pain, defined as pain with a known or unknown cause, which lasts a long time and interferes with the child's life. Many factors contribute to this syndrome, such as family functioning (especially overinvolvement of parents or modeling after parents), depression, stress, and positive reinforcement of pain behavior. The management of chronic intractable pain includes treatment for depression, stress reduction, practice of relaxation techniques, and reinforcement of non-pain behavior. The family should be included. Emphasize to the patient that the goal is not the entire disappearance of pain, but coping with the pain.

F. Psychogenic pain is defined as pain that allows a person to obtain support from the environment that otherwise might not be forthcoming. Its cause is multifactorial, including anxiety, avoidance, direct rewarding of pain behavior, or psychosis. This pain is real and can be disabling. The patient must sense that he or she is heard and believed, or an increase in pain behavior may result. Treat the specific psychological-cause or causes if they can be determined. Emphasize coping with the pain, rather than complete resolution. Include the family in therapy. Evaluate hidden stressors at school, teach relaxation techniques and behavioral skills that seem appropriate, educate, and understand, but do not encourage self-pity. Finally, remember that organic illness and organically caused pain can coexist with psychogenic pain, and be alert for indications that this is occurring.

References

Levine MD, ed. Recurrent pain in children. Pediatr Clin North Am 1984; 31:5.

McGrath PJ, Unruh AM. Pain in children and adolescents. New York: Elsevier, 1987.

Ross DM, Ross SA. Childhood pain: current issues, research and management. Baltimore: Urban & Schwarzenberg, 1988.

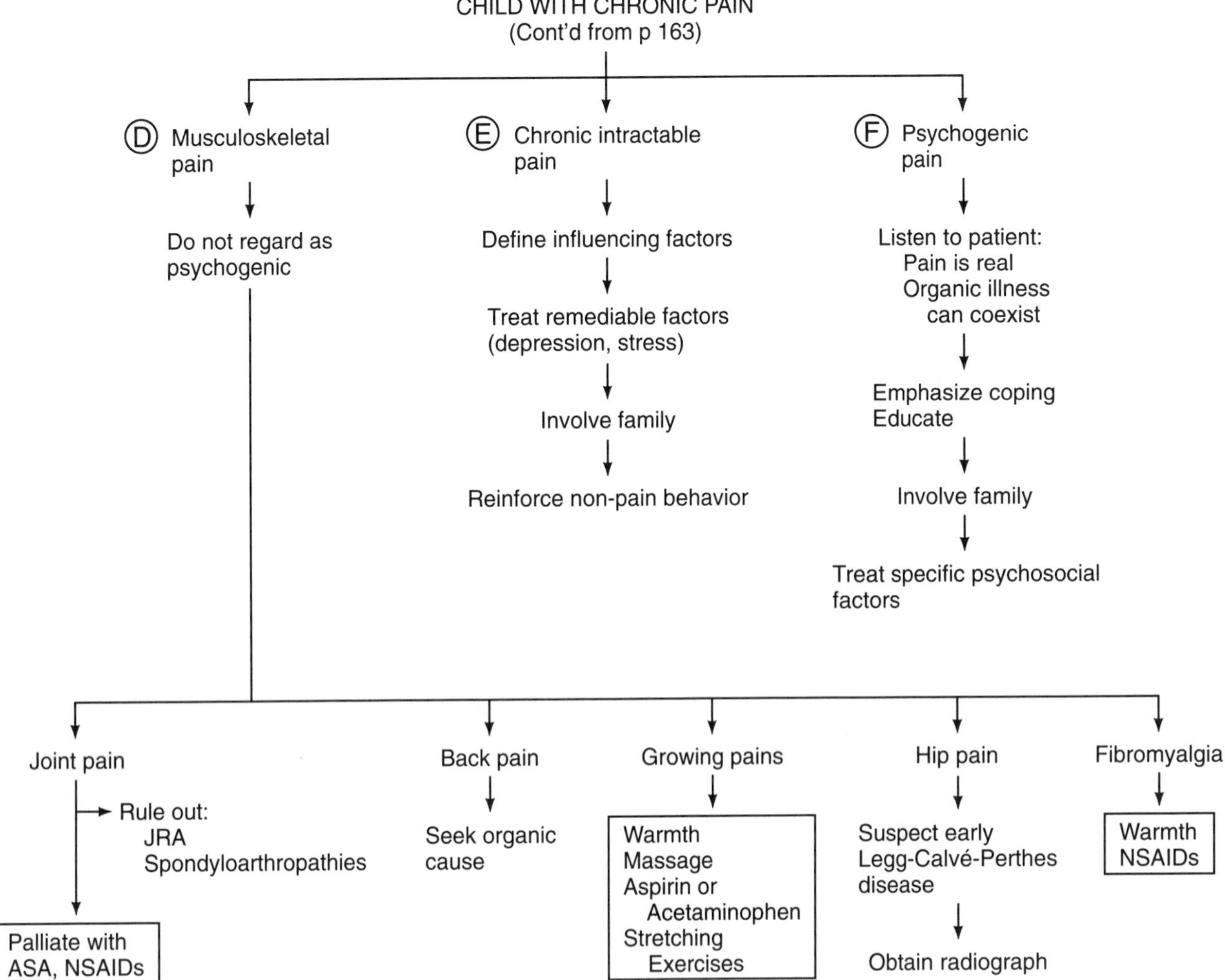
CHILD WITH CHRONIC PAIN
(Cont'd from p 163)
D Musculoskeletal pain
E Chronic intractable pain
F Psychogenic pain
Do not regard as psychogenic
Define influencing factors
Treat remediable factors (depression, stress)
Involve family
Reinforce non-pain behavior
Listen to patient:
Pain is real
Organic illness can coexist
Emphasize coping
Educate
Involve family
Treat specific psychosocial factors
Joint pain
Rule out:
JRA
Spondyloarthropathies
Palliate with ASA, NSAIDs
Back pain
Seek organic cause
Growing pains
Warmth
Massage
Aspirin or Acetaminophen
Stretching Exercises
Hip pain
Suspect early Legg-Calvé-Perthes disease
Obtain radiograph
Fibromyalgia
Warmth
NSAIDs

PAIN IN THE PEDIATRIC CANCER PATIENT

Dawn E. Webster, M.D.

Pain is a significant problem in the child with cancer. At one institution, pain occurred in 50% of hospitalized cancer patients and in 25% of outpatients. The cause of pain in patients with cancer includes tumor pain (primarily from bony invasion by cancer), pain related to painful procedures, and pain related to treatment (oral mucositis, neuropathic pain, postoperative pain, and phantom limb pain).

A. An assessment of the presence of pain should be a routine part of the evaluation of the child with cancer. A pain problem list should be generated, and a treatment plan for different causes of pain made. Frequent reassessment of pain should follow to evaluate the effectiveness of therapy. Personnel who evaluate pain must be aware that there is no "right" amount of pain for a certain amount of tissue damage.

B. If the patient reports pain, he or she should be believed. If the child does not report pain with tissue destruction, the reasons for this discrepancy must be sought (e.g., fear of a "shot," depression). Psychosocial factors that exacerbate pain in children include anxiety, depression, fear, previous pain experience, fear of lack of control, negative interpretation of situation, anxiety of parents and siblings, poor prognosis, boring environment, parental insistence on stoicism, and parental overinvolvement. These factors, if present, should be included in the pain problem list. To help assess the severity of pain, many developmentally appropriate pain scales are now available (Table 1).

C. The first line of treatment of cancer pain is the treatment of remedial causes. Tumor therapy with chemotherapy, radiation, and/or corticosteroids can palliate pain in some instances even if it does not cure the disease. In addition, abscesses, fractures, or other new organic causes of pain may be treatable by surgery or medical management.

D. Incorporate psychological techniques such as hypnosis, relaxation training, imagery, thought stopping, and child life-directed play programs into the child's care early in the disease process to help modify the emotional and psychological factors that contribute to pain and to allow time to master these techniques, some of which will be valuable when painful procedures such as bone marrow aspirations are required. Include parents in this phase of pain management, if possible.

E. For many children, the pain of procedures associated with cancer surpasses the pain of the disease and contributes to fear of treatment of the disease. An early aggressive approach to providing sedation and analgesia for procedures such as bone marrow aspirations and lumbar punctures does much to relieve the anxiety associated with these procedures. Likewise, perform venipunctures and IV catheterizations only when absolutely necessary, time so as to minimize "sticks," and have them done by the most experienced personnel, as painlessly as possible.

F. Most cancer pain can be managed pharmacologically. Use acetaminophen for mild pain. If necessary, NSAIDs may be used in patients with normal platelet counts, but they may cause gastritis. Choline-magnesium salicylate has little effect on bleeding time and causes relatively little gastritis. Aspirin is rarely indicated because of concern for bleeding problems. If these agents do not provide relief from pain, oral codeine may be added. If the oral route is unavailable, small doses of other IV narcotics may be used instead. The IV use of codeine is not recommended. Always avoid intramuscular injections. If these agents are ineffective, try narcotics such as morphine, methadone, hydromorphone, or fentanyl by the IV or, in the case of morphine, methadone, and hydromorphone, the oral route. Narcotic doses should be titrated to effect. When narcotics are in use, naloxone should always be readily available to treat respiratory depression. Narcotics have been used in many forms in children with cancer, including the oral route, single injections, continuous infusion, and patient-controlled analgesia. Do not administer narcotics on an as-needed basis, but schedule in a routine manner. Physical dependence on narcotics is common in these patients and is not usually a problem as long as withdrawal of narcotics is done gradually. Addiction in this setting is extremely rare in adults and there is no reason to believe this is not the case in children.

(Continued on page 168)

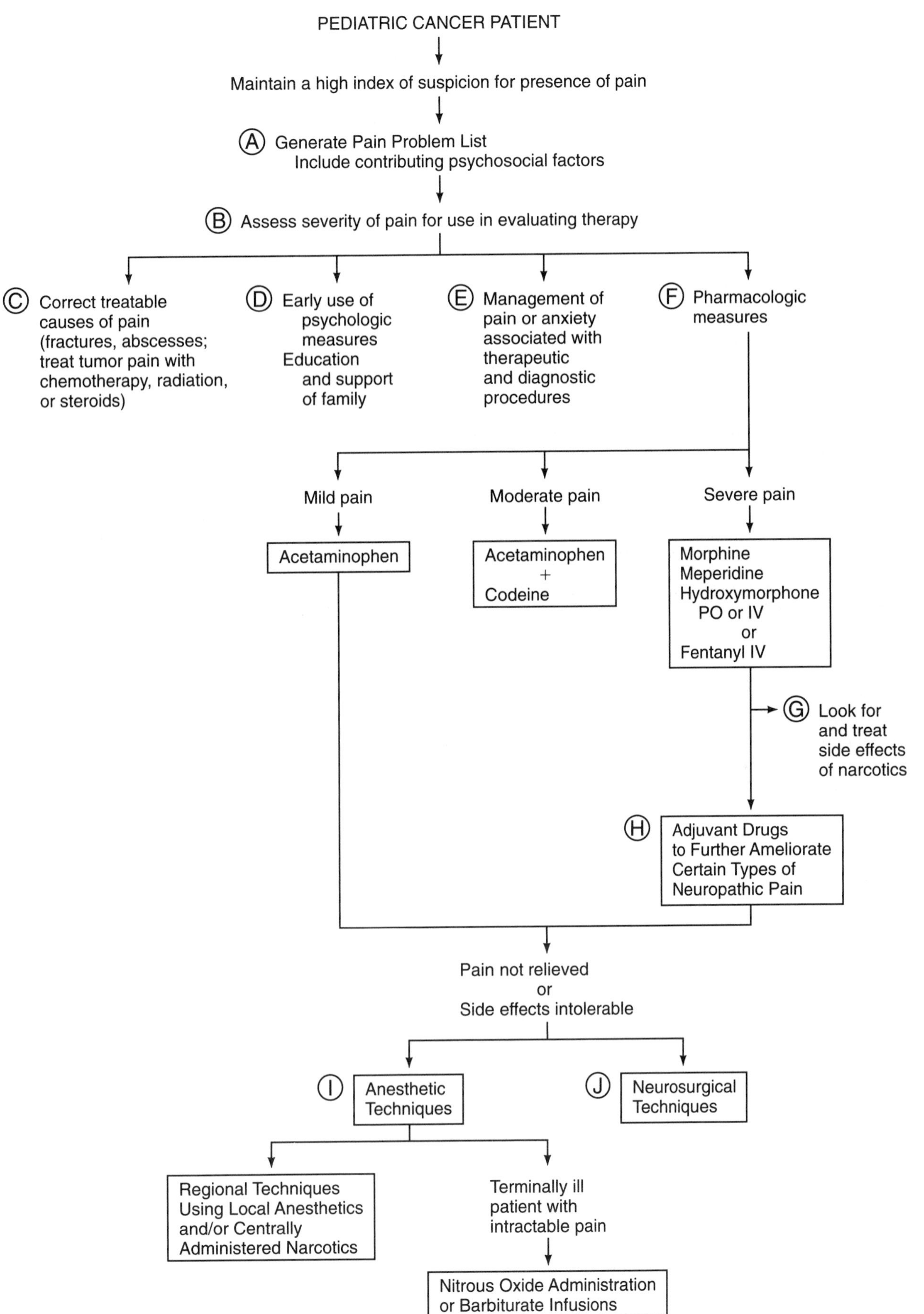
PEDIATRIC CANCER PATIENT
Maintain a high index of suspicion for presence of pain
(A) Generate Pain Problem List
Include contributing psychosocial factors
(B) Assess severity of pain for use in evaluating therapy
(C) Correct treatable causes of pain (fractures, abscesses; treat tumor pain with chemotherapy, radiation, or steroids)
(D) Early use of psychologic measures
Education and support of family
(E) Management of pain or anxiety associated with therapeutic and diagnostic procedures
(F) Pharmacologic measures
Mild pain
Moderate pain
Severe pain
Acetaminophen
Acetaminophen + Codeine
Morphine
Meperidine
Hydroxymorphone
PO or IV
or
Fentanyl IV
(G) Look for and treat side effects of narcotics
(H) Adjuvant Drugs to Further Ameliorate Certain Types of Neuropathic Pain
Pain not relieved
or
Side effects intolerable
(I) Anesthetic Techniques
(J) Neurosurgical Techniques
Regional Techniques Using Local Anesthetics and/or Centrally Administered Narcotics
Terminally ill patient with intractable pain
Nitrous Oxide Administration or Barbiturate Infusions

G. Side effects of narcotic management include respiratory depression, nausea and vomiting, constipation, pruritus, somnolence, and sleep disturbance. Question children specifically about side effects, because they often will not volunteer this information. Side effects can be treated; attempt to reach an equilibrium between acceptable levels of side effects and adequate pain relief.

H. The efficacy of narcotics may be aided by the addition of other non-narcotic medications. Anticonvulsants have been used successfully to treat shooting, stabbing neuropathic pain, and tricyclic antidepressants are useful when pain is burning or neuropathic.

I. When side effects or the treatment of side effects of narcotics prove more noxious than the analgesia achieved, or the pain remains intractable despite narcotic analgesia, several anesthetic techniques may be used. Peripheral nerve blockade may be accomplished with local anesthetics. Caudal, epidural, or subarachnoid blocks may be done with local anesthetics and/or opioids. The catheters may be tunneled under the skin to provide a route for long-term home infusions. Neurolytic blockade with phenol or alcohol should be done by someone who is skilled at these techniques. For the terminally ill child with intractable pain, barbiturate infusions or nitrous oxide inhalation may provide relief.

J. Neurostimulatory (dorsal column stimulation) and neurodestructive (cordotomy, rhizotomy) neurosurgical approaches may be useful in patients with pain localized to dermatomal distributions who suffer severe side effects from or do not respond to other measures.

TABLE 1 Best Measures for Pain Assessment by Age

	Self-Report Measures	*Behavioral Measures*	*Physiologic Measures*
Description or examples	Simple: "Oucher" scale, poker chip tool, pain thermometer, simple linear analogue, color and ladder scales More complex: numerical rating scales	Presence of crying; fussing; withdrawal; sleep disturbance; facial grimace; guarding; reduction in eating, play, or attention span	Heart rate, respiratory rate, blood pressure, palmar sweating
Drawback	Requires certain developmental skills to use	Not specific, may be difficult to discern changes	Not specific
0–3 years	N/A	Best	Secondary
Preschool	Simple self-report measures best	Helpful if self-report unavailable	Secondary
School-age children	Best; can use simple scales and numerical scales	Helpful if self-report unavailable	
Adolescents	May use visual analogue scales developed for adults; may regress to earlier stage of development in acute illness and require simpler scales	Secondary	

References

McGrath, PJ, Unruh AM. Pain in children and adolescents. New York: Elsevier, 1987.

Miser AW, Dothage JA, Wesley RA, et al. The prevalence of pain in a pediatric and young adult cancer population. Pain 1987; 29:73.

Miser AW, Miser JS. The treatment of cancer pain in children. Pediatr Clin North Am 1989; 36:979.

Report of the Consensus Conference on the Management of Pain in Childhood Cancer. Pediatrics 1990, 86(Suppl 2):5.

Schecter NL. Pain in children with cancer. In: Foley KM, ed. Advances in pain research and therapy. Vol 16. New York: Raven Press, 1990:57.

Yaster M, Deshpande JK. Management of pediatric pain with opioid analgesics. J Pediatr 1988; 113:421.

PHARMACOLOGY

DRUG INTERACTIONS

Eric B. Lefever, M.D.

Patients referred to pain management clinics frequently are taking multiple medications, both as initial treatment for their pain and for other medical conditions. The incidence of drug interactions has been estimated to be >5% in these patients. Because the number of medications available, routes of administration, and new techniques for pain management are constantly increasing, some understanding of drug interactions is necessary. A knowledge of common drug interactions allows the clinician either to choose an alternate medication or adjust the doses or schedule of drug administration. Although a comprehensive listing of possible drug interactions with medications commonly used for diagnostic and therapeutic purposes in the management of pain is clearly beyond the scope of this text, some basic principles are presented.

A. Interactions that occur when drugs are given concurrently cannot necessarily be predicted on the basis of their effects when given alone. The net pharmacologic response may result from the inhibition of one drug by another, by enhancement of the effects of either drug, or by the development of totally new effects.

B. Multiple mechanisms are responsible for drug interactions and one or more may be responsible in individual cases.

C. Numerous interactions involve the drugs' chemical or physical properties. Examples include the electrostatic interaction of heparin with protamine and the precipitation that results when acidic drugs such as thiopental are injected with more basic drugs.

D. Changes in gastrointestinal absorption affect many therapeutic agents because most are commonly taken by mouth. Mechanisms include a gastric pH that is altered by H_2 blockers, and a gastric transit time that is slowed by anticholinergics and accelerated with metoclopramide. Systemic absorption can also be affected at peripheral sites by routinely adding vasoconstrictors to injected local anesthetics, both to increase duration and decrease systemic toxicity.

E. Many drugs reversibly bind to plasma proteins. Competitors for these binding sites can have significant effects, especially with agents that are more extensively bound. NSAIDs are highly protein bound and may displace other drugs. Local anesthetics may also be affected, although they preferentially bind to glycoprotein, whereas albumin is the major binding site of most other drugs.

F. Drug biotransformation reactions occur primarily in the liver, and drug interactions can either increase or decrease specific drug metabolism and affect hepatic blood flow. Enzyme-inducing agents such as phenytoin and barbiturates, smoking, and increased hepatic blood flow increase the clearance of many drugs. Propranolol and cimetidine lower the clearance of local anesthetics, both by inhibiting enzyme systems and decreasing hepatic blood flow.

G. Agonists and antagonists exert their pharmacologic actions at specific receptors, but interactions are common because of the lack of specificity of many drugs. Tricyclic antidepressants inhibit the uptake of guanethidine into sympathetic nerve terminals, which may decrease the efficacy of guanethidine when used for intravenous regional sympathetic blocks.

H. Alterations of renal excretion are common with drugs that alter urinary pH or with medications that compete for tubular transport. The alkalinization of the urine with sodium bicarbonate or acetazolamide may increase the reabsorption of the tricyclic antidepressants.

I. Changes in the pH or electrolyte concentrations are commonly seen with diuretics and alter the absorption, distribution, and renal clearance of other drugs. Renal lithium excretion is sensitive to changes in sodium balance and is reduced with hyponatremia.

References

Hansten PD. Drug interactions. Philadelphia: Lea & Febiger, 1985.

Murad F, Gilman AG. Drug interactions. In: Gilman AG, et al, eds. Goodman and Gilman's The pharmacological basis of therapeutics. 7th ed. New York: Macmillan, 1985.

Smith NT, Corbascio AN. Drug interactions in anesthesia. 2nd ed. Phildelphia: Lea & Febiger, 1986.

Tucker GT, Mather LE. Properties, absorption, and disposition of local anesthetic agents. In: Cousins MJ, Bridenbaugh PO, eds. Neural blockade in clinical anesthesia and management of pain. 2nd ed. Philadelphia: JB Lippincott, 1988.

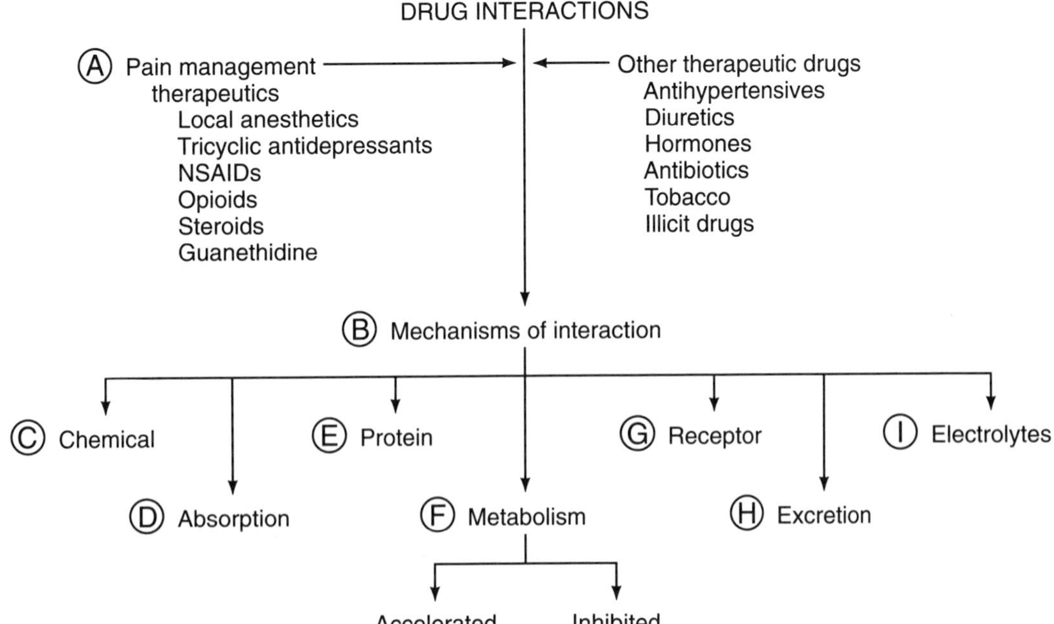
DRUG INTERACTIONS
(A) Pain management therapeutics
Local anesthetics
Tricyclic antidepressants
NSAIDs
Opioids
Steroids
Guanethidine
Other therapeutic drugs
Antihypertensives
Diuretics
Hormones
Antibiotics
Tobacco
Illicit drugs
(B) Mechanisms of interaction
(C) Chemical
(D) Absorption
(E) Protein
(F) Metabolism
Accelerated
Inhibited
(G) Receptor
(H) Excretion
(I) Electrolytes

ANAPHYLAXIS

Eric B. Lefever, M.D.

Allergic reactions are an inevitable and unpredictable consequence of the administration of therapeutic and diagnostic medications commonly used in pain management. Anaphylaxis is the most severe form of an allergic reaction.

A. The mechanisms of allergic reaction have a common final pathway. The release of histamine and other chemical mediators from mast cells and basophils produces the clinical manifestations. Anaphylaxis requires previous exposure to the drug or a chemically similar substance with the production of IgE antibodies that bind to both basophils and mast cells. With re-exposure to the drug, IgE antibodies are cross-linked and mediators are released. Complement pathways may also cause degranulation, either by C3a and C5a together or by C3a alone. Anaphylactoid reactions are a direct effect of a basic drug displacing histamine from mast cells and basophils. Contrast media reactions demonstrate a lowered incidence of anaphylactoid reactions when less basic, nonionic agents are used (p 236).

B. The magnitude of hemodynamic and pulmonary changes is not defined by the mechanism of allergy, but depends on the amount and rate of drug injected, the amount of chemical mediators liberated, the responsiveness of the vascular and bronchial smooth muscle, and the state of the autonomic nervous system. In order of frequency, symptoms are cutaneous manifestations (erythema, wheal and flare reactions); hypotension with tachycardia; and bronchospasm with hypoxemia. Histamine dilates arterioles and increases capillary permeability, leading to loss of intravascular fluid and edema formation. It also causes contraction of bronchial smooth muscle. Tachycardia results from the release of endogenous catecholamines as well as in response to hypotension. Bronchospasm is potentially the most serious feature of an anaphylactic episode, because uncorrected arterial hypoxemia will cause rapid morbidity and death.

C. A high index of suspicion must be present in the setting of sudden hypotension and bronchospasm. Alternate causes should be eliminated only after effective treatment has begun. Vasovagal reactions can be distinguished on the basis of bradycardia. Tension pneumothorax, pericardial tamponade, and dysrhythmias are diagnosed by physical examination and ECG monitoring. Although embolic phenomena and hereditary angioneurotic edema may be more difficult to diagnose definitively, they respond to supportive treatment.

D. Oxygen, equipment for airway maintenance, and resuscitative medications must be available in every treatment area. For life-threatening reactions with hypotension and bronchospasm, aggressive treatment must be initiated immediately. Obviously, administration of the suspected antigen must be stopped. Airway maintenance with 100% oxygen, intravascular fluid expansion, and epinephrine are the major components of treatment. Airway and ventilatory assistance may require immediate intubation of the trachea if significant laryngeal edema is suspected. Infuse large volumes of crystalloid rapidly. Epinephrine is the drug of choice for significant allergic reactions because it stimulates adrenergic receptors to restore vascular tone and perfusion, acts as a bronchodilator, and inhibits further release of mediators. The route of administration and dose of epinephrine must be titrated to the severity of the reaction with a dose of up to 5 μg/kg as an intravenous bolus in serious cases. Less drastic manifestations should respond to subcutaneous administration of smaller doses.

E. Secondary treatment options include antihistamines to block unoccupied histamine receptors. Use aminophylline for refractory bronchospasm. Corticosteroids, although a second-line drug because of a delayed onset of action, may attenuate secondary responses by stabilizing cell membranes and decreasing capillary permeability. Histamine receptor blockers and steroids are effective in pretreatment protocols prior to contrast agent exposure, and should be considered in patients at increased risk for allergic reactions, including those with a history of previous reaction and those with chronic atopy (asthma, hay fever). Any patient suspected of having an anaphylactic reaction should be monitored in an intensive care setting for at least 24 hours, because symptoms may recur after the initial treatment.

References

Katzberg RW. Intravascular contrast media. In: Putnam CE, Ravin CE, eds. Textbook of diagnostic imaging. Philadelphia: WB Saunders, 1988.

Lasser EC, Berry CC, Talner LB, et al. Pretreatment with corticosteroids to alleviate reactions to intravenous contrast material. N Engl J Med 1987; 317:845.

Levy JH. Anaphylactic reactions in anesthesia and intensive care. Boston: Butterworth, 1986.

Stoelting RK. Allergic reactions during anesthesia. Anesth Analg 1983; 62:341.

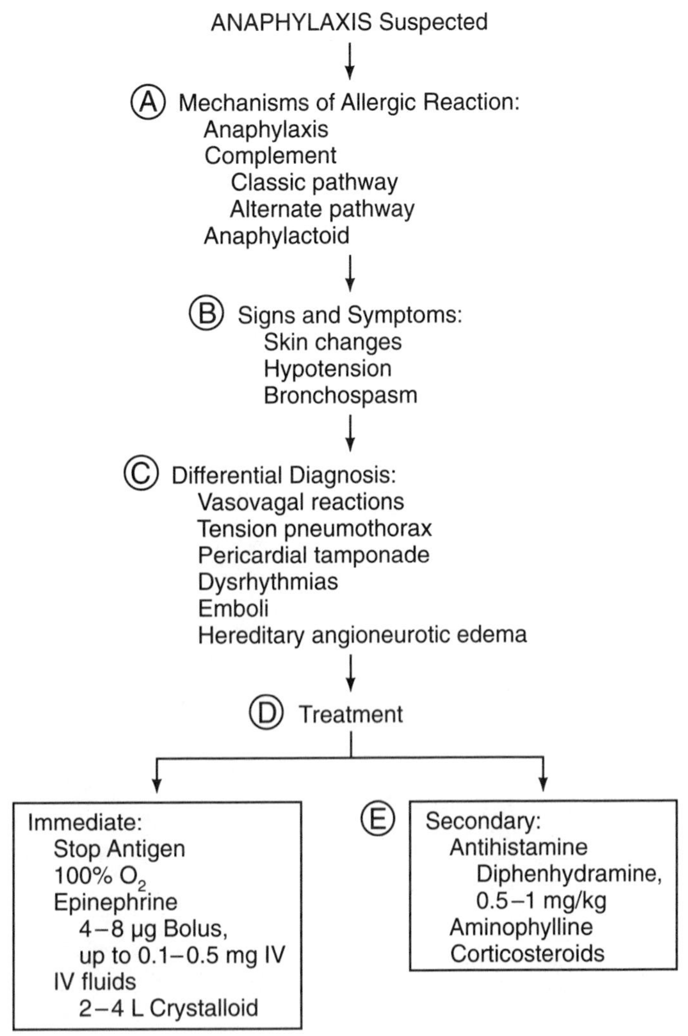
ANAPHYLAXIS Suspected
Ⓐ Mechanisms of Allergic Reaction:
Anaphylaxis
Complement
Classic pathway
Alternate pathway
Anaphylactoid
Ⓑ Signs and Symptoms:
Skin changes
Hypotension
Bronchospasm
Ⓒ Differential Diagnosis:
Vasovagal reactions
Tension pneumothorax
Pericardial tamponade
Dysrhythmias
Emboli
Hereditary angioneurotic edema
Ⓓ Treatment
Immediate:
Stop Antigen
100% O_2
Epinephrine
4–8 μg Bolus,
up to 0.1–0.5 mg IV
IV fluids
2–4 L Crystalloid
Ⓔ Secondary:
Antihistamine
Diphenhydramine,
0.5–1 mg/kg
Aminophylline
Corticosteroids

LOCAL ANESTHETIC TOXICITY

Rosemary Hickey, M.D.

Various types of toxic reaction have been reported after use of local anesthetics (LAs). The frequency of toxic reactions, however, is very low considering the widespread use of LAs.

A. To minimize systemic reactions to LAs, avoid intravascular injection, the most common cause of convulsions. Use careful, intermittent aspiration before injecting large quantities of LAs. Give a test dose and question the patient if metallic taste, numbness around the mouth, or ringing in the ears is present, indicating intravascular needle placement. Use the lowest possible effective dose and concentration to prevent toxic blood levels. Premedicate the patient with midazolam or diazepam to raise the seizure threshold.

B. Systemic toxicity may be due to unintentional intravascular injection or drug overdose. Intravascular injection produces signs of toxicity (usually convulsions) during the injection itself. A relative overdose results in toxic reactions at the time in which peak blood levels are reached, approximately 20 to 30 minutes after the injection. Factors that affect the blood concentration (site of injection, drug, dosage, addition of vasoconstrictor, speed of injection) influence the potential for systemic toxic reactions to develop.

C. LAs are relatively lipid-soluble, low-molecular-weight compounds that readily cross the blood-brain barrier. As toxic levels are reached, disturbances of CNS function are observed. Initially, LAs produce signs of CNS excitation. Early symptoms of overdose include headache, ringing in the ears, numbness in the tongue and mouth, twitching of facial muscles, and restlessness. As blood levels increase, generalized convulsions of a tonic-clonic nature occur. If sufficiently high blood levels are reached, initial signs of CNS excitation are followed by a generalized state of CNS depression. Respiratory depression and ultimately respiratory arrest may occur owing to the toxic effect of the LA on the respiratory center in the medulla. Occasionally, the excitatory phase may not be manifest, and toxicity becomes initially apparent as CNS depression.

D. Cardiovascular (CV) effects either result indirectly from inhibition of autonomic pathways during regional anesthesia (as in high spinal or epidural) or are directly due to depressant actions on the CV system. The CV system is generally more resistant than the CNS to toxicity. The CV/CNS toxicity ratio is lower for bupivacaine and etidocaine than for lidocaine. Convulsive activity may initially be associated with an increase in heart rate, BP, and cardiac output. As the blood concentration of LA further increases, CV depression occurs, resulting in a fall in blood pressure secondary to myocardial depression, impaired cardiac conduction, and eventual peripheral vasodilation. Ultimately, circulatory collapse and cardiac arrest may occur. In addition, certain agents such as bupivacaine cause ventricular arrhythmias and fatal ventricular fibrillation. The onset of CV depression with bupivacaine may occur relatively early and be resistant to usual therapeutic modalities. The pregnant patient is more sensitive to the cardiotoxic effects of bupivacaine than the nonpregnant patient.

E. Treat systemic toxicity with general supportive measures. If early signs of toxicity occur, maintain constant verbal contact, administer oxygen, encourage breathing, and monitor CV function. If convulsions occur, establish a clear airway and administer oxygen by assisted or controlled ventilation. If convulsions continue, administer thiopental (50 to 100 mg) or diazepam (2.5 to 5.0 mg) IV. Avoid large doses of thiopental, which may produce additional CV or CNS depression. If airway maintenance is jeopardized, use succinylcholine to facilitate endotracheal intubation. Muscular convulsive activity is terminated with succinylcholine, but the convulsive process in the brain is not affected. If CV depression occurs, treat hypotension by increasing IV fluids, proper positioning (elevate the legs), and vasopressors such as ephedrine.

F. Reactions to epinephrine may sometimes be confused with LA overdose. Systemic absorption of epinephrine produces palpitations and restlessness approximately 1 to 2 minutes after completion of the injection. Consider avoiding epinephrine in patients sensitive to it (e.g., hypertensive, hyperthyroid, arrhythmic patients). Do not use epinephrine for blocks of the finger, toe, or penis.

G. LAs used in recommended clinical concentrations have minimal irritating effects on the nerves, skin, and fat. Complete recovery of function occurs after regional blocks. There have been concerns, however, about potential neurotoxic effects of intrathecal chloroprocaine. Studies suggest that the combination of a low pH and the antioxidant sodium bisulfite may be responsible for the neurotoxic reactions seen after the use of large amounts of chloroprocaine solution.

H. An allergic response to LAs rarely occurs and in some instances may be confused with a vasovagal reaction or a reaction to epinephrine. Esters are more frequently associated with allergic reactions than amides because these agents are derivatives of para-aminobenzoic acid. The use of amides from multiple-dose vials may result in an allergic reaction owing to the preservative methylparaben. Intradermal skin tests can be used successfully to diagnose adverse responses, although false-positive results do occur.

I. The administration of large doses of prilocaine may lead to methemoglobinemia owing to the accumulation of a metabolite (O-toluidine) that is capable of converting hemoglobin to methemoglobin. It may betreated by IV methylene blue.

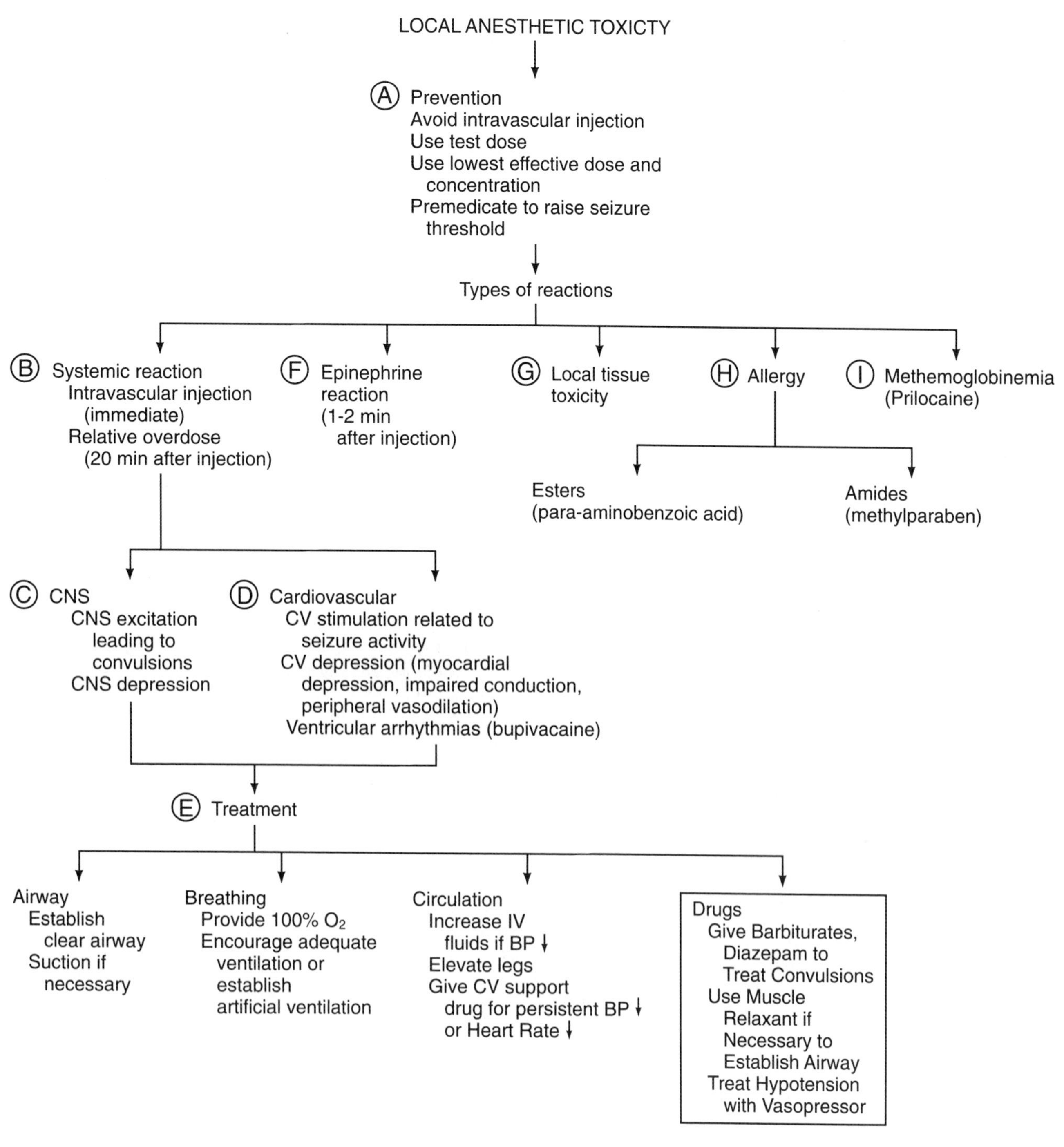

References

Covino BG. Clinical pharmacology of local anesthetic agents. In: Cousins MJ, Bridenbaugh PO, eds. Neural blockade in clinical anesthesia and management of pain. 2nd ed. Philadelphia: JB Lippincott, 1988:111.

Gissen AJ, Datta S, Lambert D, et al. Is chloroprocaine (2CP) neurotoxic? Reg Anaesth 1984; 9:37.

Kotelko DM, Shnider SM, Dailey PA, et al. Bupivacaine-induced cardiac arrhythmias in sheep. Anesthesiology 1984; 60:10.

NONSTEROIDAL ANTI-INFLAMMATORY DRUGS

Kevin L. Kenworthy, M.D., C.P.T., M.C.

The non-narcotic analgesics include acetaminophen and the NSAIDs. These agents have four major actions: analgesic, antipyretic, anti-inflammatory, and antiplatelet. Acetaminophen has no anti-inflammatory or antiplatelet activity, but it is equipotent to aspirin in analgesic and antipyretic effects. All NSAIDs inhibit the enzyme cyclooxygenase in the arachidonic acid pathway, resulting in reduced tissue prostaglandin levels. Prostaglandins are mediators of inflammation, and they facilitate nociceptor function by enhancing the effects of pain mediators such as bradykinin. NSAIDs differ from narcotic analgesics in three important ways: (1) their major site of action is peripheral, not central; (2) NSAIDs have a dose ceiling effect for analgesia; and (3) NSAIDs do not produce tolerance or physical dependence. NSAIDs have a very unpredictable individual variation in response. Therefore, therapeutic trials of about 12 to 14 days at standard doses should be given before discontinuing a particular agent.

A. Use NSAIDs to treat mild to moderate pain of either acute or chronic duration, including pain and inflammation due to trauma, surgery, or systemic disease like arthralgias or neoplasms. Other examples include headache, myalgia, dysmenorrhea, and pain from integumental structures. Because of their peripheral mechanism of action, NSAIDs are often combined with centrally acting narcotics to provide improved analgesia. NSAIDs, especially aspirin, are also used for their antipyretic and antiplatelet activity.

B. Do not use NSAIDs in pregnant or nursing patients; those with chronic hepatic or renal failure, prior anaphylactic reaction to aspirin or other NSAIDs, active gastrointestinal (GI) bleeding or other blood dyscrasias; or those who plan to undergo surgery in 1 week or less. Relative contraindications to NSAID use include bronchial asthma or nasal polyps; history of peptic ulcers, hiatal hernia, or GI bleeding; cardiovascular disease (hypertension or chronic heart failure); decreased renal blood flow or renal insufficiency; and use of potentially interacting drugs. Aspirin is specifically contraindicated in children and adolescents with a febrile illness because of the potential for Reye's syndrome.

C. Drug interactions with NSAIDs can result from protein binding competition, NSAID-mediated reduction of renal function, or hepatic enzyme induction or inhibition. The phenytoins, hydantoins, oral hypoglycemics, heparin, and oral anticoagulants may be displaced from protein binding sites by NSAIDs, resulting in increased amounts of free drug. NSAIDs may blunt the antihypertensive effects of diuretics or beta-blockers by decreasing the number of renal prostaglandins and inducing water, sodium, and potassium retention. Patients taking phenytoin, tolbutamide, phenobarbital, or warfarin may have augmented effects because of the inhibition of the hepatic metabolism by NSAIDs. Verapamil and digoxin effects may be diminished by an NSAID-induced increase in their hepatic metabolism. NSAIDs increase the blood concentration and duration of action of methotrexate, potentially resulting in toxicity.

(Continued on page 180)

NSAIDs FOR PAIN MANAGEMENT

Ⓐ Indications:
- Mild to moderate pain from trauma, surgery, or systemic disease (arthralgias, neoplasms)
- Antipyretic
- Antiplatelet activity

Ⓒ Drug-drug interactions:
- Competition for protein-binding sites (phenytoins, hydantoins, oral hypoglycemics, heparin and oral anticoagulants, methotrexate)
- NSAID-mediated reduction in renal function or urine output (diuretics, beta-blockers, anticholinesterase inhibitors)
- NSAID-altered hepatic metabolism:
  - Augmented (phenytoin, tolbutamide, phenobarbital, warfarin)
  - Diminished (verapamil, digoxin)

(Cont'd on p 181)

Ⓑ Contraindications:
- Prior reaction
- Pregnancy/nursing
- Bronchial asthma
- Nasal polyps
- Aspirin sensitivity
- Active dyspepsia
- History of:
  - Peptic ulcer disease
  - Hiatal hernia
  - Hepatic/renal failure
  - Blood dyscrasias
- One week before surgery
- Child or adolescent with febrile or viral illness (risk of Reye's syndrome)

D. Elderly patients are at increased risk for adverse reactions because of age-related changes in hepatic and renal function; fluid and electrolyte imbalances; concurrent systemic disease; and increased incidences of polypharmacy. The most frequent adverse reactions are GI-related, with dyspepsia being most common. Peptic ulceration and GI bleeding are less common. Factors that increase risk of GI side effects include age >60, history of peptic ulcers, concomitant steroid use, smoking, alcohol use, and high-dose or multiple NSAID use. Prevention and treatment of GI side effects include avoiding NSAID use in patients at risk; administering NSAIDs with food; administering antacids, H_2-blockers, Carafate, or prostaglandin agonists; and using NSAIDs with the fewest GI side-effects, such as acetaminophen, choline trisalicylate, or salsalicylate. In compromised patients, NSAID use may lead to altered renal function and nephrotoxicity. Indomethacin, aspirin, fenoprofen, and ibuprofen (in decreasing order) have been implicated as potentially renally toxic. Acetaminophen is the least toxic agent, followed by sulindac. Patients at risk should have frequent exams including urine and blood chemistries to assess renal function. Central nervous system side effects are infrequent and include headache, dizziness, confusion, somnolence, and depression.

NSAIDs inhibit platelet aggregation and affect both the intrinsic and extrinsic coagulation pathways, which may lead to bleeding. Patients should discontinue aspirin 7 to 14 days and the other NSAIDs 24 to 48 hours prior to surgery. Other hematologic reactions such as aplastic anemia, thrombocytopenia, and hemolytic anemia are very rare.

NSAIDs may cause mild elevations in liver transaminases, which typically resolve spontaneously after discontinuing the NSAID. Monitor liver function tests in patients with hepatic disease. If serum glutamic-oxaloa-acetic transaminase (SGOT) is three times the upper normal limit, NSAIDs should be discontinued. Patients with chronic hepatic failure should avoid NSAIDs.

NSAID use may also prolong or postpone labor and possibly affect closure of the fetal ductus arteriosus.

With the exception of aspirin and acetaminophen, toxicity caused by NSAID overdose is rare and typically does not require a specific antidote.

E. The selection of a specific NSAID is based on a patient's age, concurrent disease states, relative risk for organ toxicity, the clinician's experience, cost, and the likelihood of compliance. In the elderly, diabetics, and in patients with cardiovascular, renal, and hepatic disease, the mentioned precautions and monitoring must be used. In most patients the primary factor is having had a previous good response to a specific NSAID. Most authors regard prescribing NSAIDs as an "art"—not a science.

References

Beneditti C, Butler SH. Systemic analgesics. In: Bonica JJ, ed. The management of pain. 2nd ed. Philadelphia: Lea & Febiger, 1990:1660.

Brooks PM, Day RO. Nonsteroidal anti-inflammatory drugs—differences and similarities. N Engl J Med 1991; 324:1716.

Corrigan GD, Pantig-Felix L, Kanat IO. Potential complications of nonsteroidal anti-inflammatory drug therapy. J Am Podiatr Med Assoc 1989; 79:605.

Mortensen ME, Rennebohn RM. Clinical pharmacology and use of nonsteroidal anti-inflammatory drugs. Pediatr Clin North Am 1989; 36:1113.

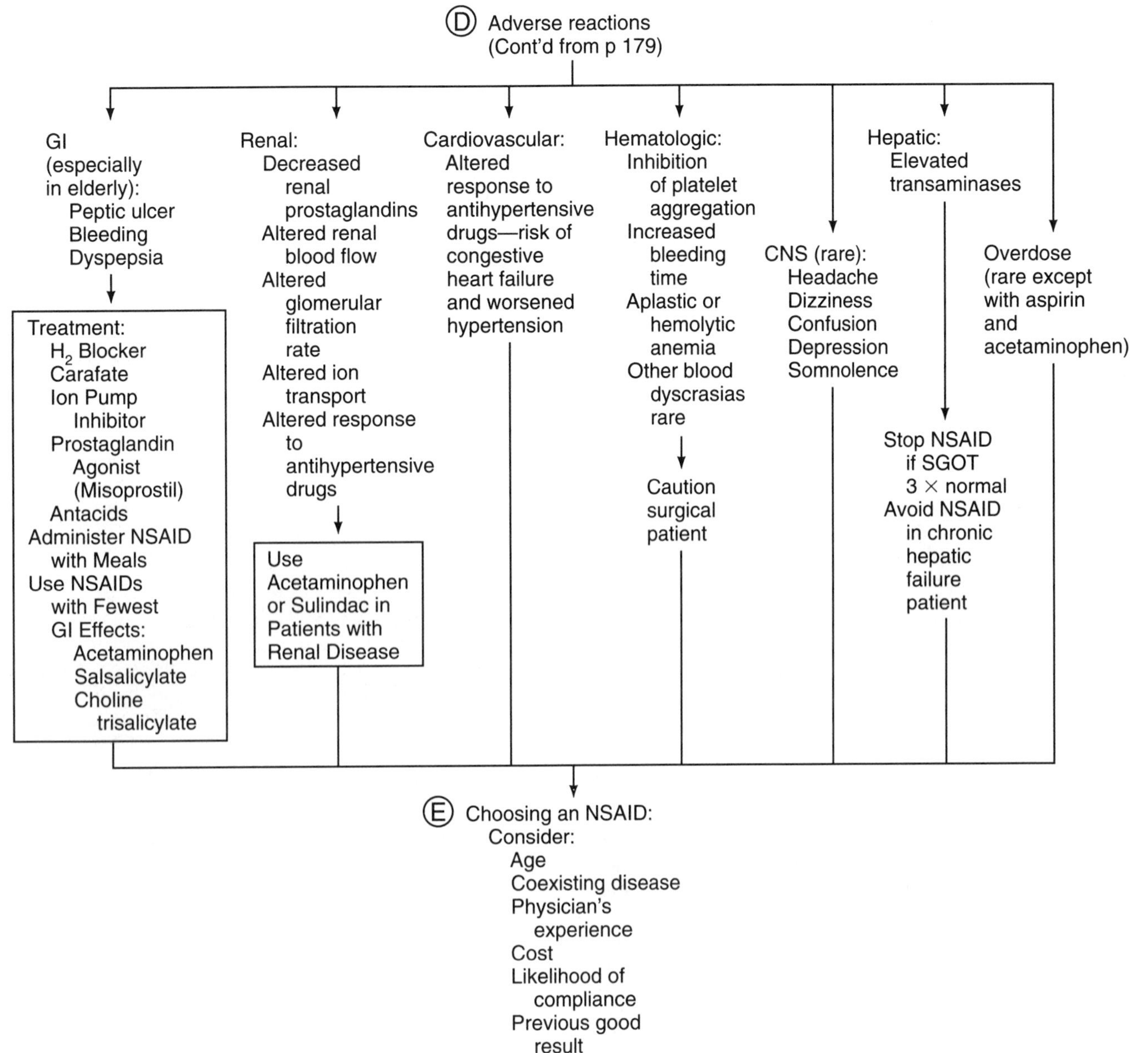

Ⓓ Adverse reactions
(Cont'd from p 179)
GI (especially in elderly):
Peptic ulcer
Bleeding
Dyspepsia
Treatment:
H_2 Blocker
Carafate
Ion Pump Inhibitor
Prostaglandin Agonist (Misoprostil)
Antacids
Administer NSAID with Meals
Use NSAIDs with Fewest GI Effects:
Acetaminophen
Salsalicylate
Choline trisalicylate
Renal:
Decreased renal prostaglandins
Altered renal blood flow
Altered glomerular filtration rate
Altered ion transport
Altered response to antihypertensive drugs
Use Acetaminophen or Sulindac in Patients with Renal Disease
Cardiovascular:
Altered response to antihypertensive drugs—risk of congestive heart failure and worsened hypertension
Hematologic:
Inhibition of platelet aggregation
Increased bleeding time
Aplastic or hemolytic anemia
Other blood dyscrasias rare
Caution surgical patient
CNS (rare):
Headache
Dizziness
Confusion
Depression
Somnolence
Hepatic:
Elevated transaminases
Stop NSAID if SGOT 3 × normal
Avoid NSAID in chronic hepatic failure patient
Overdose (rare except with aspirin and acetaminophen)
Ⓔ Choosing an NSAID:
Consider:
Age
Coexisting disease
Physician's experience
Cost
Likelihood of compliance
Previous good result

ANTIDEPRESSANTS

Roland Reinhart, M.D.

Antidepressants are often effective in the management of chronic pain syndromes. They are most useful for certain types of pain such as headache, arthritis, diabetic neuropathy, and facial pain. One of the most common sequelae of chronic pain is depression. Also, 60% of depressed patients have some pain complaint.

A. Signs and symptoms of depression should be recorded, and testing may be useful. Antidepressants alter neurotransmitter metabolites, receptor sensitivities, receptor uptake blockade, and firing rates of neurons. Which of these properties alleviate depression is unknown.

B. No one tricyclic antidepressant (TCA) has been shown to be markedly superior to any other in relieving pain. However, some antidepressants demonstrate efficacy for specific pain syndromes, and these should be tried first. The most commonly used drugs are doxepin, amitriptyline, imipramine, and clomipramine. These drugs have more serotinergic uptake inhibition than the other heterocyclic antidepressants. The choice of antidepressant is based on the pain syndrome, the patient's age and health, and the drug's side effects. Drugs with more sedation are often preferred because insomnia is a problem in many chronic pain patients.

C. Dosage of TCAs usually starts at 25 to 50 mg and is increased after the first week 25 mg every 3 to 4 days as tolerated. Of the monoamine oxidase inhibitors (MAOIs), phenelzine is most commonly used, started at 15 mg and advanced 15 mg every 2 to 3 days to a total of 45 to 60 mg/day. The dosage is reduced if serious side effects occur. Therapeutic effects are usually seen in 5 to 7 days. Single doses are as effective as divided doses, provided that side effects are tolerable. Sleep patterns improve in the first 3 days, and pain relief may improve over the first month.

D. In arthritis patients, 60 to 70% obtained relief with imipramine, 20 to 75 mg/day; amitriptyline, 75 mg/day; or clomipramine, 10 to 25 mg/day. The lower doses seemed as effective as the higher doses. However, some studies demonstrated no relief. Migraine headache occurrence was diminished by antidepressants. The prophylactic effects were seen in the first month of treatment: 80% relief with phenelzine, 45 mg/day; 50 to 100% relief with amitriptyline, 10 to 150 mg/day. Doxepin, 30 to 50 mg/day, was better than amitriptyline in one study. A 54 to 60% reduction in tension headaches occurred when doses similar to those for migraines were used. Doxepin, amitriptyline, and diazepam relieved psychogenic headache, but after 2 months only doxepin, 30 to 50 mg, was effective. Amitriptyline, 30 to 110 mg/day, reduced pain in 40 to 50% of patients with atypical facial pain; phenelzine, 45 mg/day, was effective 75% of the time and was also effective at treating the depression associated with facial pain. Amitriptyline alone at 100 mg or in combination with 2 mg fluphenazine gave 100% relief in two studies of diabetic neuropathic pain, but imipramine, 100 mg/day, gave only 58% relief. Antidepressants have had poor success in relieving back pain, perhaps because of the multiple causes of this condition. The few studies that did demonstrate improvement found that patients with the most severe symptoms tended to improve. In all studies of neoplastic pain, significant relief was accomplished with antidepressants.

E. TCAs cause anticholinergic side effects, cardiovascular complications, weight gain, and sedation in varying degrees, depending on the drug. These side effects are augmented by administration of opioid analgesics. Methadone contributes significantly to orthostatic hypotension. Elderly patients should have an ECG before administration. In a chronic pain patient with a conduction defect, trazodone might be tried first; it is sedating but without strong anticholinergic effects. Most drugs that are strongly anticholinergic are also strongly sedating. Symptomatic open-angle glaucoma and prostate hypertrophy are relative contraindications to TCAs.

Fluoxetine (Prozac), a new serotonin uptake inhibitor, causes nausea but is nonsedating. It is preferable to administer this drug in the morning; do not give with L-tryptophan, because side effects can be marked. Common side effects of MAOIs are dizziness, nausea, and weight gain. Patients on MAOIs must follow a tyramine-free diet and avoid sympathomimetics, which can cause a hypertensive crisis. Tyramine is in many foods, and fear of hypertensive crisis limits the use of these drugs. Meperidine in combination with MAOIs can cause a hyperpyrexic reaction. The platelet MAOI level should be monitored.

References

Atkinson JH, Kremer EF, Garfin SR. Psychopharmacological agents in the treatment of pain, J Bone Joint Surg 1985; 67A:337.

France R, Krishnan K. Psychotropic drugs in chronic pain. In: France R, Krishnan K, eds. Chronic pain. American Psychiatric Press, 1988.

Monks R, Merskey H. Psychotropic drugs. In: Wall PD, Melzack R, eds. Textbook of pain. 2nd ed. New York: Churchill Livingstone, 1989.

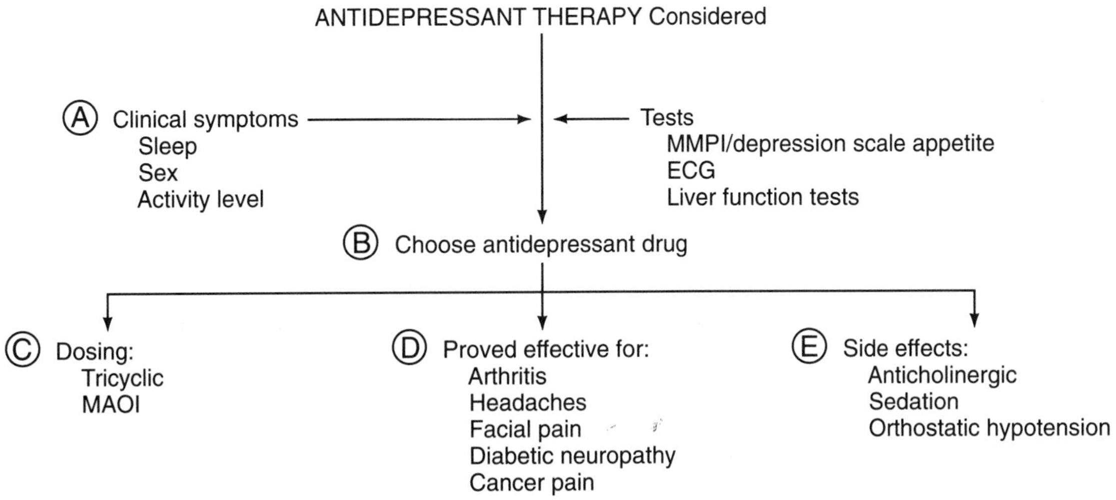

ANTIDEPRESSANT THERAPY Considered

(A) Clinical symptoms
- Sleep
- Sex
- Activity level

Tests
- MMPI/depression scale appetite
- ECG
- Liver function tests

(B) Choose antidepressant drug

(C) Dosing:
- Tricyclic
- MAOI

(D) Proved effective for:
- Arthritis
- Headaches
- Facial pain
- Diabetic neuropathy
- Cancer pain

(E) Side effects:
- Anticholinergic
- Sedation
- Orthostatic hypotension

NARCOTICS

Roland Reinhart, M.D.

Selection of an analgesic depends on the quality, intensity, duration, and underlying mechanism of pain. A general approach to systemic analgesia starts with non-narcotic analgesics and adjuvants. If pain persists, add a weak narcotic. If this is not sufficient, potent narcotics may be necessary. Unlike other analgesics, narcotics provide dose-dependent analgesia without limitation, but side effects become marked and limit drug dose at high levels. Adjuvant therapy should be continued so that the lowest effective narcotic dose may be used. Generally, chronic nonmalignant pain should be treated without narcotics because of the addictive and tolerance potential of narcotics. However, severe, recurring chronic pain of limited duration can be treated intermittently with narcotics.

A. When selecting a narcotic and dosing schedule, consider the patient's physical status. Very young, old, and malnourished patients have altered pharmacokinetics. Renal or hepatic dysfunction increases the risk of toxicity. Cancer pain may require high-dose narcotics regardless of other factors. Dosing of narcotics for severe pain should be by the clock, not on an as needed basis. The goal is to keep the patient as pain free as possible with the fewest side effects.

B. *Codeine* has high oral efficacy with a relatively lower risk of physical dependence. Tolerance, constipation, emesis, and limited potency are the major disadvantages. Adjuvant medication is often required if mild cancer pain is being treated. *Propoxyphene* is less effective than codeine. Initially it was thought to have lower potential for abuse, but this is not true. High doses may cause hallucinations.

C. *Meperidine* is often used interchangeably with morphine, but it has a shorter duration of action. Twice the oral dose is needed to equal the IM dose. Normeperidine, a metabolite, accumulates with chronic dosing, which may cause seizures. Renal failure is a contraindication to this drug. *Morphine* is the standard for pain control. It can be given PO, IV, IM, or per rectum. Tolerance and physical dependence occur after several weeks to months. Cancer pain can usually be controlled until the last days of life with oral morphine sulfate (MS). MS is given every 4 hours. MS Contin is a slow-release MS necessitating only two doses a day. *Methadone* has a long half-life and is resistant to the development of tolerance. It is a good alternative to MS, and perhaps better for chronic pain, because sustained levels are easily maintained. Adjustments of dosage to lower levels may be necessary, as this drug tends to accumulate over time. *Levorphanol* has many of the same features as methadone but is more sedating. It is useful if additional sedation is desirable. Nausea and vomiting are less than with MS. *Oxymorphone* is available as a suppository and is useful in patients with uncontrolled vomiting or other limitations to oral routes. *Hydromorphone* carries a high risk of psychological dependence. *Oxycodone* is available only in combination with aspirin or acetaminophen. It is more potent than codeine but may cause psychological dependence. A *mixed agonist-antagonist* can be helpful when side effects are a problem. Patients on other narcotics should not be abruptly switched to this category, as acute abstinence syndrome may develop. *Buprenorphine* can be given sublingually, and tolerance is slow to develop. Abstinence syndrome peaks 2 weeks after cessation. Sedation and nausea are limiting factors. *Pentazocine* has the same side effects as other opioids and produces severe withdrawal symptoms. It may cause psychotomimetic effects (seizures reversible with naloxone). *Nalbuphine* is available for IM and IV use. Chronic, high doses may accumulate, especially in liver disease, and lead to CNS irritability. Headaches may occur after 1 week of usage.

D. Respiratory depression can be fatal if the patient is overdosed. Cancer pain patients are resistant to respiratory depression because pain is a powerful respiratory stimulant. If cancer patients have a nerve block that alleviates the pain, they may be susceptible to a respiratory arrest. GI effects include a generalized slowing of gut motility leading to constipation, which should be aggressively treated. The discomfort of constipation may be more than that of the original pain. Nausea and vomiting are common. Adding hydroxyzine or perchlorperazine provides relief and often allows the narcotic dose to be reduced. Sedation may be excessive. Addition of an amphetamine can be helpful and allow for lower doses of narcotics. Seizures may occur if overdoses or toxic metabolites accumulate (see meperidine and pentazocine). Tolerance is a normal physiologic response; try switching to narcotics with a long half-life. Psychological dependence is not a factor in cancer patients but is difficult to treat in others. A discussion is beyond the scope of this chapter.

References

Benedetti C, Butler S. Systemic analgesics. In: Bonica JJ, ed. The management of pain. 2nd ed. Philadelphia: Lea & Febiger, 1990:1640.

Bonica JJ. Cancer pain. In: Bonica JJ, ed. The management of pain. 2nd ed. Philadelphia: Lea & Febiger, 1990:400.

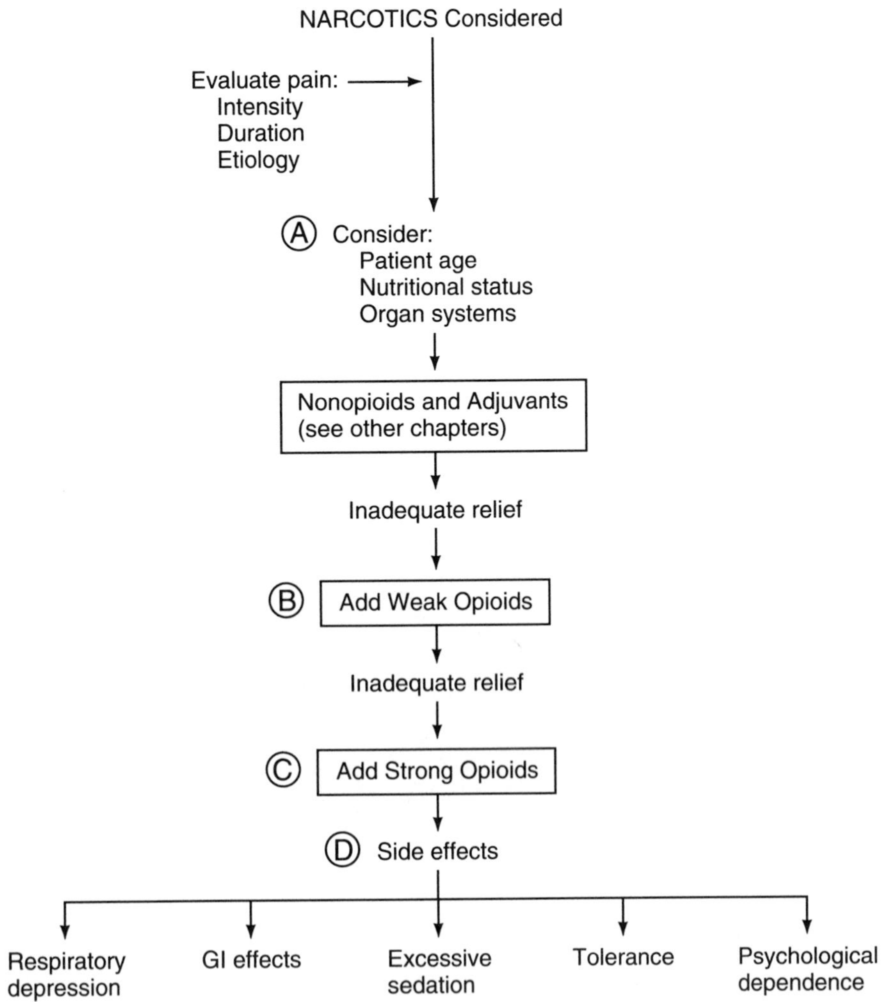
NARCOTICS Considered
Evaluate pain:
Intensity
Duration
Etiology
(A) Consider:
Patient age
Nutritional status
Organ systems
Nonopioids and Adjuvants
(see other chapters)
Inadequate relief
(B) Add Weak Opioids
Inadequate relief
(C) Add Strong Opioids
(D) Side effects
Respiratory depression
GI effects
Excessive sedation
Tolerance
Psychological dependence

THERAPEUTIC MODALITIES

Narcotic Detoxification
Physical Therapy
Vocational Rehabilitation
Transcutaneous Electrical Nerve Stimulation
Psychological Interventions
Hypnosis
Biofeedback
Placebo Analgesia
Acupuncture
Continuous Neural Blockade
Intravenous Regional Blockade
Epidural Steroid Injection
Intrathecal Narcotics
Neurolytic Nerve Block
Complications of Neurolytic Blocks
Implantable Infusion Pumps
Dorsal Column Stimulation
Cryoanalgesia
Neurosurgical Procedures for Pain

NARCOTIC DETOXIFICATION

David Vanos, M.D.

In the management of patients with chronic pain, narcotics often are not useful except in certain circumstances such as acute or cancer pain. It is often necessary to wean patients off narcotics in order to better evaluate and treat their pain. In such a case, physical dependence and psychological dependence must be considered.

A. Physical dependence is demonstrated when abrupt discontinuation of the medication leads to physical signs of withdrawal, or the abstinence syndrome. These symptoms may include anxiety, irritability, chills, hot flashes, salivation, lacrimation, sweating, diarrhea, nausea, vomiting, abdominal cramps, insomnia, and occasionally multifocal myoclonus. Shorter half-life narcotics (e.g., morphine sulfate) have an earlier onset, more intense symptoms, and a shorter course (24 to 72 hours), whereas with longer half-life agents (e.g., methadone) symptoms may be delayed several days and are milder in intensity.

B. Psychological dependence, otherwise known as "addiction," is the desire to use the drug for purposes other than pain relief. Usually this is coupled with drug-seeking behavior and an active effort on the part of the patient to obtain the drug. Psychologic interventions may be helpful in dealing with this aspect. It is important to note that not all patients taking narcotics for pain experience psychological dependence.

C. The goal of weaning a patient off narcotics is to avoid producing significant physical withdrawal symptoms. This can be accomplished in the outpatient setting when the daily narcotic usage is low to moderate. It requires a cooperative, motivated patient. The reasons for discontinuing narcotics, the expected effects, and future therapeutic plans should be explained carefully to the patient. Outpatients should be given a written schedule to follow. Family support can be very helpful.

D. Patients taking large amounts of narcotics, taking narcotics obtained from different sources, or with drug-seeking behavior often require a formal inpatient detoxification program.

E. Usually a reduction of 75% of the patient's daily dosage of narcotic can be accomplished every 2 days without provoking signs of the abstinence syndrome. (Note: 75% is a guideline; a lower percentage may be chosen as the reduction fraction.) This can be continued until the total daily dose of narcotic is equivalent to 30 to 45 mg of oral morphine sulfate. After 2 days at this level, the medication may be stopped. Methadone may be considered for oral therapy; figure an equivalent dosage to the currently used narcotic, take 25% of this as a starting point, and then follow the same schedule as above.

F. Random drug screening will aid the clinician in determining patient compliance. Inform the patient of the possibility of drug screening at the beginning of the weaning process.

References

Bonica JJ. The management of pain. 2nd ed. Philadelphia: Lea & Febiger, 1990:1671.

Payne R. Principles of analgesic use in the treatment of acute pain and chronic cancer pain. A concise guide to medical practice. American Pain Society. c/o American Pain Society, 1615 L Street, NW, Suite 925, Washington, DC 20036.

Tywcross RG, McQuay HF. Opioids. In: Wall PD, Melzack R, eds. Textbook of pain. 2nd ed. New York: Churchill Livingstone, 1989:694.

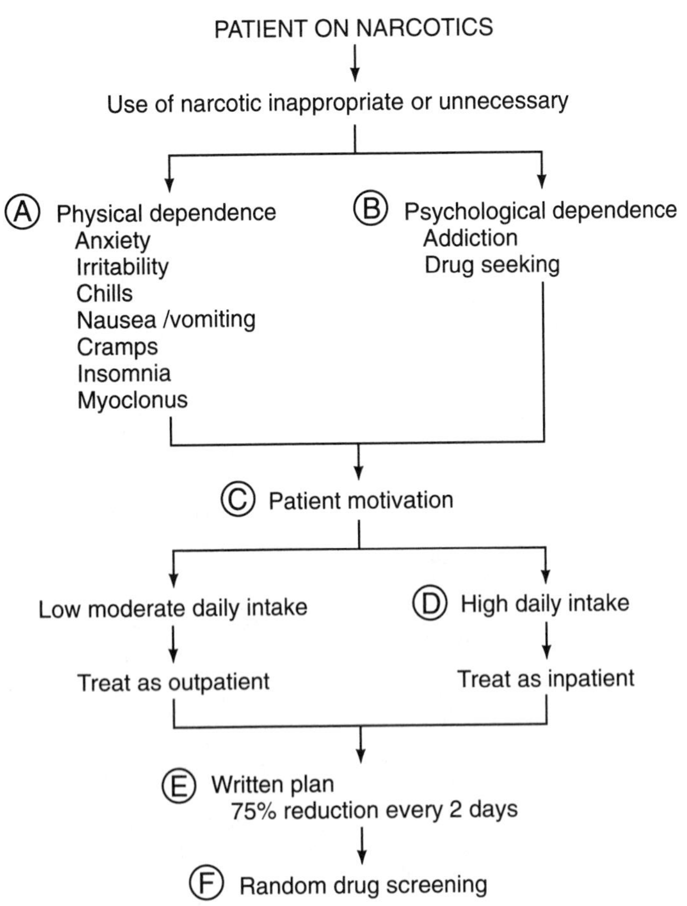
PATIENT ON NARCOTICS
Use of narcotic inappropriate or unnecessary
(A) Physical dependence
Anxiety
Irritability
Chills
Nausea /vomiting
Cramps
Insomnia
Myoclonus
(B) Psychological dependence
Addiction
Drug seeking
(C) Patient motivation
Low moderate daily intake
Treat as outpatient
(D) High daily intake
Treat as inpatient
(E) Written plan
75% reduction every 2 days
(F) Random drug screening

PHYSICAL THERAPY

James Griffin, P.T., A.T.C.

A. Heat is probably the most commonly used modality in physical therapy. Heat increases blood flow and tissue distensibility, decreases muscle spasm, and produces analgesia, apparently through the action of cutaneous receptors. It is indicated for chronic stiffness, spasm, and pain and is generally helpful before stretching or exercise. Hot packs, heating pads, paraffin baths, or whirlpools can be used to deliver heat. A modality called fluidotherapy uses particles of finely ground cellulose suspended in hot air (120° F) circulating through a cabinet. The limb is inserted in the cabinet and range-of-motion exercise may be done during treatment. Contraindications to the use of heat are the presence of sensory impairment, circulatory insufficiency, malignancy, and infection. Care should also be taken with elderly patients in whom sensation and judgment may be suspect.

B. Ultrasound is produced by electrical stimulation of a quartz or artificial crystal, which vibrates in response. At 1 MHz, tissue penetration to 5 cm occurs. The rapid vibration of the tissue by the sound waves produces heat, with the maximum effect occurring at the junction of bone and muscle. Ultrasound can be effective in treating frozen shoulder, postamputation pain, decubitus ulcers, and reflex sympathetic dystrophy. It is safe for use with implants and does not increase their temperature. Contraindications include malignancy, circulatory impairment, pregnancy, use over the eye, impaired sensation, and infection.

Shortwave or microwave diathermy produces heating of the tissue to a depth of 3 to 4 cm. Indications are the same as for ultrasound. The advantage of the diathermies is the depth of penetration they provide. Care must be taken during treatment to keep metal out of the electromagnetic field, and patients with any metallic implant should not be treated. Areas of high fluid volume, such as the eyes or joint effusions, may overheat. Pregnancy, ischemic tissue, and pain or sensory deficit are other contraindications.

C. Cold decreases pain, spasm, swelling, and nerve conduction velocity. It is generally used for acute injury or acute exacerbation of chronic injuries but may also be effective for chronic pain. Ice bags, ice massage, or reusable cold packs are most commonly used for cold application. Treatment time is 10 to 20 minutes, or until the area is numb. After treatment, the area should be red or pink, cool, and insensitive to touch. Care must be taken when treating extremities or over superficial nerves. Contraindications include impaired sensation or circulation and cold intolerance. Cold sprays, such as ethyl chloride or fluoromethane, are used in conjunction with stretching for the treatment of myofascial pain. Contrast baths, using two containers or whirlpools, are advocated in the treatment of the extremities for sprains, strains, arthritis, and some cases of peripheral vascular disease.

D. Traction in various modes is effective for the treatment of cervical and lumbar disc disorders, muscle spasm, hypomobility, and osteoarthritis of the lumbar and cervical spine. Gravity traction for the low back can achieve distraction forces of up to 40% of the person's body weight. Manual traction can be done for both the cervical and lumbar spine as a screen for effectiveness of treatment or in patients who do not tolerate mechanical traction. Autotraction is a modality developed in Sweden that uses gravity traction and three-dimensional positional traction to treat lumbar disc problems. Intermittent mechanical traction is most commonly used. Lumbar traction can be administered with the patient in the supine or prone position with varying degrees of flexion. Cervical traction requires a minimum pull of 25 pounds to achieve separation of the posterior elements of the cervical spine, with the neck in 25° to 30° of flexion. Distraction of the atlanto-occipital and atlantoaxial joints requires only 10 pounds of pull in a neutral position, and symptomatic relief may be achieved at lower levels. Contraindications to traction are instability secondary to tumor, disease, or infection; vascular compromise; and situations in which movement is contraindicated. Relative contraindications are recent sprain or strain, osteoporosis, hiatal hernia, pregnancy, and increased neurologic symptoms with treatment. Patients with claustrophobia may not tolerate the restrictive nature of this treatment.

E. Electrical stimulation is provided with either direct current (DC) or alternating current (AC). DC devices are now commonly used only to stimulate denervated muscle and to drive medication subcutaneously (iontophoresis). Most devices on the market use some form of AC current. AC devices produce low total current and do not produce thermal or chemical effects. Most AC devices produce a high voltage output (>150 volts) with a monophasic wave form, and allow adjustment of intensity, pulse rate, and pulse width. Clinical guidelines for high voltage stimulation are available for treating acute and chronic conditions including pain, joint effusion, muscle spasm, muscle disuse atrophy, circulatory disorders, and wound healing. "Interferential current" supposedly avoids the cutaneous discomfort of traditional electrical stimulation by using a high-frequency carrier current that cannot be felt on the skin and is cancelled out at the site of treatment, leaving a lower therapeutic frequency. Electrical stimulation should not be used in patients with pacemakers, across the pregnant uterus, to stimulate the carotid sinus, and in patients with systemic infection or malignancy.

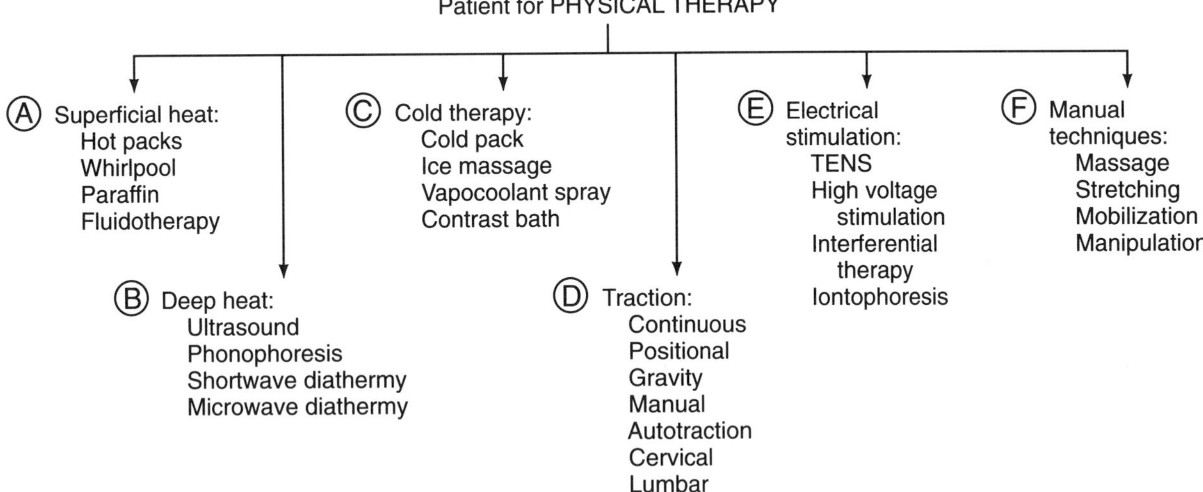

Transcutaneous electrical neuromuscular stimulation (TENS) is considered a special form of electrical stimulation (p 194), although any electrical stimulation is TENS. Numerous clinical usage guides are available.

Phonophoresis is the use of ultrasound to drive medication through the skin. Iontophoresis is the use of DC current to achieve the same purpose. Local anesthetic and steroid medications are typically used. Both of these methods are effective for superficial bursitis, tendinitis, ligamentous strain, and trigger point treatment, and may be useful in patients who cannot tolerate an injection. Contraindications include drug allergies and side effects, as well as any of the precautions for ultrasound or electrical stimulation.

F. Several manual techniques can be applied as part of the treatment of pain. Massage, in its many forms, can enhance circulation and promote venous and lymphatic return. Specific manual techniques can stretch the skin, fascia, and connective tissues to increase motion and pliability (myofascial release) or treat pain (acupressure). Stretching, whether performed manually or done by the patient, is important in treating muscle pain. Joint hypomobility can be assessed and treated with manual techniques. Repetitive oscillation of a joint can increase range and improve "quality" of motion of a joint. Manipulation is mobilization with impulse in which the motion barrier is met and thrust through to achieve more normal joint motion. Manipulation is possible in many joints of the body and is advocated as the treatment for specific musculoskeletal disorders in the low back and foot. Contraindications for soft tissue techniques include open wounds, recent surgery, and infection. For joint mobilization and manipulative techniques the contraindications also include osteoporosis, pregnancy, and active inflammatory processes in the joint. Additional contraindications are tumor, malignancy, segmental instability, and neurologic deficit.

References

Alon G. Principles of electrical stimulation. In: Nelson RM, Currier DP, eds. Clinical electrotherapy. Los Altos, CA: Appleton & Lange, 1987.

Cummings J. Iontophoresis. In: Nelson RM, Currier DP, eds. Clinical electrotherapy. Los Altos, CA: Appleton-Lange, 1987.

Greenman PE. Principles of manual medicine. Baltimore: Williams & Wilkins, 1989.

Griffin J, Karselis P. Physical agents for physical therapists. Springfield, IL: Charles C Thomas, 1982.

Kirkaldy-Willis WH. A comprehensive outline of treatment. In: Kirkaldy-Willis, ed. Managing low back pain. 2nd ed. New York: Churchill Livingstone, 1988.

Klein J, Pariser D. Transcutaneous electrical nerve stimulation. In: Nelson RM, Currier DP, eds. Clinical electrotherapy. Los Altos, CA: Appleton & Lange, 1987.

Kloth L. Shortwave and microwave diathermy. In: Michlovitz S, ed. Thermal agents in rehabilitation. Philadelphia: FA Davis, 1986.

Michlovitz S. Biophysical principles of heating and superficial heat agents. In: Michlovitz S, ed. Thermal agents in rehabilitation. Philadelphia: FA Davis, 1986.

Newell SG, Woodle A. Cuboid syndrome. Phys Sports Med 1981; 1:71.

Ottoson D, Lundberg T. Treatment by transcutaneous electrical nerve stimulation. New York: Springer-Verlag, 1988.

Saunders D. Lumbar traction. In: Grieve GP, ed. Modern manual therapy of the vertebral column. New York: Churchill Livingstone, 1986.

Savage B. Interferential therapy. Boston: Faber and Faber, 1984.

Travell JG, Simmons DG. Myofascial pain and dysfunction. Baltimore: Williams & Wilkins, 1983.

VOCATIONAL REHABILITATION

Paul T. Ingmundson, Ph.D.

Many patients referred for treatment in pain management programs have unresolved disability or worker's compensation claims originating with on-the-job injuries. Such patients are frequently caught up in a system in which they have incentives to exaggerate symptoms of disability in order to avoid employment or return to an unpleasant work environment. A narrow focus on medical problems without an appreciation for the social and economic context in which the pain complaint is presented can result in a perpetuation of chronic disability and inappropriate demands for additional medical services. Alternatively, a brief assessment of occupational status and referral to rehabilitation resources may facilitate a return to productive and independent living.

A. The vocational rehabilitation referral begins with a comprehensive diagnosis, including any applicable psychiatric and substance abuse diagnosis. A comprehensive list of diagnoses assists the vocational rehabilitation specialist in treatment planning and also may facilitate access to programs with entry criteria keyed to specific disabilities.

B. A statement of prognosis and a functional assessment are required for rational rehabilitation planning. Self-limiting pain symptoms generally do not necessitate access to rehabilitation resources, but chronic pain symptoms may require permanent changes in work activities. Statements of limitations and anticipated length of disability need to be as specific as possible. Statements of anticipated needs for ongoing medical treatment are also a necessary part of the prognostic assessment.

C. The vocational rehabilitation specialist's work starts once the physician has provided the applicable diagnostic and prognostic referral information. Assessment procedures often include tests of aptitude, such as the General Aptitude Test Battery (GATB), as well as surveys of interests, such as the Strong Campbell Interest Inventory (SCII).

D. The vocational rehabilitation specialist must simultaneously assess the patient's intrinsic resources and the family and community resources that can be enlisted in assisting in the rehabilitation process, including special entitlements (e.g., veteran's benefits).

E. Retraining may take the form of entry into a general secondary or college level education program, or retraining in specific occupational skills. The choice of retraining program is dictated by the patient's interests, aptitudes, strengths, and disabilities; the available training resources; and, it is hoped, the demands of the local labor market.

F. In addition to job placement, a variety of possible outcomes need to be considered. Some patients are able to return to their previously established career paths after an injury or illness. Others need retraining in different skills compatible with their disabilities, but are able to return to the competitive labor market. Some patients do not have the resources to compete in the general labor market even after extensive rehabilitation and may need to be directed into supported employment, such as Goodwill Industries or various government-sponsored programs. Still other patients are not able to return to gainful employment but may be able to participate in activities such as volunteer work. For some patients the goals of rehabilitation are limited to increasing their capacity to maintain whatever autonomy may be possible in managing their activities of daily living.

References

Caplan B. Rehabilitation psychology desk reference. Rockville, Md, Aspen, 1987.

Goldenson RM, Dunham JR, Dunham CS (eds). Disability and rehabilitation handbook. New York: McGraw-Hill, 1978.

Wright GN. Total rehabilitation. Boston: Little, Brown, 1980.

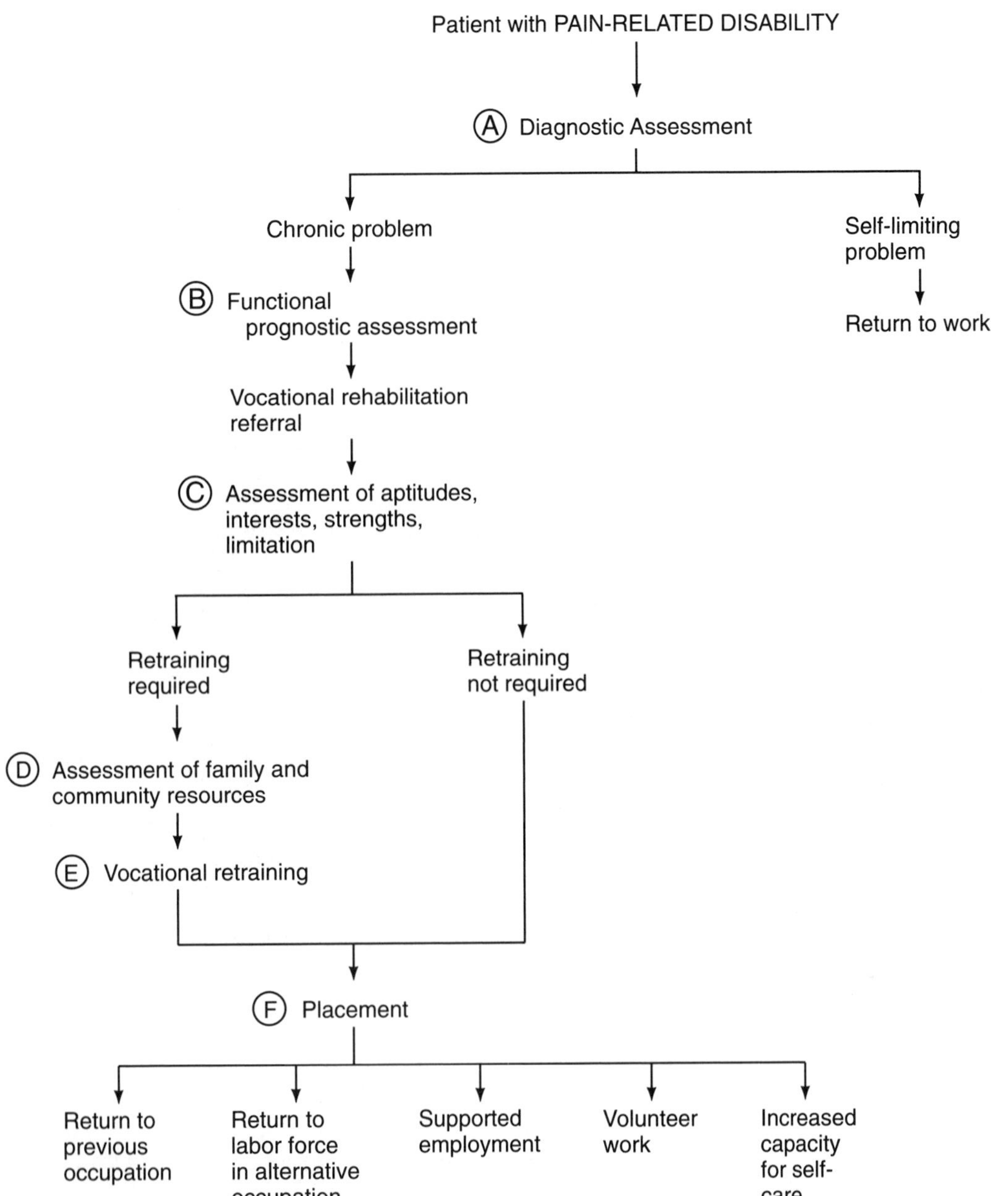
Patient with PAIN-RELATED DISABILITY
A Diagnostic Assessment
Chronic problem
Self-limiting problem
Return to work
B Functional prognostic assessment
Vocational rehabilitation referral
C Assessment of aptitudes, interests, strengths, limitation
Retraining required
Retraining not required
D Assessment of family and community resources
E Vocational retraining
F Placement
Return to previous occupation
Return to labor force in alternative occupation
Supported employment
Volunteer work
Increased capacity for self-care

TRANSCUTANEOUS ELECTRICAL NERVE STIMULATION

James Griffin, P.T., A.T.C.

As a tool for the treatment of pain, transcutaneous electrical nerve stimulation (TENS) can be used for a wide variety of acute and chronic conditions. These include, but are not limited to, acute and chronic musculoskeletal pain, postoperative pain, dental pain, headaches, peripheral neuropathies, reflex sympathetic dystrophy, postherpetic neuralgia, and cancer pain. TENS is thought to work by temporarily inhibiting transmission from small afferent nerves to second-order neurons in the spinal cord by non-noxious stimuli. TENS may also access the body's endogenous opioids, as the analgesia produced by some forms of TENS stimulation has been shown to be reversible by naloxone, an opioid antagonist. TENS is safe and nonaddictive. Contraindications include pregnancy, use over the carotid sinus, and the presence of a cardiac pacemaker. The last-named may not be an absolute contraindication, because there are case reports of the safe use of TENS with a pacemaker. The immediate effectiveness of TENS in pain control has been shown to be 60 to 80% in some studies, but this falls off over time. Estimates of the effect of TENS on chronic conditions after 1 year fall to 25 to 30%.

Modern TENS units are small portable devices powered by a 9-volt battery. Most units have two channels, each controlling a pair of electrodes affixed to the body at the desired locations. The output of each channel, except for intensity, is identical and can be altered by varying the stimulation parameters of the unit. Commercial units allow the clinician to alter intensity, pulse width, and pulse rate and may offer any or all of such features as an automatic modulation mode, a dedicated burst or acupuncture mode, an automatic timer, a battery life indicator, and other stimulation or convenience options. Given the cost of such devices (over $600 retail), a 5-year or lifetime warranty is desirable and available from some manufacturers.

TENS units produce a small electrical current ranging up to 120 mA, depending on the unit selected. Most commercial devices automatically alter the voltage output to account for variations in skin resistance, and produce a constant current. Depending on the unit, the pulse rate can be altered between 2 and 200 pulses/sec and pulse width can be varied from 9 to 500 μsec. Most TENS units now offer a modulation setting that automatically alters pulse rate, width, and/or intensity around previously selected parameters. This feature is said to diminish the body's tendency to accommodate to a constant stimulus, one reason why the effect of TENS is theorized to fall off over time. Waveform varies with the TENS unit selected and generally is not an adjustable parameter. There is no consensus on an optimal waveform and there may be little difference in waveforms once they have penetrated the tissue.

A. High-frequency or conventional TENS is the stimulation mode most commonly used. This employs a pulse rate of 50 to 100 Hz and a short pulse width of 20 to 60 μsec. Treatment time may vary from 30 minutes to several hours per day at a perceptible, comfortable level of stimulation. Studies in a clinical pain population show that a subthreshold stimulus is also effective for initial TENS trials. Conventional TENS has proved effective for a wide variety of conditions and is the treatment of choice for acute or postsurgical situations and a starting point for chronic pain conditions.

B. Other stimulus modes may be more effective for chronic pain conditions. Acupuncture-like TENS uses a low frequency (1 to 4 Hz) and wide pulse (150 to 250 μsec). Intensity is at a level to produce a strong, visible muscle contraction in the related myotome. Treatment time is 20 to 30 minutes once or twice a day. Analgesia takes longer to produce but lasts longer than with conventional TENS.

C. Burst or pulse train TENS is similar to acupuncture-like TENS. This employs a series of four to ten high-frequency pulses (70 to 100 Hz) delivered one to four times/sec. Stimulation intensity is to the point of muscle contraction.

D. Brief, intense TENS employs a high frequency (above 100 Hz) and wide pulse width (150 to 250 μsec) at the highest intensity the patient can tolerate for 1 to 15 minutes. It is proposed that this stimulus mode may disrupt the "pain memory" or act centrally in some other way.

E. If none of the above modes produce acceptable analgesia, the clinician may try to "tune in" an optimal setting by first holding the pulse width constant at about 100 μsec and sweeping through the pulse rate in small increments to find an ideal setting. The process is then repeated for pulse width, maintaining the pulse rate at the previously determined level.

F. Microcurrent TENS devices are being marketed that purport to use microamperage current to produce pain relief for conditions treated with traditional TENS. Numerous anecdotal claims are made for these devices, but no current research validates their effectiveness.

(Continued on page 196)

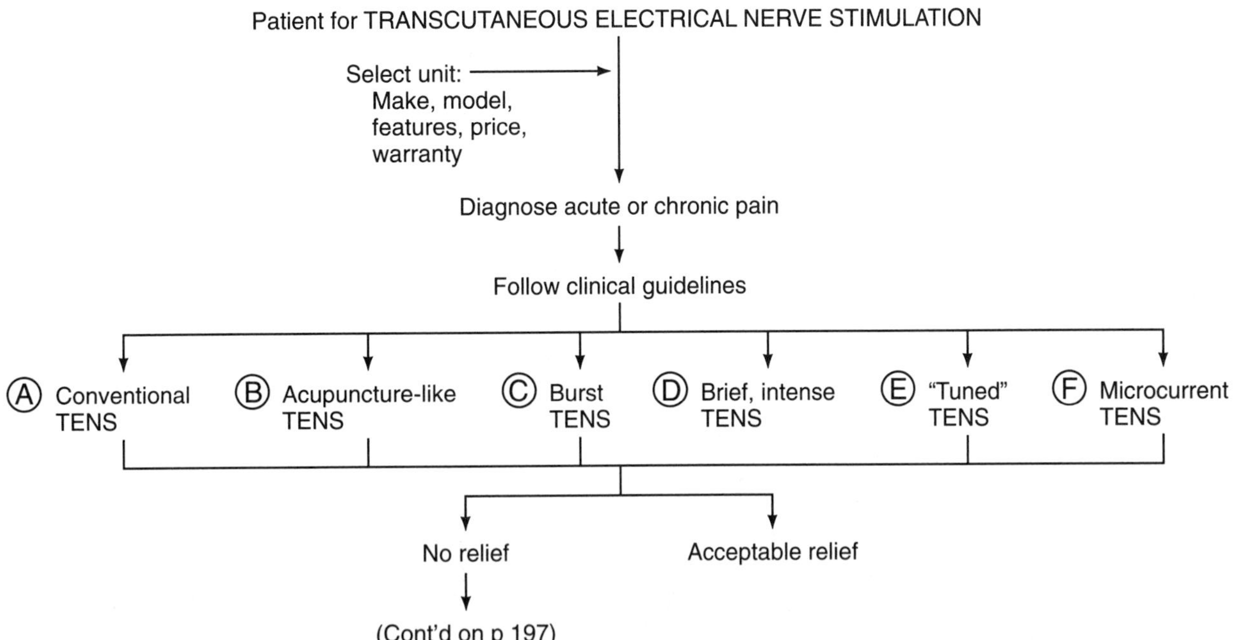
Patient for TRANSCUTANEOUS ELECTRICAL NERVE STIMULATION
Select unit:
Make, model,
features, price,
warranty
Diagnose acute or chronic pain
Follow clinical guidelines
Ⓐ Conventional TENS
Ⓑ Acupuncture-like TENS
Ⓒ Burst TENS
Ⓓ Brief, intense TENS
Ⓔ "Tuned" TENS
Ⓕ Microcurrent TENS
No relief
Acceptable relief
(Cont'd on p 197)

G. Successful electrode placement can be achieved using a number of methods shown by research to be effective. Most common is to place the electrodes on or bracketing the painful site. Both electrodes from each channel may be on one side of the painful area or in a crisscross pattern.

H. Electrodes may be placed in the dermatome, myotome, or sclerotome in which the painful site is located. Specific sites in a region may be targeted, e.g., a trigger point, or the placement may be on the anterior and posterior aspect of the dermatome, as in the thoracic region.

I. Acupuncture points, trigger points, or motor points may be effective stimulation sites. There is a high percentage of correlation between acupuncture points and trigger points, and between acupuncture points and the superficial areas of peripheral nerves. Acupuncture and trigger point charts are available to guide the clinician. Acupuncture points may be located with a probe, indicating areas of decreased tissue resistance. This may also be accomplished by clinicians using themselves in the circuit to locate such points.

J. Stimulation of peripheral nerves can be achieved at their most superficial site to obtain analgesia distally. Electrodes can be placed paraspinally and distally in the corresponding dermatome to treat radicular pain.

K. Electrodes may be placed contralaterally in appropriate stimulus sites if the ipsilateral side is too irritable to allow electrode placement, e.g., as in reflex sympathetic dystrophy.

L. If pain with motion is a major difficulty, the clinician may wish to try a series of electrode locations and have the patient perform the offending action(s) with stimulus of the selected points. Stimulus sites may be any combination of the points described above. This method can be time consuming but is of great functional significance to the patient.

M. Authorities differ in their recommendations of duration and frequency of stimulation during the day. Relief has been obtained experimentally with treatment from 30 minutes twice a week to constant stimulation. Because TENS stimulation has a carry-over effect, a treatment cycle that gives relief with scheduled "on" and "off" periods should be established. It is theorized that accommodation to TENS may be delayed or prevented by avoiding constant use. Intermittent use may also slow or prevent depletion of endogenous pain-relieving substances accessed by TENS stimulation.

N. TENS electrodes are available in several types. Carbonized silicon electrodes are durable and inexpensive but require the use of conductive gel and some sort of adhesive gel or patch. There are single- and multi-use disposable electrodes that are pre-gelled, self-adhering, sterile (for postoperative pain), and available in a variety of sizes and shapes. These are convenient but more expensive. Any of these electrodes may cause skin irritation, and the individual's skin chemistry or strenuous activity may result in failure to maintain a good bond. A trial of several electrode types may be necessary to find the best one for the patient.

Successful use of TENS requires skill and perseverance on the part of clinician and patient. Initially, pain relief may require several hours or days of TENS use, because some individuals respond in a cumulative fashion. More than one trial may be required to obtain the ideal combination of stimulus parameters and electrode location. If satisfactory results cannot be obtained in a single office visit, patients should try further suggested stimulus modes or sites at home for several days to maximize the chance of success. Although many clinical guidelines are available, success with TENS depends on individualizing electrode type and placement, stimulation parameters, and stimulation time to the patient's requirements.

References

Barr JO, Nielsen DH, Soderbert GL. Transcutaneous electrical nerve stimulation characteristics for altering pain perception. Phys Ther 1986; 66:1515.

Beriant SR. Method of determining optimal stimulation sites for transcutaneous electrical nerve stimulation. Phys Ther 1984; 64:924.

Gersh MR. Microcurrent electrical stimulation: Putting it in perspective. Clin Management 1989; 9:51.

Gersh MR, Wolf SL. Applications of transcutaneous electrical nerve stimulation in the management of patients with pain. Phys Ther 1985; 65:314.

Klein J, Pariser D. Transcutaneous electrical nerve stimulation. In: Nelson RM, Currier DP, eds. Clinical electrotherapy. Norwalk, CT: Appleton & Lange, 1987:209.

Lamm K. Optimal placement techniques for TENS: A soft tissue approach. Tucson, AZ: Kenneth E. Lamm, 1986.

Leo KC, Dostal WF, Bossen DG, et al. Effect of transcutaneous nerve stimulation characteristics on clinical pain. Phys Ther 1986; 66:200.

Ottoson D, Lundeberg T. Pain treatment by transcutaneous electrical nerve stimulation. New York: Springer-Verlag, 1988.

Shade SK. Use of transcutaneous electrical nerve stimulation for a patient with a cardiac pacemaker. Phys Ther 1985; 65:206.

Woolf CF: Segmental afferent fiber induced analgesia: Transcutaneous electrical nerve stimulation (TENS) and vibration. In: Wall PD, Melzack R, eds. Textbook of pain. New York: Churchill Livingstone, 1989:884.

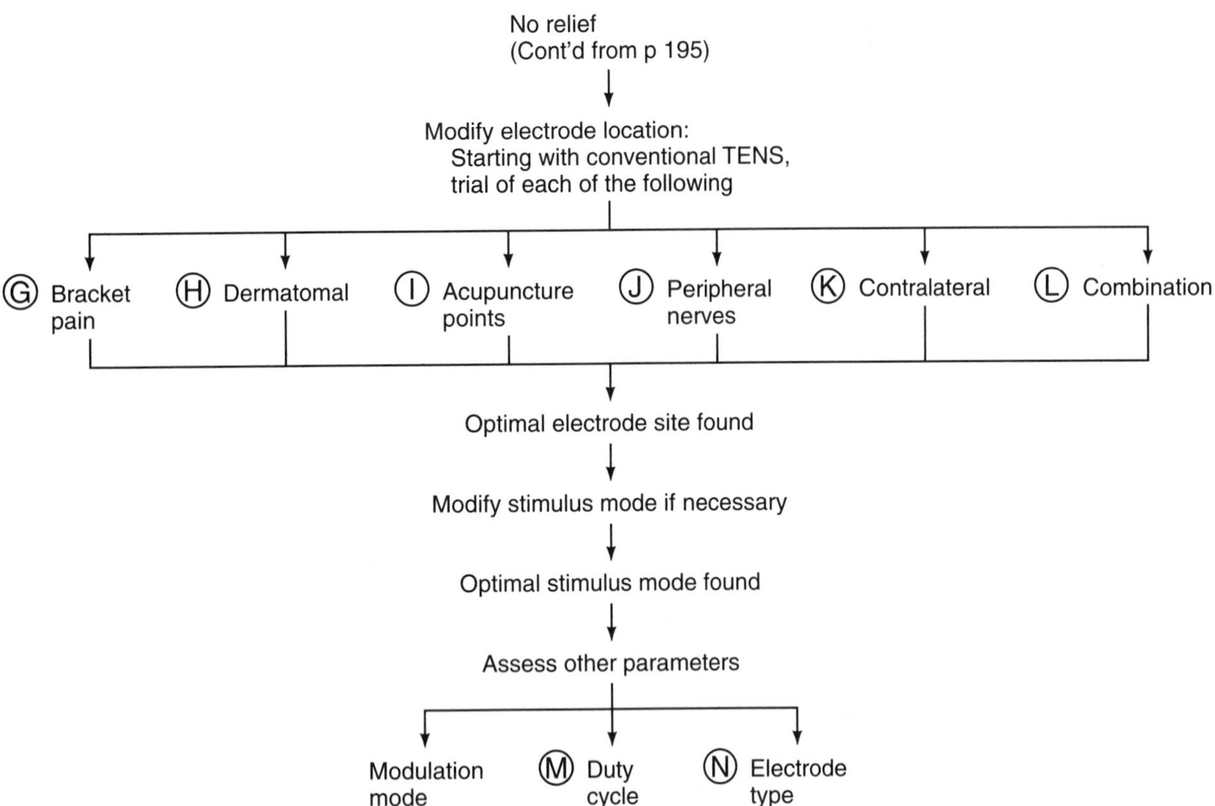
No relief
(Cont'd from p 195)
Modify electrode location:
Starting with conventional TENS,
trial of each of the following
(G) Bracket pain
(H) Dermatomal
(I) Acupuncture points
(J) Peripheral nerves
(K) Contralateral
(L) Combination
Optimal electrode site found
Modify stimulus mode if necessary
Optimal stimulus mode found
Assess other parameters
Modulation mode
(M) Duty cycle
(N) Electrode type

PSYCHOLOGICAL INTERVENTIONS

Lawrence S. Schoenfeld, Ph.D.

The comprehensive evaluation of patients with pain results in the identification of dysfunctional factors in four primary areas: motivation, cognition, affect, and physical (somatic) well-being. Each of these factors contributes to pain perception and can be modified through psychological interventions. Successful pain treatment programs must identify the dysfunctional components and initiate appropriate psychological intervention strategies to decrease pain perception and abnormal illness behavior.

A. Primary and secondary gains through interpersonal manipulations and/or the avoidance of responsibilities through pain behavior need direct resolution for the patient to improve. Job-related stress, social acceptance, sexual dysfunction, and marital difficulties may contribute significantly to pain and are addressed through behavior modification, supportive psychotherapy, marital or sex therapy, and vocational rehabilitation (p 192).

B. Dysfunctional beliefs, attributions, and expectations often perpetuate pain behavior. Cognitive coping skills can be easily taught to the patients.

C. Depression, anxiety, and anger often magnify pain. Relaxation therapies, including biofeedback and hypnosis, serve as useful anxiolytic interventions (pp 200 and 202). Antidepressant medication, exercise, and cognitive behavior therapy have antidepressant, analgesic, and sleep-normalizing properties. Traditional psychotherapy may assist the patient in facilitating compliance with rehabilitation plans.

D. Narcotic and anxiolytic drug abuse requires detoxification and appropriate psychological support (p 188). Myofascial pain and disuse can be reduced through operant behavior modification strategies, exercise, biofeedback, and psychotropic medication.

References

France R, Krishnau KRR, eds. Chronic pain. Washington, DC: American Psychiatric Press, 1988.

Turk D, Meichenbaum D, Genest M. Pain and behavioral medicine. New York: Guilford Press, 1983.

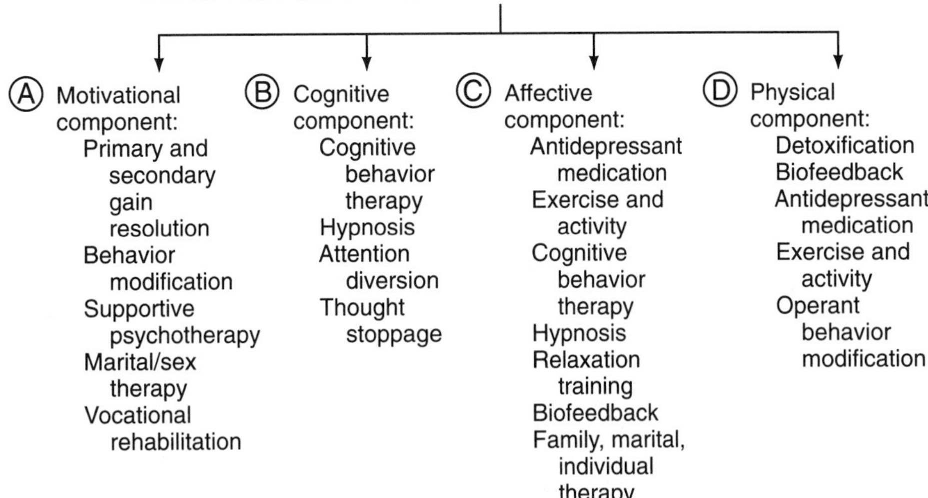
Chronic Pain Patient in Need of PSYCHOLOGICAL INTERVENTIONS
A Motivational component:
Primary and secondary gain resolution
Behavior modification
Supportive psychotherapy
Marital/sex therapy
Vocational rehabilitation
B Cognitive component:
Cognitive behavior therapy
Hypnosis
Attention diversion
Thought stoppage
C Affective component:
Antidepressant medication
Exercise and activity
Cognitive behavior therapy
Hypnosis
Relaxation training
Biofeedback
Family, marital, individual therapy
D Physical component:
Detoxification
Biofeedback
Antidepressant medication
Exercise and activity
Operant behavior modification

HYPNOSIS

Lawrence S. Schoenfeld, Ph.D.

Hypnosis is a pain-attenuating procedure that does not cause significant side-effects or a reduction in mental status. The mechanism by which hypnotic pain relief is achieved remains unclear. For most patients with chronic pain, hypnosis serves as an adjunct to other interventions by enhancing the relaxation response and augmenting self-control strategies. Some patients are able to achieve total pain control through self-hypnosis.

A. Hypnosis requires the patient to engage in sustained or focused attention or concentration. When the ability to sustain focused attention is compromised, hypnosis provides little or no therapeutic value and may further frustrate the patient, thus diminishing motivation and compliance. An initial clinical evaluation should exclude those patients with psychosis, organic brain syndrome, mental retardation, and severe depression. Patients with significant depression should receive antidepressant treatment prior to a trial of hypnosis.

B. Provide patients with a full explanation of hypnosis for pain control and have them undergo a trial hypnotic induction to establish susceptibility to hypnosis and to desensitize them to the procedure. The use of formal hypnotic susceptibility scales such as the Stanford Hypnotic Susceptibility Scale and Hypnotic Induction Profile is not necessary and may interfere with the use of hypnosis for pain control. Both direct and indirect hypnotic induction techniques are useful for pain control.

C. Patients with low susceptibility to hypnosis may still find hypnosis useful to facilitate the relaxation response and as a strategy for attention diversion. The relaxation response and attention diversion provide the patient with perceived control over aspects of the pain.

D. Those patients who demonstrate moderate to high ability to be hypnotized are able to modify the perception of pain to a significant degree. These patients undergo repeated induction and are provided with direct and indirect suggestions that facilitate dissociation, analgesia, and anesthesia. Pain perception can be moved to alternate locations in the body and pain characteristics can be altered to increase tolerance. Suggest life-enhancing attitudes to facilitate other treatment modalities.

E. After an introduction to hypnosis, the patient may choose to use this procedure for pain management. An audio recording of the procedure can help the patient practice hypnosis daily. Often, patients can use self-hypnosis after repeated tape-recorded inductions. Some patients are able to learn self-hypnosis for pain control after a single trial of hypnosis. Repeat follow-up to reinforce the use of hypnosis in facilitating compliance and attending to modifications of the pain experience.

References

Barber J. Rapid induction analgesia: a clinical report. Am J Clin Hypn 1977; 19:138.

Crasilneck H, Hall J. Clinical hypnosis: principles and applications. New York: Grune & Stratton, 1975.

Edmonston WE Jr. Hypnosis and relaxation. New York: John Wiley and Sons, 1981.

Orne M. Hypnotic methods for managing pain. In: Bonica J, ed. Advances in pain research and therapy. Vol. 5. New York: Raven Press, 1983:847.

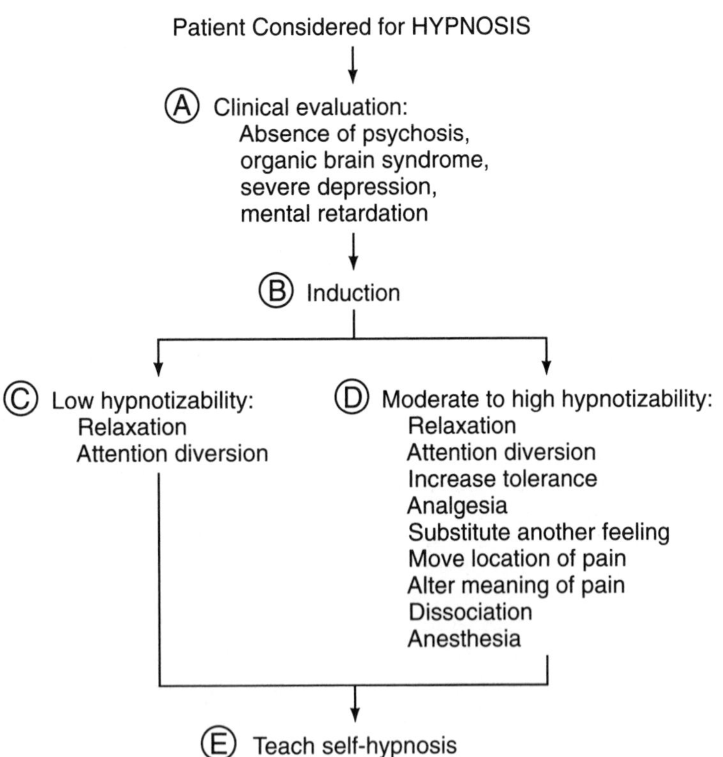
Patient Considered for HYPNOSIS
(A) Clinical evaluation:
Absence of psychosis,
organic brain syndrome,
severe depression,
mental retardation
(B) Induction
(C) Low hypnotizability:
Relaxation
Attention diversion
(D) Moderate to high hypnotizability:
Relaxation
Attention diversion
Increase tolerance
Analgesia
Substitute another feeling
Move location of pain
Alter meaning of pain
Dissociation
Anesthesia
(E) Teach self-hypnosis

BIOFEEDBACK

Paul T. Ingmundson, Ph.D.

Biofeedback is a therapeutic procedure in which a physiologic parameter, typically one under autonomic influence, is detected, amplified, and "fed back" to the patient, usually in the form of a visual signal or audiotone. The feedback procedure enables the patient to exert some conscious, self-regulatory control over a process that is usually deemed "involuntary."

A. The selection of candidates for biofeedback is typically preceded by an assessment process. In many cases, patients are selected for conservative treatment because more invasive approaches have failed or are deemed inappropriate. Psychologic testing may be helpful in identifying patients with concentration difficulties secondary to depression that may limit their capacity to participate in self-regulatory approaches to treatment. Patients with elevated scores on the MMPI Hypochondriasis and Hysteria scales have been shown to experience poorer outcomes, and younger patients sometimes may have more favorable outcomes than older individuals. Patients with previously untreated depression should usually be referred for treatment of the mood disturbance before biofeedback training. Hypochondriacal trends are not a definitive contraindication to biofeedback treatment, but may suggest a pattern of illness behavior or secondary gain that needs to be modified before a self-regulatory approach, such as biofeedback, has a reasonable chance for success.

B. The next step in the implementation of a biofeedback procedure is the choice of a target response. The most popular modalities are skin temperature for disorders in which dysregulation of blood flow has been implicated, and EMG for disorders in which elevated levels of muscle tension are thought to play a role. Other parameters (EEG alpha rhythm) have also been used, although skin temperature and EMG appear to be by far the most popular approaches. Disorders of blood flow (Raynaud's disease, vascular headaches) typically are treated with skin temperature feedback procedures. Disorders associated with musculoskeletal pain (back pain, temporomandibular joint [TMJ] disorders, tension headaches) are generally treated with EMG feedback. The choice between modalities is not always clear, and the generalized relaxation effects obtained with both procedures suggest that common mechanisms may be involved in many cases.

C. After determining that EMG is the procedure of choice, the biofeedback clinician must next choose the appropriate site for electrode placement. Frontalis EMG is used in most patients with anxiety disorders as well as those with tension headaches. Patients referred for chronic lower back pain may undergo frontalis EMG monitoring, although feedback from electrodes placed over the erector spinae muscles can also be used. Trapezii and cervical paraspinal muscles are sometimes monitored in patients with neck or shoulder pain. Masseter muscles are frequently monitored in patients with bruxism or TMJ disorders.

D. Most EMG biofeedback is performed with the patient in a static, resting posture. An alternative approach, however, involves providing EMG feedback during dynamic movement. This procedure is currently available in relatively few laboratories, but may provide a bridge between traditional biofeedback procedures and other forms of physical therapy.

E. Biofeedback treatment typically consists of the establishment of baseline levels, a series of five to ten treatment sessions, and post-treatment baseline observations. Interestingly, changes in the physiologic parameters of interest do not always correlate highly with the subjective relief of symptoms. Some theorists have suggested that the treatment works by reducing general levels of anxiety or tension, rather than by specific changes in blood flow or muscle activity. Others have suggested that the procedure permits patients to obtain a greater sense of mastery or control over their symptoms.

F. Home biofeedback units are available, but most clinical applications aim at teaching patients either a generalized or specific response that they can invoke after training without the use of peripheral instrumentation.

References

Blanchard EB, Ahles TA. Biofeedback therapy. In: Bonica JJ. The management of pain. 2nd ed. Philadelphia, Lea and Febiger, 1990:1722.

Keefe FJ. EMG-assisted relaxation training in the management of chronic low back pain. Am J Clin Biofeedback 1981; 4:93.

Wolf SL, Nacht M, Kelly JL. EMG biofeedback training during dynamic movement for low back pain patients. Behav Ther 1982; 13:395.

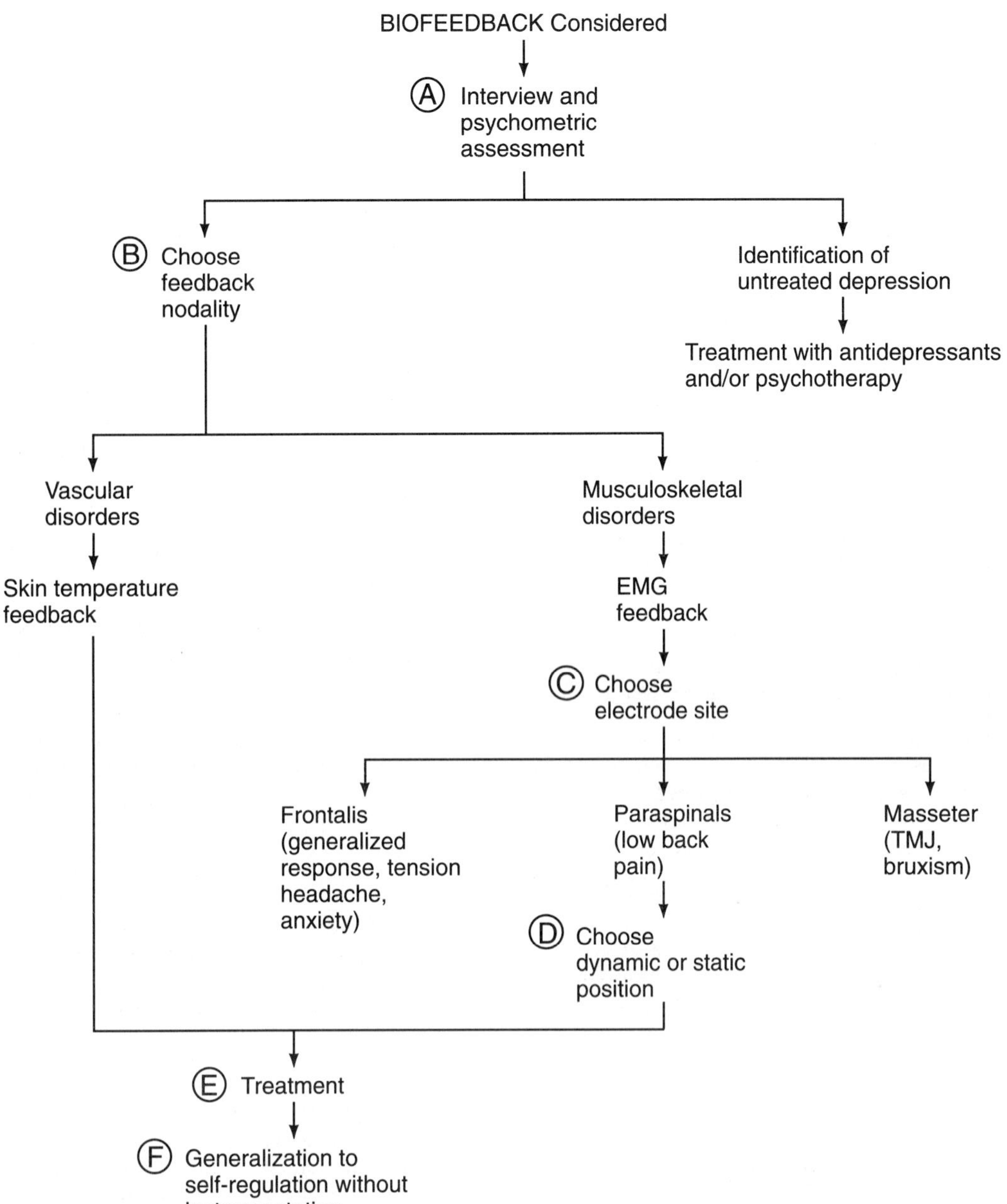
BIOFEEDBACK Considered
(A) Interview and psychometric assessment
(B) Choose feedback nodality
Identification of untreated depression
Treatment with antidepressants and/or psychotherapy
Vascular disorders
Musculoskeletal disorders
Skin temperature feedback
EMG feedback
(C) Choose electrode site
Frontalis (generalized response, tension headache, anxiety)
Paraspinals (low back pain)
Masseter (TMJ, bruxism)
(D) Choose dynamic or static position
(E) Treatment
(F) Generalization to self-regulation without instrumentation

PLACEBO ANALGESIA

Joan Hoffman, R.N., M.S.N.

Placebo consistently produces analgesia in 30% to 40% of patients with varying painful conditions. Patients with more intense pain and those with high anxiety levels have been shown to be more likely to respond favorably to placebo administration. A patient who reports analgesia with placebo in one situation does not necessarily report analgesia with placebo in every situation. A response to placebo cannot be used to determine whether a patient's pain is "real." The response to any treatment is a result not only of pharmacologic effect, but also a nonpharmacologic phenomenon that can be termed "placebo effect." A knowledge of placebo effect (Table 1) can assist in maximizing the therapeutic response to prescribed treatments. Also, before performing a neurolytic block, a block using a placebo should be performed to help establish the pharmacologic efficacy of the block.

A. Consider the possibility that what was considered a placebo treatment has a specific pharmacologic effect.

B. Although the placebo response is not well understood, several theories explain how placebos can consistently produce such a significant response. One theory is that the response is mediated by endorphin release. In several studies the administration of naloxone reversed placebo analgesia at least partially, which supports this theory.

C. A conditioned response, according to operant and classical conditioning theory, is based on a person's previous experience with treatment. Previous similar treatments that were extremely effective could cause a placebo treatment to be associated with an effective outcome. Likewise, previous experience with negative outcome could condition a patient to have a negative response to placebo.

D. A person's specific expectations for what will happen in a given situation are a primary determinant of what he or she will experience, according to expectancy theory. Conditioning, verbal persuasion, modeling, and observation are methods by which to develop expectations. The interactions between patient and caregiver, enthusiasm and expected results communicated to the patient, and information the patient receives from other sources all contribute to the patient's expectancy. Side effects commonly associated with placebos could also be explained by this theory.

E. Reduction of anxiety by administration of a placebo may contribute to its effectiveness. With experimentally induced pain, patients with higher levels of anxiety are more likely to be placebo responders. Further clinical research is needed to clarify the role of anxiety reduction in placebo response.

TABLE 1 Strategies to Maximize Placebo Effect

Develop open and supportive communication with patient
Express confidence and enthusiasm in treatment
Inform patient fully about expected benefits
Prescribe treatment congruent with patient's beliefs and previous experience when appropriate

References

Beecher HK. Measurement of subjective responses: quantitative effect of drugs. New York: Oxford University Press, 1959.

Evans FJ. Expectancy, therapeutic instructions and the placebo response. In: White L, Tursky B, Schwartz GE, eds. Placebo: theory, research and mechanisms. New York: The Guilford Press, 1985.

Grevert P, Albert LH, Goldstein A. Partial antagonism of placebo analgesia by naloxone. Pain 1983; 16:129.

Levine JD, Gordon NC, Bornstein JC, Fields HL. Role of pain in placebo analgesia. Proc Natl Acad Sci USA 1979; 76:3528.

Levine JD, Gordon NC, Fields HL. The mechanism of placebo analgesia. Lancet 1978; 2:654.

Liberman R. An experimental study of the placebo response under three different situations of pain. J Psychiatr Res 1964; 2:233.

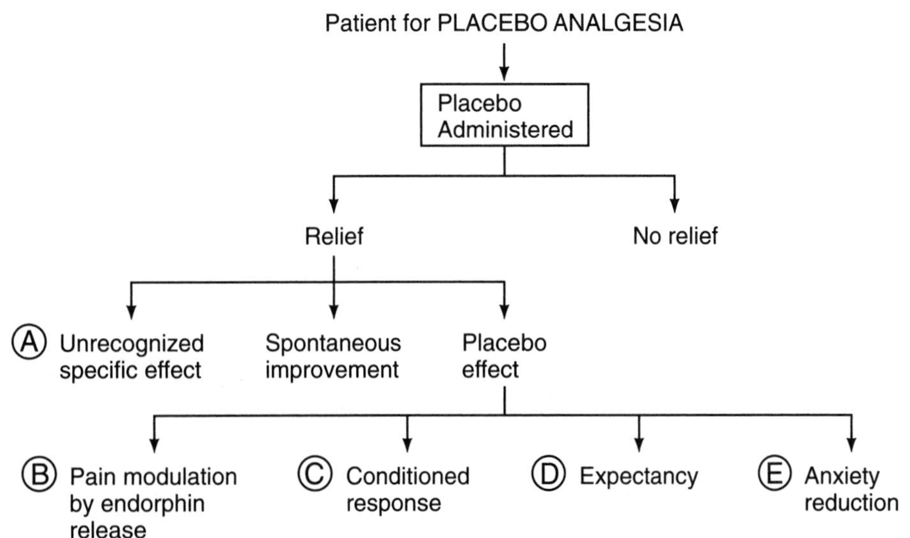
Patient for PLACEBO ANALGESIA
Placebo Administered
Relief
No relief
(A) Unrecognized specific effect
Spontaneous improvement
Placebo effect
(B) Pain modulation by endorphin release
(C) Conditioned response
(D) Expectancy
(E) Anxiety reduction

ACUPUNCTURE

Gregory J. Meredith, M.D., M.P.H.
Richard Rosenthal, M.D.

Acupuncture is a form of East Asian medicine dating back over 4500 years and traditionally involving the insertion of gold or silver needles in various points throughout the body. It was believed that disease states were caused by an imbalance in the natural energy of life, which the Chinese called Chi. By the insertion of acupuncture needles into points along meridians where Chi was believed to flow, life's energy would be drawn into a correct balance and disease would be cured. Throughout the centuries, various modifications have been made to acupuncture.

China in the late 1940s turned to acupuncture rather than Western medicine as an inexpensive method of medically treating the millions of sick and injured. When Nixon "opened" China in the early 1970s, acupuncture became a household word in the West, but the media quickly sensationalized it as the ultimate panacea. This was easily disproved by the medical community. The extensive research of the past two decades has shown that acupuncture is neither a panacea nor a fraud, but for a select group of patients with certain, specific disorders, acupuncture is often effective. Several mechanisms have been proposed to explain the alleviation of pain by acupuncture. These include the gate theory, the release of endorphins in the CNS stimulated by the manipulation of acupuncture points, and the muscle contracture theory.

A. Specific patients who may be candidates for acupuncture treatment include those with complaints relating to chronic musculoskeletal pain, fibromyalgia syndrome, spondylotic radiculopathy, facet joint syndrome, muscle tension headache and neck pain, lower back pain, and perhaps discogenic pain in its early phase. Some studies have shown that disorders resulting from a hypoactive parasympathetic nervous system (and consequently an unopposed sympathetic tone) (e.g., Raynaud's syndrome, asthma, and dysmenorrhea) may be amenable to acupuncture.

B. For acupuncture to be employed, specific points on the body must be located and stimulated. Charts are available that identify the common acupuncture sites. The most effective focal points for acupuncture are often where the affected muscle and its tendon meet. These points correspond to the traditional acupuncture points and also to the trigger points described in fibromyalgia syndrome and the points used in manipulative therapy described in osteopathic medicine. Once these points have been stimulated, the corresponding muscle usually has a small, brief, slightly painful spasm.

C. There are several possible methods for stimulating these points. A needle may be carefully inserted into and twisted within a point. An alternative approach may be to connect a small 9-volt intermittent current to the needle after it is inserted. This is similar to transcutaneous electrical nerve stimulation (TENS). Needles may be heated by burning moxa herb on their bases. The injection of normal saline or local anesthetics into an acupuncture point has been described in the treatment of myofascial pain (p 46), whereas simple pressure to the point (acupressure) is often effective for less severe pain. Points are stimulated for 10 to 20 minutes once a week for perhaps 4 weeks. If patients are properly selected and treatment is properly employed, acupuncture has proved very effective.

D. Despite the relatively benign nature of acupuncture, there is an ever-increasing list of complications associated with its use. Probably the most common is infection, either from the spread of coexisting local infection at the site of insertion or from person to person by unsterilized needles. Transmission of hepatitis B has been described, and HIV infection is a possibility. Needles have been reported to break off subcutaneously and require surgical removal. Pneumothorax from needles placed too deep in the chest has been described.

References

Annual Meeting Report: Acupuncture. J Tenn Med Assoc 1981; 75:202.

Bao JZ. Acupuncture treatment of Raynaud's disease: Report of 43 cases. J Tradit Chin Med 1988; 8:257.

Gray R, Maharajh GS, Hyland R. Pneumothorax resulting from acupuncture. Can Assoc Radiol J 1991; 42:139.

Gunn CC, Milbrandt WE. Acupuncture loci: A proposal for their classification according to their relationship to known neural structures. Am J Chin Med 1976; 4:183.

He LF. Involvement of endogenous opioid peptides in acupuncture analgesia. Pain 1987; 31:99.

He JA, Ma RY, Ahu L, Wang Z. Immediate relief and improved pulmonary functional changes in asthma symptomocomplex treated by needle warming moxabustion. J Tradit Chin Med 1988; 8:164.

Kent GP, Brondum J, Keenlyside RA, et al. A large outbreak of acupuncture-associated hepatitis B. Am J Epidemiol 1988; 127:591.

Melzack R. Myofascial trigger points: Relation to acupuncture and mechanism of pain. Arch Phys Med Rehabil 1981; 62:114.

Travell J, Simons D. Myofascial pain and dysfunction: The trigger point manual. Baltimore: Williams & Wilkins, 1983.

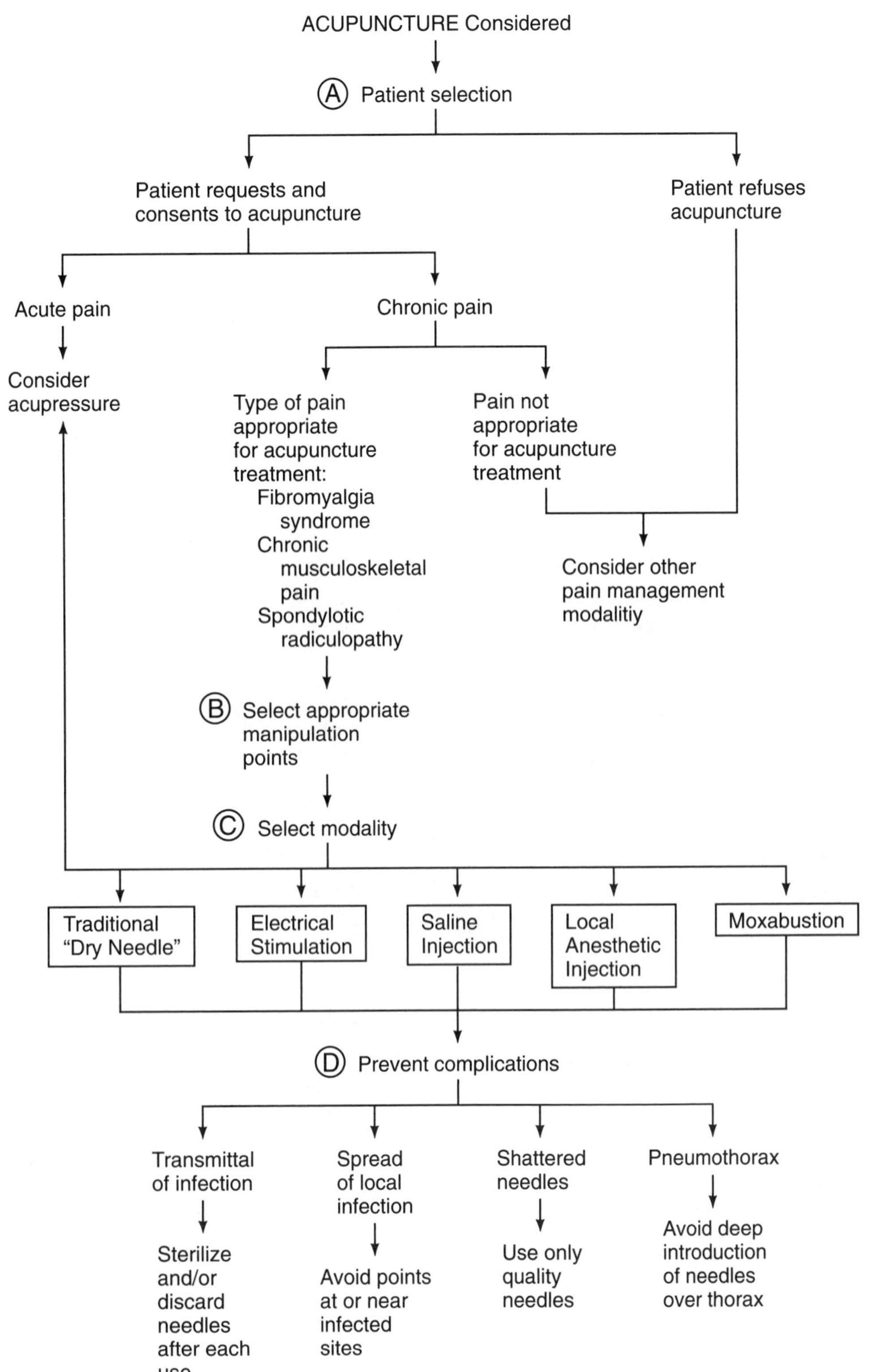

ACUPUNCTURE Considered
(A) Patient selection
Patient requests and consents to acupuncture
Patient refuses acupuncture
Acute pain
Chronic pain
Consider acupressure
Type of pain appropriate for acupuncture treatment:
Fibromyalgia syndrome
Chronic musculoskeletal pain
Spondylotic radiculopathy
Pain not appropriate for acupuncture treatment
Consider other pain management modalitiy
(B) Select appropriate manipulation points
(C) Select modality
Traditional "Dry Needle"
Electrical Stimulation
Saline Injection
Local Anesthetic Injection
Moxabustion
(D) Prevent complications
Transmittal of infection
Spread of local infection
Shattered needles
Pneumothorax
Sterilize and/or discard needles after each use
Avoid points at or near infected sites
Use only quality needles
Avoid deep introduction of needles over thorax

CONTINUOUS NEURAL BLOCKADE

Rosemary Hickey, M.D.

In continuous neural blockade techniques, a catheter is placed to allow repeated and/or continuous infusions of local anesthetics or narcotics. Indications for continuous techniques include surgical procedures of long duration (major vascular and nerve injury repair), repeated surgical procedures, the necessity to provide prolonged sympathetic block or analgesia, and provision of analgesia for postoperative pain. Also, continuous infusion techniques may allow the use of a more dilute local anesthetic solution, thus avoiding high peak blood concentrations that may be seen with intermittent techniques.

A. Before performing continuous neural blockade, confirm that there are no contraindications to regional anesthesia, such as anticoagulation, infection or tumor at the block site, and patient refusal. If the patient's clinical status permits, give premedication to reduce pain (narcotics), relieve anxiety, and raise the seizure threshold (benzodiazepines). For continuous epidural techniques in obstetric patients, withhold or reduce premedication to avoid effects on the fetus.

B. For upper extremity block, use continuous brachial plexus techniques. Place a catheter in the brachial plexus sheath using either the interscalene (ISB), supraclavicular (SCB), subclavian perivascular (SPB), infraclavicular (ICB), or axillary (AB) block techniques. An ICB technique has the advantage of a relatively deep catheter insertion, resulting in minimal catheter movement. A special cannula-over-needle and catheter set for continuous plexus anesthesia is available (Contiplex). Using sterile technique, identify the brachial plexus sheath by paresthesias, fascial click, or loss of resistance or with the assistance of a nerve stimulator (p 234). If a nerve stimulator is used, identify the point of maximal contraction of the hand or arm before injection and use low current (<2 mA) to obtain contractions. Pass the catheter directly into the fascial sheath or first distend the space with a small volume of local anesthetic solution. In order to maintain stability of the catheter and promote proximal spread of the local anesthetic, introduce the catheter through the cannula a distance of several centimeters. Alternatively, a guidewire may be passed into the sheath and the catheter passed over the guidewire. Secure the catheter in place by suturing it to the skin or using a transparent adherent dressing. Verify the absence of intravascular placement by careful aspiration and test doses prior to each injection.

C. Complications related to brachial plexus block include phrenic nerve block (ISB, SCB, SPB), pneumothorax (ISB, SCB, SPB), Horner's syndrome (ISB, SCB, SPB), recurrent laryngeal nerve block (ISB, SCB, SPB), epidural block (ISB), and subarachnoid block (ISB).

D. For lower extremity or abdominal block, use continuous epidural, spinal, or caudal techniques. Continuous techniques may also be used to block the femoral, the sciatic, and other peripheral nerves when a more discrete area of analgesia is desired. For epidural and caudal techniques, insert an 18-gauge Tuohy needle into the epidural space and thread an epidural catheter through the needle so that the catheter is advanced 2 to 3 cm within the epidural space. For continuous spinal techniques, an epidural needle and catheter can be advanced into the subarachnoid space, or alternatively use a smaller-gauge needle and catheter set designed specifically for continuous spinal anesthesia. The smaller-gauge needle and catheter carry the advantage of a lower incidence of spinal headache secondary to a smaller dural puncture site, but may have the disadvantages of more difficulty with insertion and catheter kinking.

E. Epidural, spinal, and caudal techniques may result in headache, backache, and hypotension secondary to sympathetic block. Avoid accidental dural puncture during performance of an epidural anesthetic with an 18-gauge needle, because this is associated with headache in a high percentage of patients. Treat postspinal headache with bed rest, analgesics, and copius amount of oral and/or IV fluids. Caffeine sodium benzoate (500 mg added to 1 L of IV fluids) may also be of benefit. If these conservative measures fail, an epidural blood patch may be necessary.

F. Choose the local anesthetic based on duration of anesthesia desired, potential toxicity (p 176), and type of block desired (sympathetic, sensory, motor). Choose subarachnoid or epidural narcotics when selective regional anesthesia is desired without the production of autonomic or motor blockade. These agents (fentanyl, morphine, meperidine, and sufentanil) act at presynaptic and postsynaptic receptors in the substantia gelatinosa of the spinal cord and may be used singly or in combination with local anesthetics.

G. Complications of local anesthesia include intravascular injection, local anesthetic overdose, and allergy. Avoid these complications by careful aspiration before injection, use of a test dose, and keeping local anesthetic doses below the maximal safe limits recommended.

H. Side effects of subarachnoid and epidural narcotics include respiratory depression, nausea and vomiting, urinary retention, and itching. Respiratory depression is a biphasic phenomenon initially due to systemic absorption (within the first hour of injection) and later (6 to 8 hours) to central migration of the drug. Treat respiratory depression with IV naloxone and general supportive measures (oxygen, airway maintenance, close surveillance of respiratory function).

I. Complications that may be associated with continuous neural blockade include those related to catheter

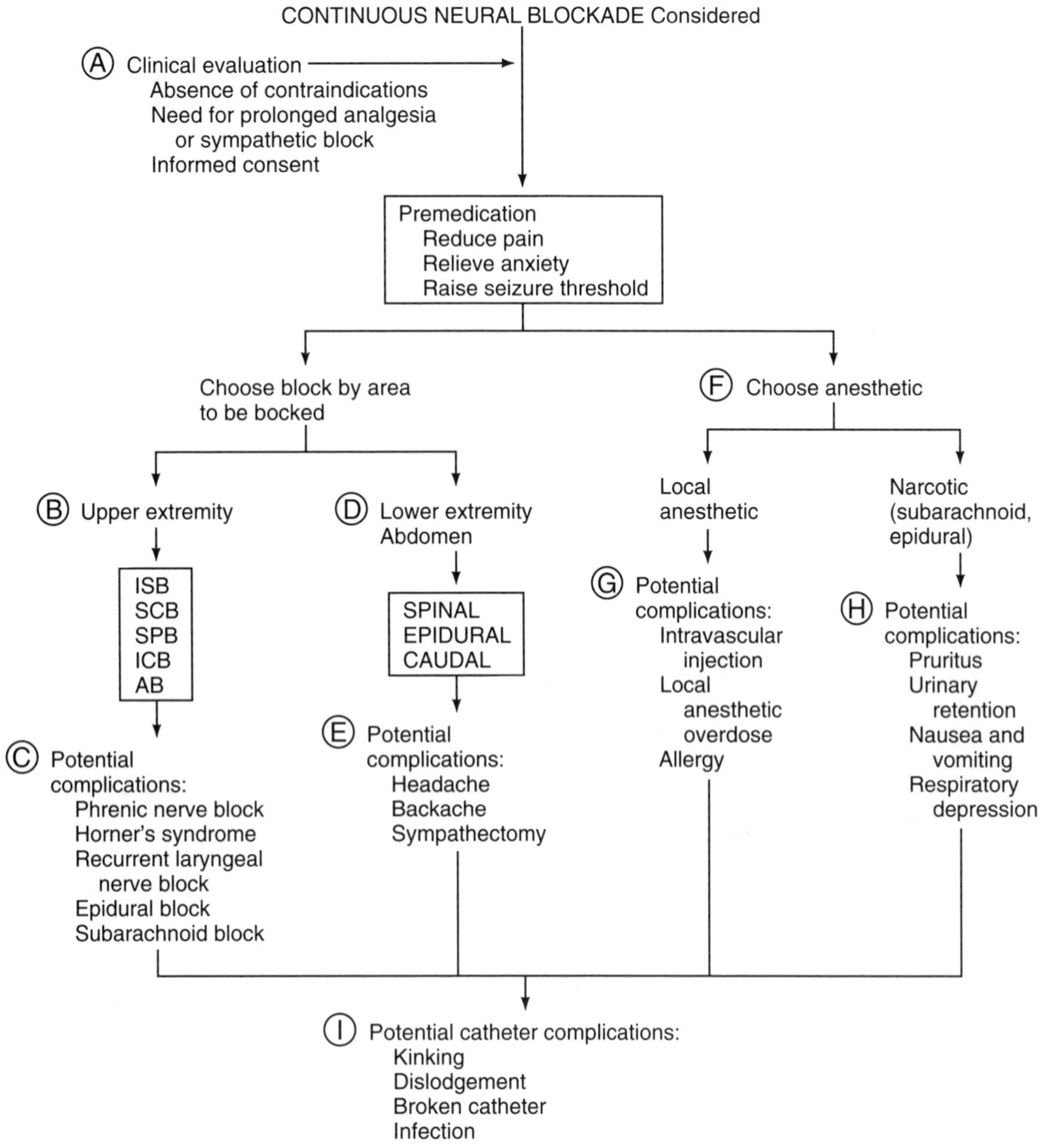

insertion and those associated with the particular type of block. Catheter complications include kinking or dislodgement of the catheter, broken catheters, and the introduction of infection.

References

Jarvis AP, Greenawalt JW, Fagraeus L. Intravenous caffeine for post-dural puncture headache. Reg Anesth 1986; 11:42.

Kirkpatrick AF, Bednarczyk LR, Hime GW, et al. Bupivacaine blood levels during continuous interscalene block. Anesthesiology 1985; 62:65.

Rawal N. Postoperative pain and its management. In: Raj PP, ed. Practical management of pain. 2nd ed. St. Louis: Mosby–Year Book, 1992:367.

Rosenblatt RM. Continuous femoral anesthesia for lower extremity surgery. Anesth Analg 1980; 59:631.

Smith BE, Fischer HBJ, Scott PV. Continuous sciatic nerve block. Anaesthesia 1984; 39:155.

INTRAVENOUS REGIONAL BLOCKADE

James N. Rogers, M.D.

Intravenous regional blockade (IVRB) is one of the earliest forms of regional anesthesia. It provides analgesia in a limb with an IV injection of local anesthetic while blood flow to and from the limb is occluded.

A. IVRB is very reliable, with a high success rate. It is easy to perform and safe, and provides rapid onset and a controllable duration of action. Recovery is rapid. It is most suited for hand and forearm surgery, reduction of forearm fractures, and foot procedures.

B. Disadvantages of IVRB include tourniquet pain, which limits the duration of the procedures; the need for exsanguination of the limb; and the risk of toxic reactions to the local anesthetic. Pain management after the procedure is necessary because of the rapid recovery of full sensation.

C. After obtaining informed consent, secure peripheral IV access in the most distal vein available in the limb to be blocked. An orthopedic, pneumatic tourniquet is placed above the IV line and the site of the proposed procedure. A second IV line should be placed in the contralateral limb to provide IV access during the procedure. The limb should be exsanguinated using an Esmarch bandage, wrapping snugly from distal to proximal. The tourniquet is then inflated to 50 to 100 mm Hg above the patient's systolic blood pressure. The bandage is then removed.

D. Injection, which should be slow, usually consists of 40 ml of 0.5% lidocaine for the upper limb and 50 ml for the lower limb. The skin usually becomes mottled, and muscle relaxation and analgesia usually appear rapidly.

E. Tourniquet release should be achieved incrementally: e.g., release for 5 seconds, reinflate for 15 seconds, and repeat this cycle four to five times to minimize the toxic effects of the local anesthetic. Give an ECG and monitor pulse and blood pressures. Resuscitation equipment should be readily available.

F. IV regional sympathetic blockade may be used in the management of reflex sympathetic dystrophy. Guanethidine, with its high affinity for sympathetic nerve endings, provides a long-lasting sympathetic block, often lasting days to weeks. For upper extremity blockade, use 20 mg in 0.5% lidocaine; for lower extremity blockade, use 40 mg.

References

Brown BR. Discussion on: The site of action of intravenous regional anesthesia. Anesth Analg 1972; 51:776.

Davies JAH, Gill SS, Weber JCP. Intravenous regional analgesia. Anaesthesia 1984; 39:416.

Driessen JJ, van der Werken C, Nicolai JPA, Crul JF. Clinical effects of regional intravenous guanethidine (Ismelin) in reflex sympathetic dystrophy. Acta Anaesthesiol Scand 1983; 27:505.

Hannington-Kiff JG. Intravenous regional sympathetic block with guanethidine. Lancet 1974; 1:1019.

Holmes CM. Intravenous regional neural blockade. In Cousins MJ, Bridenbaugh PO, eds. Neural blockade in clinical anesthesia and management of pain. 2nd ed. Philadelphia: JB Lippincott, 1988:443.

McKain CW, Bruno JU, Goldner JL. The effects of intravenous regional guanethidine and response. J Bone Joint Surg 1983; 6:808.

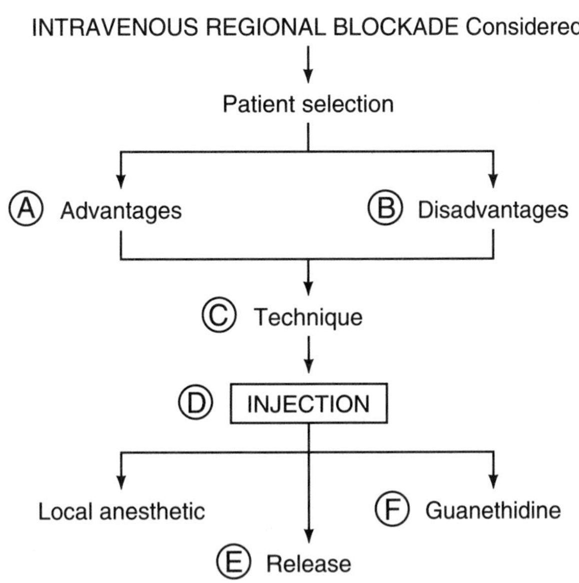
INTRAVENOUS REGIONAL BLOCKADE Considered
Patient selection
Ⓐ Advantages
Ⓑ Disadvantages
Ⓒ Technique
Ⓓ INJECTION
Local anesthetic
Ⓕ Guanethidine
Ⓔ Release

EPIDURAL STEROID INJECTION

Jeffery J. Baeuerle, M.D.

Epidural steroid injection (ESI) is one form of nonsurgical therapy for cervical, thoracic, or lumbar pain. It is most effective for cervical and lumbosacral radiculopathy associated with intervertebral disc herniation, bulging, or degeneration, which produces irritation of an adjacent nerve root. ESI has been used to treat pain caused by degenerative joint disease, scoliosis, spondylolysis, spondylolisthesis, postlaminectomy syndrome, and facet abnormalities as well. It has also been successfully used in the treatment of herpes zoster pain as well as postherpetic neuralgia. The main criterion for successful epidural steroid therapy is the presence of nerve root inflammation, which can be relieved by the steroid.

A. All patients should previously have been evaluated by an orthopedic surgeon or neurosurgeon to rule out serious neurologic dysfunction. Malignancy must also be ruled out as the cause of pain. No contraindication to epidural placement (e.g., infection, coagulation abnormality, or patient refusal) must exist. Patients have better success with epidural steroid therapy if they have had no prior surgery and their pain has lasted <6 to 12 months.

B. The ESI should be placed at or near the level of the nerve root derangement. Patients are usually given a series of three injections, each separated by 2 weeks, and should experience pain relief or improvement in symptoms within 6 days after an injection. If there is no response after three injections, other modalities should be explored. The steroids most often injected into the epidural space are methylprednisolone acetate (80 mg) and triamcinolone diacetate (50 mg). Dilution of the corticosteroid with either local anesthetic or preservative-free normal saline (6 to 10 ml) provides an adequate distribution of steroid, although many clinicians use a 2 cc volume of undiluted steroid with good success and without increased side effects. Local anesthetic provides muscle relaxation and pain relief as well as confirmation of steroid placement in the epidural space.

C. Use the C-7 spinous process as a landmark and either the C6-7 or C7-T1 interspace for access to the cervical epidural space. The hanging drop technique and the midline approach are commonly used to identify the epidural space. Deposit steroid as close as possible to the involved nerve roots. The laminar approach to the epidural space can allow steroid to be deposited at nerve roots on one particular side.

D. If the patient has had a laminectomy, the caudal approach may be used, although a greater volume of diluent (20 to 40 ml) would be required to reach the level of disease. A reproduction of pain on injection is a good indicator of an inflammatory process in the epidural space and carries a greater potential for a successful outcome. An epidural catheter may be placed to gain access to the inflamed nerve root.

E. Epidural steroids have been successfully used to treat the pain associated with acute herpes zoster infections as well as postherpetic neuralgia. When therapy is initiated in the acute phase of a herpes zoster infection, the development of postherpetic neuralgia may be prevented. Use a paramedian approach to gain access to the thoracic epidural space.

F. Complications, although rare, can result from technical problems of epidural placement, the steroid and its preservative, or infection. Accidental dural puncture, the most common technique-related complication, may lead to post–dural puncture headache. When a dural puncture goes undetected and an intrathecal steroid injection is administered, aseptic meningitis, adhesive arachnoiditis, pachymeningitis, or conus medullaris syndrome may result, although many clinicians have deliberately used intrathecal steroids without problem in the past. When a dural puncture occurs, an intrathecal steroid injection should probably not be initiated. Each milliliter of methylprednisolone acetate contains approximately 30 mg of polyethylene glycol, which has been associated with nerve damage in experimental models. Dilution with preservative-free normal saline or local anesthetic lowers the concentration of the polyethylene glycol substantially. Exacerbation of back pain is less likely when a volume of 6 to 10 ml is injected slowly. Epidural steroids affect the hypothalamus-pituitary-adrenal axis, resulting in depression of plasma cortisol levels for approximately 3 to 5 weeks. Epidural steroids have caused iatrogenic Cushing's syndrome, congestive heart failure secondary to fluid retention, and changes in blood glucose levels in susceptible patients. When a cervical epidural injection is performed, vasovagal syncopal episodes may occur.

References

Benzon HT. Epidural steroid injections for low back pain and lumbosacral radiculopathy. Pain 1986; 24:277.

Manchikanti L. Management of postherpetic neuralgia. Anesth Rev 1990; 17:31.

Nelson DA. Dangers from methylprednisolone acetate therapy by intraspinal injection. Arch Neurol 1988; 45:805.

Rowlingson JC, Kirschenbaum LP. Epidural analgesic techniques in the management of cervical pain. Anesth Analg 1986; 65:939.

Tuel SM, Meythaler JM, Cross LL. Cushing's syndrome from epidural methylprednisolone. Pain 1990; 40:81.

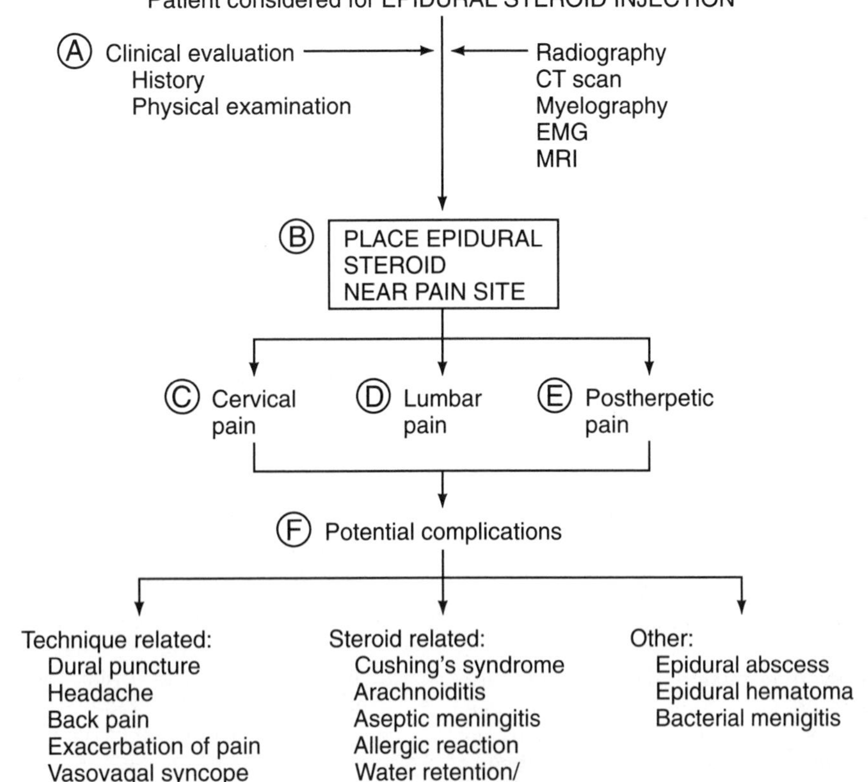
Patient considered for EPIDURAL STEROID INJECTION
(A) Clinical evaluation
History
Physical examination
Radiography
CT scan
Myelography
EMG
MRI
(B) PLACE EPIDURAL STEROID NEAR PAIN SITE
(C) Cervical pain
(D) Lumbar pain
(E) Postherpetic pain
(F) Potential complications
Technique related:
Dural puncture
Headache
Back pain
Exacerbation of pain
Vasovagal syncope
Steroid related:
Cushing's syndrome
Arachnoiditis
Aseptic meningitis
Allergic reaction
Water retention/ weight gain
Other:
Epidural abscess
Epidural hematoma
Bacterial menigitis

INTRATHECAL NARCOTICS

Kelly Gordon Knape, M.D.

Like epidural narcotics, the administration of narcotics via the cerebrospinal fluid (subarachnoid or intrathecal [IT] administration) provides excellent analgesia of long duration with small doses. The opioid receptors can be accessed directly by this route, thereby improving time of onset over the epidural route. The receptors in the substantia gelatinosa of the dorsal horn and those in the periaqueductal gray matter can be reached by lumbar puncture (LP) or intraventricular injection, respectively.

A. Contraindications to IT narcotics include those of LP or subarachnoid block (SAB) for spinal anesthesia: evidence of increased intracranial pressure (ICP) without previous CT scan, infection at puncture site, and patient refusal. In patients with recurrent herpetic infections, there may be a recrudescence after IT morphine. In view of the potential for respiratory depression, this regimen should be used with caution in patients with severe respiratory disease (COPD) or documented elevation of ICP, and avoided when there is a true narcotic allergy and a history of excessive side effects. Young patients, especially laboring parturients, are at high risk for developing "spinal" or postdural puncture headache (PDPH).

B. IT narcotics provide good analgesia for the pain of contractions (avoiding the problems of sympathectomy and motor blockade associated with epidural anesthesia) as well as for post–cesarean section pain. Multiparous patients may require only a single injection because of shorter labors. Primiparous patients can be dosed early in the active phase to avoid repeated dosing with systemic analgesics (and neonatal depression); an epidural catheter can be placed at the same time and activated later. Narcotics can be administered using small-gauge (24G or 25G) Sprotte or Whitacre needles to lessen the incidence of PDPH. Small-gauge (28G or 32G) continuous spinal catheters may reduce the incidence of PDPH in this high-risk group by initiating a sterile inflammatory response that acts to seal the hole. Fentanyl or sufentanil may be used alone, especially with continuous techniques, but are usually mixed with preservative-free (PF) morphine to accelerate the onset while providing longer duration.

C. Postoperative pain can be efficiently managed with superior results by adding narcotics to the local anesthetic used in subarachnoid techniques. Single-shot "spinals" for abdominal surgery and lower extremity procedures can provide approximately 24 hours of analgesia when PF morphine is added. Fentanyl may improve the quality of intraoperative anesthesia but its duration is too short to provide postoperative analgesia unless it is readministered via a continuous spinal catheter. IT catheters can be repeatedly used with sterile technique but are usually removed after 24 hours because of the risk of infection. Also, cauda equina syndrome has been reported after use of local anesthetics with these catheters.

D. Patients with terminal cancer pain that has been refractory to other regimens can receive excellent analgesia with IT narcotics as an adjunct or as the sole alternative. Patients who normally require large doses of systemic narcotics will need much lower doses, although higher or more frequently than for acute pain. Implanted continuous-infusion devices are reserved for patients with terminal disease or malignancy. When all less-invasive therapies have failed, intraventricular (intracranial) dosing is a humane option.

E. The recommended single dose of PF morphine for both labor and postoperative pain is 0.005 mg/kg, or usually 0.25 mg, to a maximum of 0.5 mg for most adults, although the elderly do well with a lower dose of 0.1 mg. The duration is approximately 24 hours. With a catheter in place, morphine can be readministered as often as every 8 hours. Fentanyl and sufentanil are more appropriate for continuous techniques, especially during labor, and can be given as often as hourly. Analgesia may be inadequate for delivery, in which case a local anesthetic is added to produce a true "saddle block." For chronic pain, larger or more frequent doses may be needed by which the total daily requirement can be determined. Thereafter, larger, less frequent doses can be used to meet the total daily dose. There is no maximal dose, but only moderate increases are needed once the requirement is determined.

F. Side effects are similar to those from epidural administration, but more frequent. Pruritus is the most common, although the mechanism is unclear, and spinally mediated urinary retention is not unusual, especially in males. Respiratory depression is possible, but is unlikely with monitoring, proper dosing, and avoidance of systemic narcotics and other depressants. Chronic pain patients, especially those with a long history of narcotic use, are tolerant, so that side effects are rare. The substantial decrease in narcotic exposure that results may precipitate withdrawal, but this is uncommon.

G. The best treatment for side effects is prevention by using small doses and titrating upward as needed (with an IT catheter). Larger doses increase side effects more than they prolong the duration. IV naloxone, in titrated doses of 40 μg, is effective without affecting analgesia. Owing to its brief duration, a naloxone infusion may be needed for persistent symptoms. Longer-acting butorphanol and nalbuphine can be used to both prevent and treat side effects, and are also safe to use for "breakthrough" pain. Non-narcotic

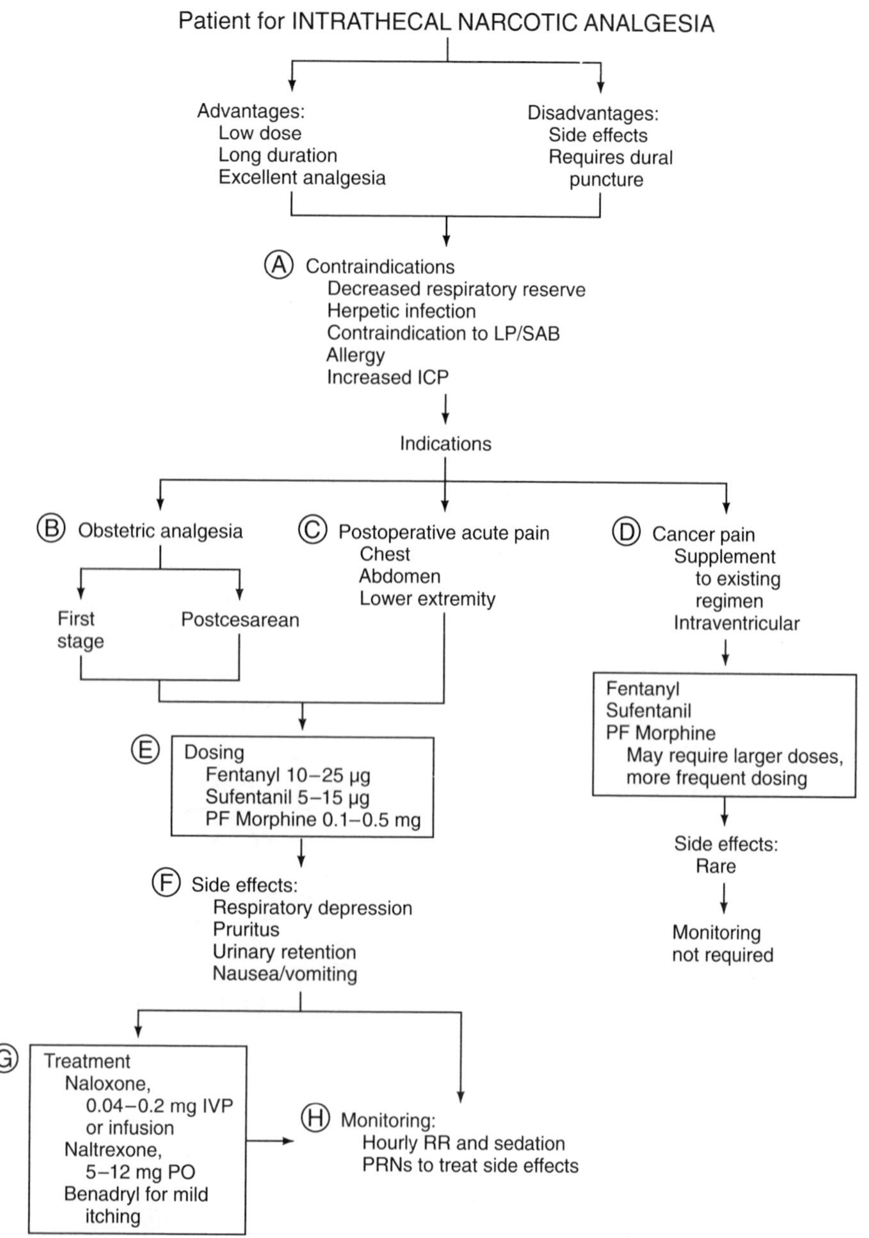

analgesics, especially NSAIDs, can also be used to augment analgesia safely.

H. The monitoring standard consists of hourly respiratory rates (RR) and level of consciousness or sedation scoring by personnel trained in this technique, although opioid-tolerant patients may be monitored less frequently. Owing to CO_2 retention secondary to rostral spread, sedation precedes change in RR. Electronic RR monitoring is acceptable, although false alarms are frequent. Pulse oximetry is useful, but desaturation may be a late sign in patients on supplemental O_2 owing to "apneic oxygenation."

References

Gwirtz KH. Intraspinal narcotics in the management of postoperative pain. Anesthesiol Rev 1990; 17:16.

Kirson LE, Goldman JM, Slover RB. Low dose intrathecal morphine for postoperative pain control in patients undergoing transurethral resection of the prostate. Anesthesiology 1989; 71:192.

Lazorthes Y, Verdie JC, Caute B, et al. Intracerebroventricular morphinotherapy for control of chronic cancer pain. Prog Brain Res 1988; 77:395.

Leight CH, Evans DE, Durkan WJ. Intrathecal sufentanil for labor analgesia: Results of a pilot study. Anesthesiology 1990; 73:A981.

Leighton BL, DeSimone CA, Norris MC, Ben-David B. Intrathecal narcotics for labor revisited: The combination of fentanyl and morphine intrathecally provides rapid onset of profound, prolonged analgesia. Anesth Analg 1989; 69:122.

Waldman SD. The role of spinal opioids in the management of cancer pain. J Pain Sympt Manag 1990; 5:163.

Yagamuchi H, Watanabe S, Motokawa K, et al. Intrathecal morphine dose response data for pain relief after cholecystectomy. Anesth Analg 1990; 70:168.

NEUROLYTIC NERVE BLOCK

Richard Rosenthal, M.D.

Neurolytic nerve blocks were quite popular earlier in the 20th century. However, their use has recently been supplanted by the improved use of analgesics as well as newer surgical techniques. For instance, radiofrequency neurolysis may provide more accurate and safer results than chemical neurolysis. Nevertheless, there remains a place for the latter in a select group of patients, usually those who have severe pain due to cancer and other nonoperable, chronically painful conditions and whose life expectancy is less than 1 year.

A. Careful patient selection is the key to a rewarding outcome. The patient's pain should be unresponsive to other forms of treatment. Psychological testing is also important in completely evaluating the patient before considering a neurolytic block. If a block is chosen, it is usually only part of a multidisciplinary approach. Antidepressants and analgesics, psychological and social counseling, and physical modalities for pain relief are important adjuncts to therapy. Extensive communication with the patient is necessary, explicitly detailing the risks and benefits, before proceeding with the block.

B. Diagnostic blockade with local anesthetics is crucial in predicting the success of a neurolytic block. Several should be performed with local anesthetics of varying duration. One of the blocks should be a placebo to identify placebo responders. The duration and extent of the pain relief should correspond to the agent used. The local anesthetic blocks confirm the anatomic nature of the pain and allow the patient to experience the effects of the neurolytic block with little risk. The relief of pain may be replaced with numbness or dysesthesia in the affected part, which is as distressing as the original pain.

C. If the diagnostic blocks have provided only short-term pain relief and the patient is satisfied with risks, a neurolytic block can be performed by a physician experienced in the planned procedure. Informed consent in writing is mandatory.

D. Multiple chemicals are used to perform these blocks, but alcohol and phenol are the most widely used in the United States. Both agents indiscriminately affect both motor and sensory nerves. Phenol can be used intrathecally, epidurally, for paravertebral somatic and peripheral nerve blocks, and for sympathetic blocks. It is poorly soluble in water and is often added to glycerine to achieve concentrations >7% phenol. Phenol can be added to radiographic contrast to allow fluoroscopic visualization of the spread of the agent. Phenol in glycerine is hyperbaric in CSF. The drug has a local anesthetic effect, resulting in less pain after the injection. The effects of the block cannot be evaluated for 24 to 48 hours, to allow time for the local anesthetic effect to dissipate. Phenol toxicity can occur. Systemic doses >8.5 g cause convulsions and CNS depression. Renal toxicity can also occur. Doses <100 mg are unlikely to result in serious toxicity.

E. Alcohol is used primarily intrathecally and for sympathetic blockade, celiac plexus blockade, and chemical hypophysectomy. Alcohol is hypobaric to CSF, is readily soluble in body tissues, and produces painful burning on injection. It requires 12 to 24 hours before the effects of the block can be assessed.

F. Subarachnoid blockade is usually reserved for patients with unilateral pain limited to a few spinal cord segments. The aim is to perform a chemical posterior root rhizotomy. Patient positioning and the appropriate choice of agent (baricity) is needed for a successful block. Good results should occur in about 50% of patients. Serious complications include paraplegia and bowel/bladder paresis.

G. Epidural neurolytic blockade can be used in patients with bilateral pain. A catheter should be placed at the correct level and small doses of phenol (1 ml) injected daily until pain relief lasts more than 24 hours.

H. Celiac plexus blocks can provide excellent relief of pain associated with abdominal malignancies, particularly pancreatic cancer. Both catheter and single-injection techniques have been used successfully. Excessive spread of the solution may cause paraplegia, but fluoroscopic guidance can reduce this risk. Postural hypotension, urinary difficulty, and failure of ejaculation may also occur.

I. Neurolytic lumbar sympathetic blocks (LSBs) can be used in patients with sympathetically mediated pain of the lower extremities or in patients with vascular compromise. Bilateral blocks should be avoided in males, because they can interfere with ejaculation.

J. Neurolytic somatic nerve blocks are seldom used, except in terminally ill cancer patients, because of the high incidence of postblock neuralgia and limb weakness.

K. Cranial nerve blocks are often performed for trigeminal neuralgia. Chemical hypophysectomy may provide relief of diffuse pain due to hormone-dependent metastatic cancer.

L. The duration of a neurolytic block can be anywhere from weeks to months and depends on the type of block and the skill of the physician. Failure of the block may be the result of incorrect placement of the neurolytic agent, or the source of the pain may be other than expected (e.g., psychogenic or central). Again, diagnostic blocks with local anesthetics/placebo reduce the risk of a missed diagnosis.

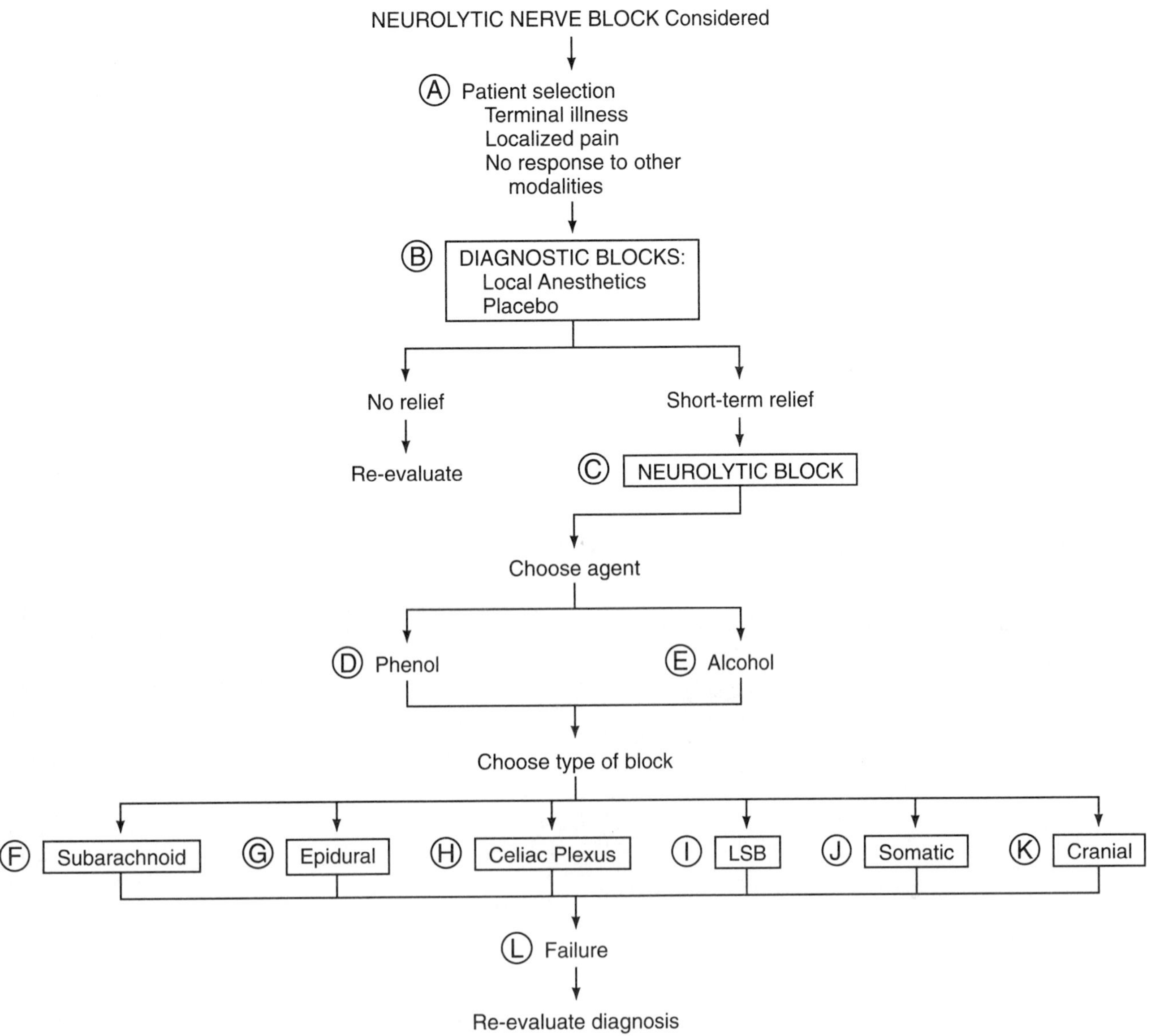

References

Black RG, Bonica JJ. Analgesic blocks. Postgrad Med 53:105.

Bonica JJ. Management of pain. 2nd ed. Philadelphia: Lea & Febiger, 1990:1980.

Cousins MJ, Bridenbaugh PO. Neural blockade in clinical anesthesia and management of pain. Philadelphia: JB Lippincott, 1980:1053.

Racz GB, ed. Techniques of neurolysis. Boston: Kluwer Academic, 1989.

Wall PD, Melzack R, eds. Textbook of pain. 2nd ed. New York: Churchill Livingstone, 1989:768.

COMPLICATIONS OF NEUROLYTIC BLOCKS

Anthony Pellegrino, M.D.

Neurolytic blocks are usually performed in patients with severe intractable pain. Most of these patients have contraindications to specific neurosurgical procedures (e.g., poor physical status). Neurolytic blocks may be useful by means of many techniques (sympathetic, central, or peripheral), but complications can occur.

A. Medicolegal aspects of pain management should always be a concern. Legal action may be taken for many reasons. Most lawsuits have been because (1) of complications caused by the injection, (2) the patient did not consent to the procedure, (3) the procedure was carried out inexpertly, (4) the wrong procedure was performed, or (5) treatment was inadequate. Therefore, one must always discuss the indications, explain the procedure and its complications, and have a written consent signed, in front of a witness, *before* proceeding with the block. Any complications must be immediately addressed and handled by the physician or appropriate health care provider.

B. Complications associated with neurolytic paravertebral sympathetic blocks are primarily the result of spread of the neurolytic agent to surrounding anatomic structures. Radiopaque contrast media and fluoroscopy can be very helpful during placement of needles. Spillovers can easily involve intercostal and somatic nerves (especially the genitofemoral and lumboinguinal nerves). Motor and sensory dysfunction can occur. Intravascular or intrathecal injection may occur and result in inability to move an extremity, hypotension, or dyspnea. Other complications include neuritis, puncture of the kidneys, inability to ejaculate, and backache.

C. As in paravertebral sympathetic blocks, many of the complications of neurolytic celiac plexus blocks are due to the close proximity of surrounding structures. Again, radiopaque dye and fluoroscopy are useful in ensuring correct needle placement. Intrathecal injection, with disastrous consequences, is always possible. Other complications include pneumothorax, intravascular injection, pain at the level of the injection for 1 to 2 days, temporary increase in GI motility, neuritis, temporary difficulty in urination, failure of ejaculation, and paraplegia.

D. Trigeminal nerve neurolytic blocks have resulted in temporary oculomotor, abducens, and glossopharyngeal palsy. Corneal anesthesia and permanent anesthesia of the cheek and nose is common. Nasal ulceration, blindness, corneal ulceration, and trigeminal motor weakness can also occur. The proximity of important structures makes them susceptible to hemorrhage or diffusion of neurolytics. Mandibular nerve blocks can result in paresis or paralysis of the muscles of mastication, resulting in deviation. Facial nerve blocks can cause permanent paralysis of facial muscles. Complications of the glossopharyngeal nerve block include dysphagia, sloughing, fibrosis, carotid artery or internal jugular vein thrombosis, and facial nerve block. It is generally recommended that injection be performed under fluoroscopic control, since many nerves are so close in this region (e.g., vagus, hypoglossal, accessory).

E. Neurolytic blocks of the cervical plexus may result in intrathecal or intravascular injection, esophageal and/or spinal accessory nerve damage, and prolonged Horner's syndrome. Neurolytic blocks of the brachial plexus are seldom performed because of the high frequency of upper extremity paralysis and vessel thrombosis. Complications of a neurolytic stellate ganglion block include temporary hoarseness and dysphagia from recurrent laryngeal nerve block, persistent Horner's syndrome, and spread to the brachial plexus and paravertebral and subarachnoid spaces.

F. Intercostal neurolytic blocks can cause subcutaneous and cutaneous sloughing of tissue and severe neuritis, especially after alcohol injection.

G. Central neurolytic block complications depend on which part of the spinal cord is being blocked. Complications may be temporary but can persist. Numbness, bladder paresis, headache, muscle and bowel paresis, paresthesia, and hyperesthesia have been reported to last 72 hours or less after an intrathecal injection of a neurolytic agent. Meningismus is rare but can occur. Cauda equina syndrome and anterior and posterior spinal artery thrombosis have also been reported.

H. Alcohol injection via the epidural route may result in severe neuritis. Grunwald used 6 to 10% phenol in 221 cancer patients. He found urinary incontinence in 57 patients (17 for longer than 2 weeks), bowel incontinence in 21 (8 for longer than 2 weeks), and muscular weakness in 14 (3 for longer than 2 weeks). Hypertonic saline has resulted in permanent paraplegia.

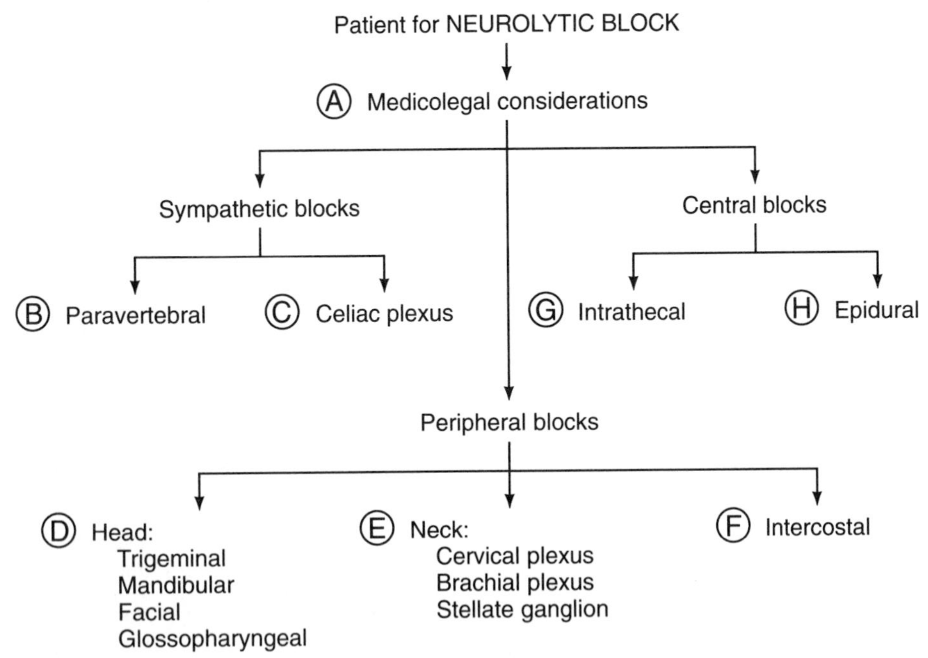

References

Benson HT. Convulsions secondary to intravascular phenol; a hazard of celiac plexus block. Anesth Analg 1979; 58:150.

Bonica JJ. Management of pain. 2nd ed. Philadelphia: Lea & Febiger, 1990.

Cherry DA. Chemical lumbar sympathectomy. Curr Concepts Pain 1984; 2:12.

Grunwald I: Neurolise com fenol: Uso da via peridural no tratamento da dor de cancer. Rev Bras Anestes 1976; 26(4):628.

Reid W, Watt JK, Gray TG. Phenol injection of sympathetic chain. Br J Surg 1970; 47:45.

Swerdlow M. Medicolegal aspects of complications following pain relieving block. Pain 1982; 13:321.

Swerdlow M. Complications of neurolytic neural blockade. In: Cousins MJ, Bridenbaugh PO, eds. Neural blockade in clinical anesthesia and management of pain. 2nd ed. Philadelphia: JB Lippincott, 1988:719.

IMPLANTABLE INFUSION PUMPS

Mark E. Romanoff, M.D.

Most implantable infusion pumps are used for epidural or intrathecal narcotic infusions for pain control in terminal cancer patients. Before implanting these pumps one must determine the feasibility of using this type of system versus an implanted reservoir or an open system. Open systems have the spinal catheter tunnelled and exteriorized. Closed systems have all components (spinal catheter, reservoir, or pump) implanted under the skin of the patient. The risk of infection is higher in open systems. Closed systems have the advantages of lower infection risk, less catheter breakage, and improved mobility but are significantly more expensive, may be more difficult to inject, and require surgery to remove or replace.

Reservoir systems are less costly to insert than pump systems. They require multiple injections, so needles, syringes, and medications must be prepared each day. Daily support personnel are needed if the patient cannot perform these functions. Implantable pumps are more bulky than reservoirs but allow relatively infrequent injections (usually every 10 to 14 days). A continuous infusion, as opposed to intermittent injections, may improve pain control and decrease side effects.

Most studies have shown good to excellent pain relief in 50% to 80% of patients. Systemic narcotic consumption (oral or IV) usually decreases by 50% to 75%. Mobility improves and patient satisfaction is enhanced. The initial fusion of intrathecal morphine is commonly 1 to 6 mg per day, although up to 150 mg per day have been used. After 6 to 9 months of use the efficacy of pain relief appears to decrease markedly. The characteristics of implantable infusion pumps are shown in Table 1.

A. Candidates for implantation should have narcotic-sensitive pain but be unable to continue oral medications due to side effects (nausea, vomiting, CNS effects). Relative contraindications include coagulopathy, systemic infection, local infection at the site of implantation, psychological abnormalities, and the lack of adequate support personnel (family, hospice, nursing, or emergency medical care immediately available). A life expectancy >3 months is usually necessary to justify the cost of the system. A trial of epidural or intrathecal narcotics is required before implantation. A reduction of pain ≥ 50% should be achieved before proceeding.

B. Epidural placement requires a larger dosage and volume of narcotic than intrathecal placement, necessitating more frequent reservoir refilling; most implantable infusion pump systems, therefore, are used with an intrathecal catheter. The rest of this chapter describes intrathecal catheter characteristics.

C. Insertion is performed in an operating room environment under aseptic technique. Local or regional anesthesia may be used for patient comfort. The patient is placed in the lateral decubitus position and the area of needle insertion (most commonly, L2-3 midline) and the location of pump implantation (upper lateral abdomen) are prepped and draped. A 3 to 4 cm incision is made over the interspace and a Tuohy needle is inserted into the subarachnoid space. The catheter is threaded approximately 8 to 10 cm under fluoroscopy to the correct level. A 15-20 cm incision is made in the flank and a pocket is opened down to the abdominal fascia. The catheter is tunnelled to the pocket and attached to the pump. All connections are checked, kinks removed, and free flow of CSF is demonstrated through the catheter. The pump is placed in the pocket, secured, and the pocket is closed. Often, a dose of narcotic is given into the side port before closing the skin.

D. The reported complication rate of these systems is 5% to 15%. Most complications arise from systemic or central effects of the narcotic. Mechanical failures, catheter migration, and infection often occur.

(Continued on page 222)

TABLE 1 Characteristics of Implantable Infusion Pumps*

Pump	*Cost ($)*	*Weight (g)*	*Dimensions (mm)*	*Power Source*	*Reservoir Size (cc)*	*Flow Rate*	*Side Port*	*Programmable*
Infusaid[†] 100	3654	187	87 × 28	2-phase Charging fluid	47	1–6 cc/day	–	–
400	4795	208	87 × 28	Charging fluid	47	1–6 cc/day	+	–
600	In clinical trials	100	63 × 22	Charging fluid	22	0.75 cc/day or 1.4 cc/day	+	–
1000	In clinical trials	272	90 × 23	Charging fluid Lithium battery	25	0.001–0.5 cc/hr	+	+
Medtronics[‡] 8610/8611	12,600§	175	70 × 28	Lithium battery	18	0.004–0.9 cc/hr	+	+

*Adapted from Kwan JW. Use of infusion devices for epidural or intrathecal administration of spinal opioids. Am J Hosp Pharm 1990; 47:S18–23.
[†]Personal communication 1/91 with Infusaid, Inc., Norwood MA.
[‡]Personal communication 1/91 with Medtronics, Minneapolis MN.
§Includes programmer.

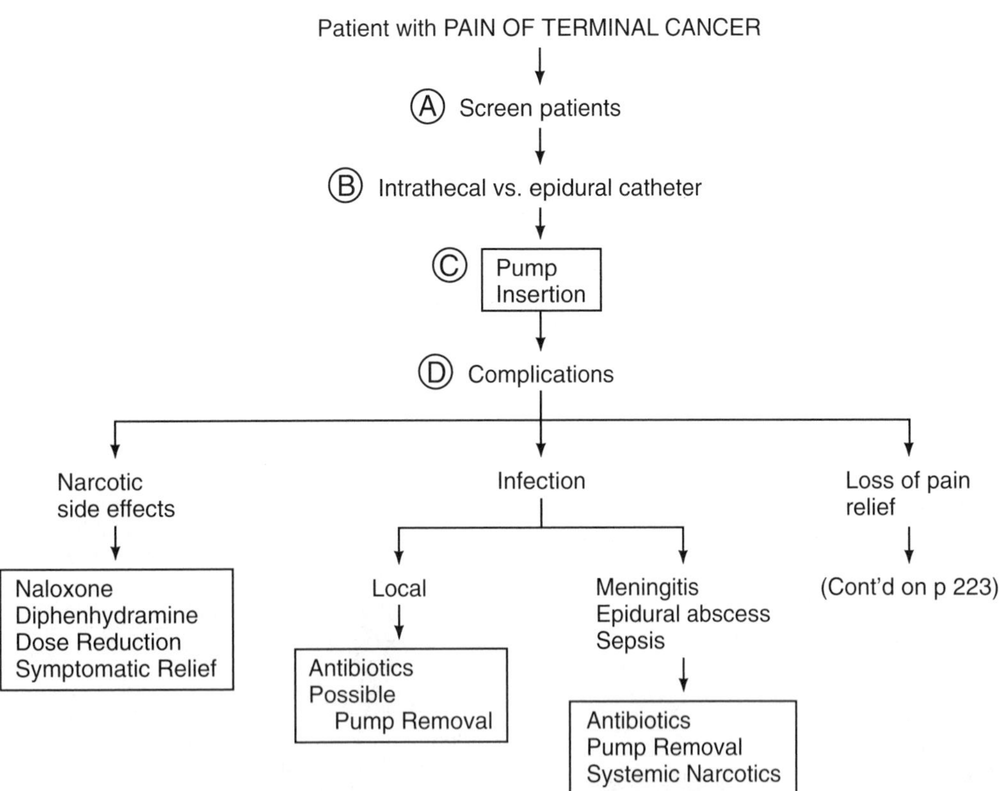
Patient with PAIN OF TERMINAL CANCER
(A) Screen patients
(B) Intrathecal vs. epidural catheter
(C) Pump Insertion
(D) Complications
Narcotic side effects
Infection
Loss of pain relief
Naloxone
Diphenhydramine
Dose Reduction
Symptomatic Relief
Local
Meningitis
Epidural abscess
Sepsis
(Cont'd on p 223)
Antibiotics
Possible
Pump Removal
Antibiotics
Pump Removal
Systemic Narcotics

E. The loss of pain relief can have numerous causes. An improper injection technique can lead to narcotic being deposited subcutaneously and not into the reservoir. Errors in the preparation of the narcotic may reduce the concentration of drug infused. Hardware failure and tolerance can also occur.

F. Injection of metrizamide into the side port of the pump can help delineate catheter disconnections, kinks in the catheter, and the location of the distal tip of the catheter. CSF fistulas may be seen as extravasation from the distal catheter tip into the subcutaneous area. If a fistula is suspected, a technetium-99m pyrophosphate intrathecal injection can be used for identification.

G. If the signs of a spinal anesthetic are seen with the injection of a local anesthetic through the side port, the catheter system is most likely intact and another trial of the pump is recommended. If the local anesthetic does not produce spinal anesthesia, the system should be removed.

H. Tolerance and a progressive increase in narcotic requirements have been reported in every study that has followed patients for longer than 2 weeks. Tolerance can be caused from an increasing tumor load, or from pharmacodynamic or pharmacokinetic changes of the narcotic. The most common treatment is an increase in the dosage of narcotic. Most infusion pumps have fixed rates, so the concentration of narcotic needs to be increased to increase the dosage. Concentrations of morphine sulfate of up to 60 mg per cubic centimeter have been used without toxicity. Other strategies include discontinuing the narcotic (drug "holiday," use of local anesthetics), using other narcotic receptors (D-ala^2-d-lev^{5}enkephalin [DADL] and nalbuphine, for delta and kappa stimulation, respectively), and stimulating other receptors with clonidine (alpha$_2$) or gamma-aminobutyric acid (GABA). Neurodestructive procedures may also be contemplated if pain relief remains unsatisfactory.

References

Cherry DA. Drug delivery systems for epidural administration of opioids. Acta Anaesth Scand 1987; 31(suppl 85):54.

Greenberg HS. Continuous spinal opioid infusion for intractable cancer pain. In: Foley KM, Inturrisi CE, eds. Advances in pain research and therapy. Vol. 8. New York: Raven Press, 1986:351.

Greenberg HS, Taren J, Ensminger WD, Doan D. Benefit from and tolerance to continuous intrathecal infusion of morphine for intractable cancer pain. J Neurosurg 1982; 52:360.

Hassenbusch SJ, Pillay PK, Magdinec M, et al. Constant infusion of morphine for intractable cancer pain using an implanted pump. J Neurosurg 1990; 73:405.

Kwan JW. Use of infusion devices for epidural or intrathecal administration of spinal opioids. Am J Hosp Pharm 1990; 47:S18.

Madrid JL, Fatela LV, Alcorta J, et al. Intermittent intrathecal morphine by means of an implantable reservoir: a survey of 100 cases. J Pain Symptom Management 1988; 3:67.

Onofrio BM, Yaksh TL. Long-term pain relief produced by intrathecal morphine infusion in 53 patients. J Neurosurg 1990; 72:200.

Ventafridda ES, Caraceani A, De Conno F. Intraspinal morphine for cancer pain. Acta Anaesth Scand 1987; 31(suppl 85):47.

Waldman SD. Implantable drug delivery systems: practical considerations. J Pain Symptom Management 1990; 5:169.

Waldman SD. The role of spinal opioids in the management of cancer pain. J Pain Symptom Management 1990; 5:163.

Waldman SD, Feldstein GS, Allen ML. A troubleshooting guide to the subcutaneous epidural implantable reservoir. J Pain Symptom Management 1986; 1:217.

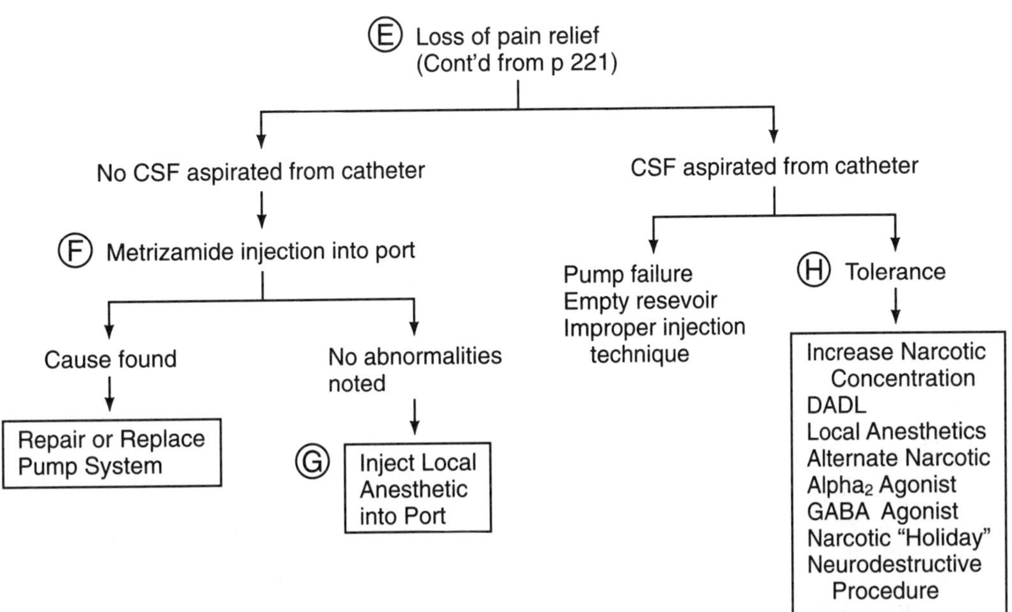

E Loss of pain relief
(Cont'd from p 221)
No CSF aspirated from catheter
F Metrizamide injection into port
Cause found
Repair or Replace Pump System
No abnormalities noted
G Inject Local Anesthetic into Port
CSF aspirated from catheter
Pump failure
Empty resevoir
Improper injection technique
H Tolerance
Increase Narcotic Concentration
DADL
Local Anesthetics
Alternate Narcotic
Alpha2 Agonist
GABA Agonist
Narcotic "Holiday"
Neurodestructive Procedure

DORSAL COLUMN STIMULATION

Marc B. Hahn, D.O.

Electrical dorsal column stimulation (DCS) of the spinal cord is a nondestructive modality used to treat some chronic pain syndromes. The physiologic mechanism of action is poorly understood. The most accepted mechanism to date involves the stimulation of inhibitory pathways in the dorsal columns. Indiscriminate patient selection, combined with the unreliability of the original hardware, initially led many experts to question the efficacy of this procedure. However, with proper patient selection and the advent of reliable, technically advanced stimulators and electrodes, the efficacy has markedly increased. Currently, DCS electrodes are placed percutaneously into the epidural space and separated from the dorsal columns by the dura.

The primary painful conditions that respond to DCS therapy are neurogenic (arising from the nervous system). These painful conditions are usually associated with some sensory dysfunction. Pain associated with peripheral vascular disease also responds well to DCS. Nociceptive pain (caused by a pathologic process that stimulates nerve endings), supraspinal pain (e.g., thalamic infarct), and some deafferentation pain (secondary to afferent nerve destruction) usually do not respond to DCS.

A successful preoperative trial of transcutaneous electrical nerve stimulation (TENS) may aid in appropriate patient selection. However, a failure of TENS does not necessarily obviate a trial of DCS.

A. DCS is most commonly used to treat pain in patients who have undergone multiple back operations. It is most effective for postoperative patients with true adhesive arachnoiditis or cauda equina syndrome. Subjectively, these patients complain of radicular pain along with low back symptoms. Objectively, these patients may have abnormal EMG or nerve conduction findings, as well as radiographic evidence of cauda equina syndrome. Low back pain alone is not an indication for DCS.

B. Other neurogenic pain syndromes also respond to DCS. Postamputation (phantom limb) pain may respond well initially, but efficacy may decrease with time. Reflex sympathetic dystrophy (RSD) appears to respond favorably to DCS, and diabetic neuropathies and some plexus lesions may also respond.

C. Pain secondary to peripheral vascular disease is a promising new application for DCS. In addition to alleviation of pain, patients may also demonstrate an increase in walking distances, healing of small trophic ulcers, or increase in capillary blood flow.

D. Before a trial of DCS, all patients should be given an adequate trial of conventional therapies and/or accepted surgical interventions. Patients should also be evaluated by a mental health professional to determine the influences of psychosocial issues on their pain complaints. Prior clearance by a mental health professional will help ensure proper patient selection. Because DCS is expensive and invasive, it should not be a first-line therapy.

E. Place the electrodes under sterile conditions using fluoroscopic guidance. Most lead electrodes can be placed percutaneously into the epidural space through a blunt needle. To treat pain in the lower extremities, place the electrode between thoracic vertebrae 8 and 10, and for the upper extremities, between the middle cervical vertebrae. In the patient with unilateral pain, orient the electrode toward the involved side. Many electrodes have multiple contacts so that stimulation can be varied. General stimulator adjustments include intensity, rate, and pulse width. Vary electrode placement, stimulator adjustments, electrode selection, and polarity until the paresthesia created by the DCS closely shadows the painful region. Anchor the electrode and cover with a sterile dressing. Continue test stimulation for 3 to 7 days. Test stimulation can range between 30 minutes every 8 hours to constant stimulation during waking hours. Make stimulator adjustments as needed. The patient will probably not receive total pain relief. Therefore, the patient must decide if the pain relief is sufficient to warrant internalization of the hardware.

F. Couple the anchored electrode to either an antenna or a pulse generator, which is placed in a subcutaneous pocket. Tape an external antenna connected to a stimulator over the subcutaneous antenna to achieve DCS through induction. The totally implanted pulse generator is programmed by a computerized interrogation unit, and the patient can turn the unit on and off with a small magnet. The epidural electrode will become fibrosed in place over 4 to 6 weeks. In the interim, the patient should avoid strenuous activity, twisting, and lifting. Despite these precautions, the electrode may migrate.

G. Reprogramming the parameters of the stimulator or changing the electrode combinations may recapture the proper stimulation. If this is unsuccessful, consider replacing the percutaneous electrode. Surgical placement of a flat electrode through a laminotomy minimizes the chance of movement.

H. Follow patients at least twice a year to ensure proper functioning of the hardware. Some studies suggest a decreased efficacy of DCS with time. It is also unrealistic to expect complete pain relief with DCS.

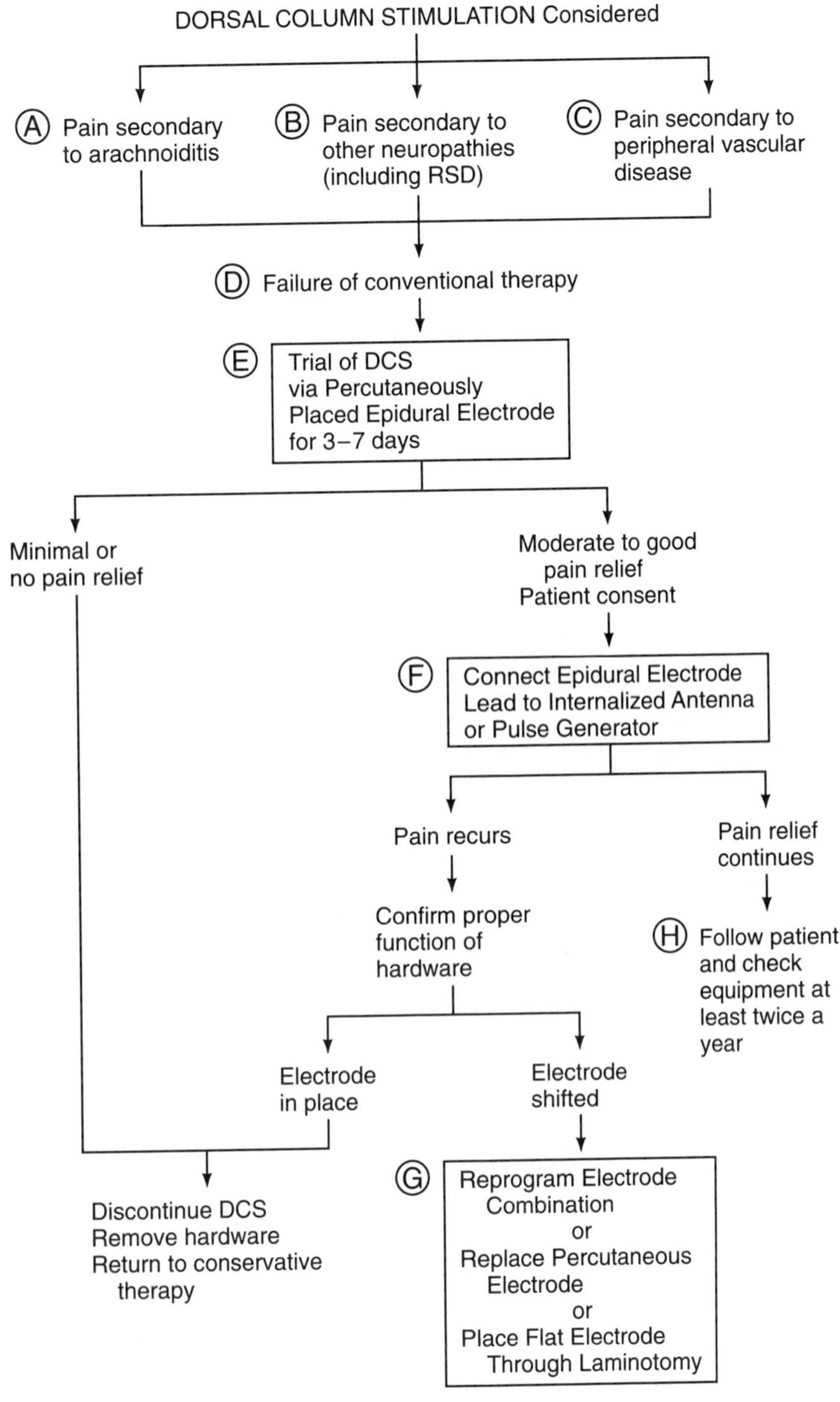

References

Jacobs, M, Jorning P, Beckers R, et al. Foot salvage and improved microvascular blood flow as a result of epidural spinal cord electrical stimulation. J Vasc Surg 1990; 12:354.

Long DM. Patient selection and the results of spinal cord stimulation for chronic pain. In: Hosobuchi Y, Corbin T, eds. Indications for spinal cord stimulation: proceedings of a symposium. New York: Excerpta Medica, 1981.

Myerson BA. Electrostimulation procedures: effects, presumed rationale and possible mechanisms. Adv Pain Res Ther 1983; 5:495.

Robaina FJ, Rodriquez JL, Martin MA. TENS and spinal cord stimulation for pain relief in RSD. Stereotact-Funct Neurosurg 1989; 52:53.

Shealy CN, Mortimer JT, Reswick JB. Electrical inhibition of pain by stimulation of the dorsal column. Anesth Analg 1967; 46:489.

Siegfried J, Lazorthes Y. Long-term follow-up of dorsal column operations. Appl Neurophysiol 1982; 45:201.

CRYOANALGESIA

Donald B. Tallackson, M.D.
Robert E. Middaugh, M.D.

The term *cryoanalgesia* was coined in 1976 to describe pain relief from the destruction of peripheral nerves after exposure to extreme cold. How freezing produces cellular and, specifically, neural destruction remains controversial. Different degrees of destruction result in different clinical outcomes. First-degree, or neurapraxia, produces minimal damage and usually disrupts function for approximately 2 weeks. Second-degree, or axonotmesis, destroys both the axon and myelin sheath and may provide pain relief for several months. Finally, third- through fifth-degree, or neurotmesis, results in destruction of both neural and stromal tissues. Regeneration and return of function at this stage becomes unpredictable.

A. Patients with pain of diverse origin are candidates for cryoanalgesia; however, they must have the ability to effect analgesia with selective placement of the relatively large cryoprobe where it will produce minimal collateral damage. Acute pain problems that have been managed with cryoanalgesia include postoperative pain from thoracotomy or inguinal hernia repair procedures. Selected chronic pain problems are also responsive to cryotherapy. Chest wall pain can be controlled with specific intercostal nerve blocks. Certain facial pain syndromes, such as tic douloureux, and suprascapular and other specific neuralgias have been treated with good success. Cryoanalgesia has also been effective in treating facet syndrome and coccydynia. Access the sacral canal for relief of perineal neuropathies or phantom limb pain. Use local applications with such conditions as trigger points, pain neuromas, or painful superficial scars. If the cryoprobe can be reliably placed on the sensory nerve transmitting the painful impulses with negligible risk of involving other important structures (i.e., motor nerves), cryoanalgesia can be an effective treatment.

B. Before performing any neurolytic block percutaneously, perform a diagnostic block. After needle placement is confirmed with the method of choice (e.g., fluoroscopy), inject a small amount of local anesthetic. This allows one to confirm the production of adequate analgesia without significant side effects. If failure is encountered in either category, reassess correct needle placement and/or consider alternative modalities.

C. Cryoanalgesia may be performed with direct placement of the probe after surgical isolation of the selected nerve, or indirectly, with percutaneous insertion of a relatively large-bore needle tip adjacent to the selected nerve. Fluoroscopy and electrical nerve stimulation are routinely used to verify placement. With the probe tip in correct position two 2-minute freeze-thaw cycles may be used, each attaining temperatures of $-60°$ C. The patient may initially experience some discomfort, but it should quickly dissipate if the probe is accurately placed. Axonotmesis is not accomplished if the pain continues. Thus, the cryoprobe must be repositioned and the procedure repeated. Specific times, temperatures, and precautions may vary for different blocks. These factors are well described in the literature and should be reviewed.

D. When cryotherapy is used on a superficial lesion, full-thickness skin damage may occur, resulting in depigmentation. Intercostal nerve blocks may be complicated by a pneumothorax. Possible damage to adjacent structures must always be carefully considered. Duration and degree of pain relief is not always predictable and often only lasts for weeks to months; therefore, patients may need repeated treatments. Finally, the equipment is expensive and requires experience for optimal results. Advantages of cryoanalgesia include the lack of neuritis or neuroma formation and prolonged pain relief with reversible effects (unlike chemical neurolysis). This procedure is usually accomplished with minimal tissue damage and no systemic side effects. It can routinely be performed as an outpatient procedure and is readily learned by practitioners experienced with nerve block techniques. As improvements in technology produce smaller probes with built-in nerve stimulators, indications for cryotherapy will continue to expand.

References

Glynn CJ, Lloyd JW, Barnard JD. Cryoanalgesia in the management of pain after thoracotomy. Thorax 1980; 35:325.

Lloyd JW, Barnard JDW, Glynn, CJ. Cryoanalgesia: a new approach to pain relief. Lancet 1976; 2:932.

Myers R, et al. Biophysical and pathological effects of cryogenic nerve lesions. Ann Neurol 1981; 10:478.

Sunderland S. A classification of peripheral nerve injuries producing loss of function. Brain 1951; 74:491.

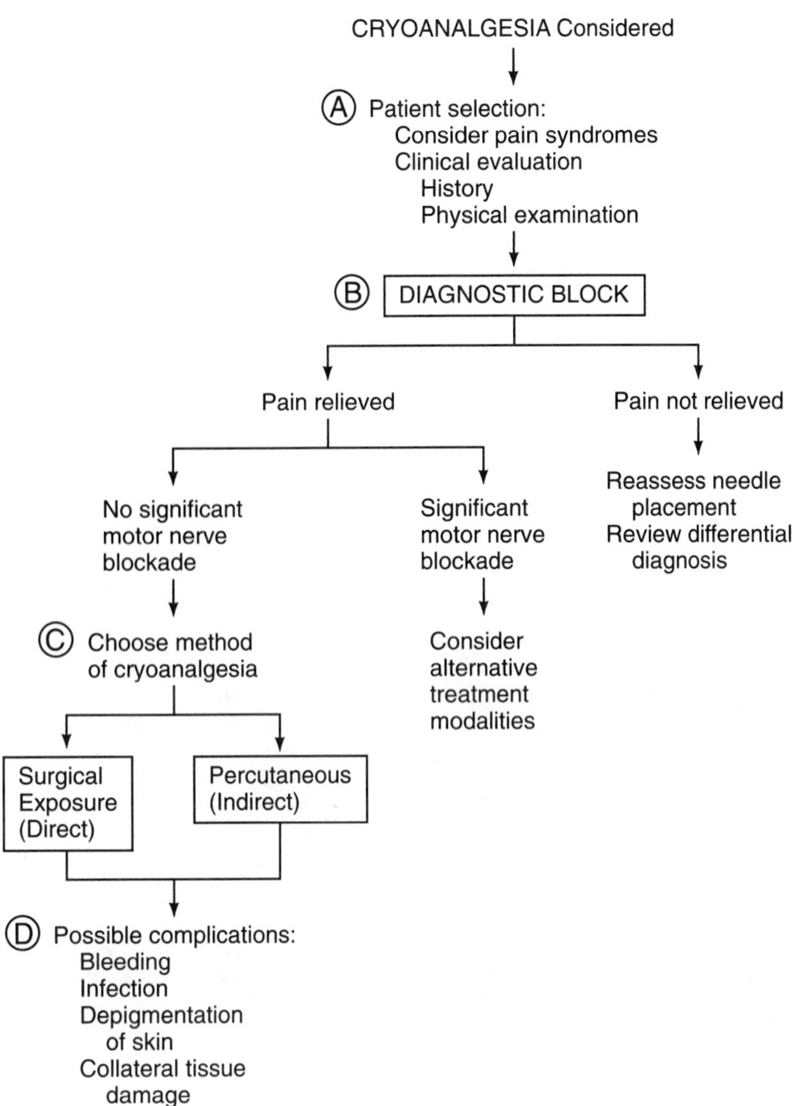

CRYOANALGESIA Considered
Ⓐ Patient selection:
Consider pain syndromes
Clinical evaluation
History
Physical examination
Ⓑ DIAGNOSTIC BLOCK
Pain relieved
Pain not relieved
No significant motor nerve blockade
Significant motor nerve blockade
Reassess needle placement
Review differential diagnosis
Ⓒ Choose method of cryoanalgesia
Consider alternative treatment modalities
Surgical Exposure (Direct)
Percutaneous (Indirect)
Ⓓ Possible complications:
Bleeding
Infection
Depigmentation of skin
Collateral tissue damage

NEUROSURGICAL PROCEDURES FOR PAIN

Somayaji Ramamurthy, M.D.

Neurosurgical techniques can be valuable if used in highly selected patients.

A. A thorough history, physical examination, and diagnostic work-up are important in patient selection.

B. All patients before undergoing neurosurgical procedures should receive a multidisciplinary pain evaluation. Pay special considerations to psychological factors, drug-seeking behavior, and secondary gain factors. Give an adequate trial to noninvasive modalities and nonsurgical approaches, including nerve blocks and physical and psychological methods.

C. Patients who have pain due to malignancy that is not controlled by oral medications, including narcotics, NSAIDs, tricyclic antidepressants, and neuraxial narcotics, should be considered for operative procedures. If there is localized pain, a diagnostic nerve block is performed. If the patient obtains complete pain relief from a nerve root block or a sympathetic block, perform repeated blocks to make sure the patient receives good pain relief consistently and is not a placebo responder. This also gives the patient an opportunity to evaluate the numbness, weakness, and other effects of interruption of neural pathways. Dorsal rhizotomy and sympathectomy in the lumbar and thoracic area can provide excellent pain relief. Patients who have diffuse pain may benefit from cordotomy, myelotomy, thalamotomy, or cingulotomy. Patients with diffuse pain secondary to metastatic breast or prostate cancer have received excellent relief from hypophysectomy with the use of alcohol injection, cryo or thermal lesions, or even an open surgical procedure.

D. Patients with trigeminal neuralgia who are unresponsive to carbamazepine, phenytoin, and other anticonvulsants, or those who are unable to tolerate these drugs because of side effects, are candidates for neurosurgical procedures. Glycerol rhizotomy and radiofrequency lesion are very effective. Even though there may be recurrence, these procedures seem to give excellent pain relief without significant sensory loss and sparing the motor function of the mandibular nerve. Microvascular decompression has a high success rate but involves posterior fossa exploration with significant surgical risk.

E. Patients who have pain from nonmalignant conditions may be considered either for ablative surgery or stimulation techniques, depending on the type, extent, and location of the pain.

F. Patients with a long life span who have pain from a nonmalignant condition are not good candidates for neuroablative surgery. There is a significant pattern of recurrence, and any impairment of function secondary to weakness or bladder/bowel incontinence can seriously impair the quality of life. Dysesthesias and anesthesia dolorosa can produce discomfort worse than that of the original pain. Patients with localized pain unresponsive to all other therapies may benefit from dorsal root rhizotomy. This may spare the motor function, but if more than five to six roots are sectioned this can result in loss of proprioception and motor incoordination. Patients who have diffuse pain, especially unilateral, may benefit from cordotomy. Patients with significant respiratory impairment are not suitable candidates for this procedure. Percutaneous cordotomy is preferred to open cordotomy. Patients with deafferentation pain may benefit from dorsal root entry zone (DREZ) lesions. Pain from avulsed spinal nerve roots, postherpetic neuralgia, phantom pain, and postradiculopathy pain have been reported to be alleviated by this procedure.

G. When pain is in a single nerve distribution, peripherally implanted nerve stimulators have provided effective relief in patients with causalgia and other peripheral types of pain. If there is diffuse pain over large areas of the body, dorsal column stimulation through an electrode placed in the epidural space with an implanted battery or through an RF generator can be effective. It relieves various types of pain, especially in patients with postlaminectomy pain, phantom limb pain, or reflex sympathetic dystrophy. In patients with more diffuse pain, deep brain stimulation can be very effective.

References

Bonica JJ, ed. Management of pain. Philadelphia: Lea & Febiger, 1990:2040.

Coffey RJ. Surgical technique in pain management. In: Raj PP, ed. Practical management of pain. 2nd ed. St Louis: Mosby–Year Book, 1992:877.

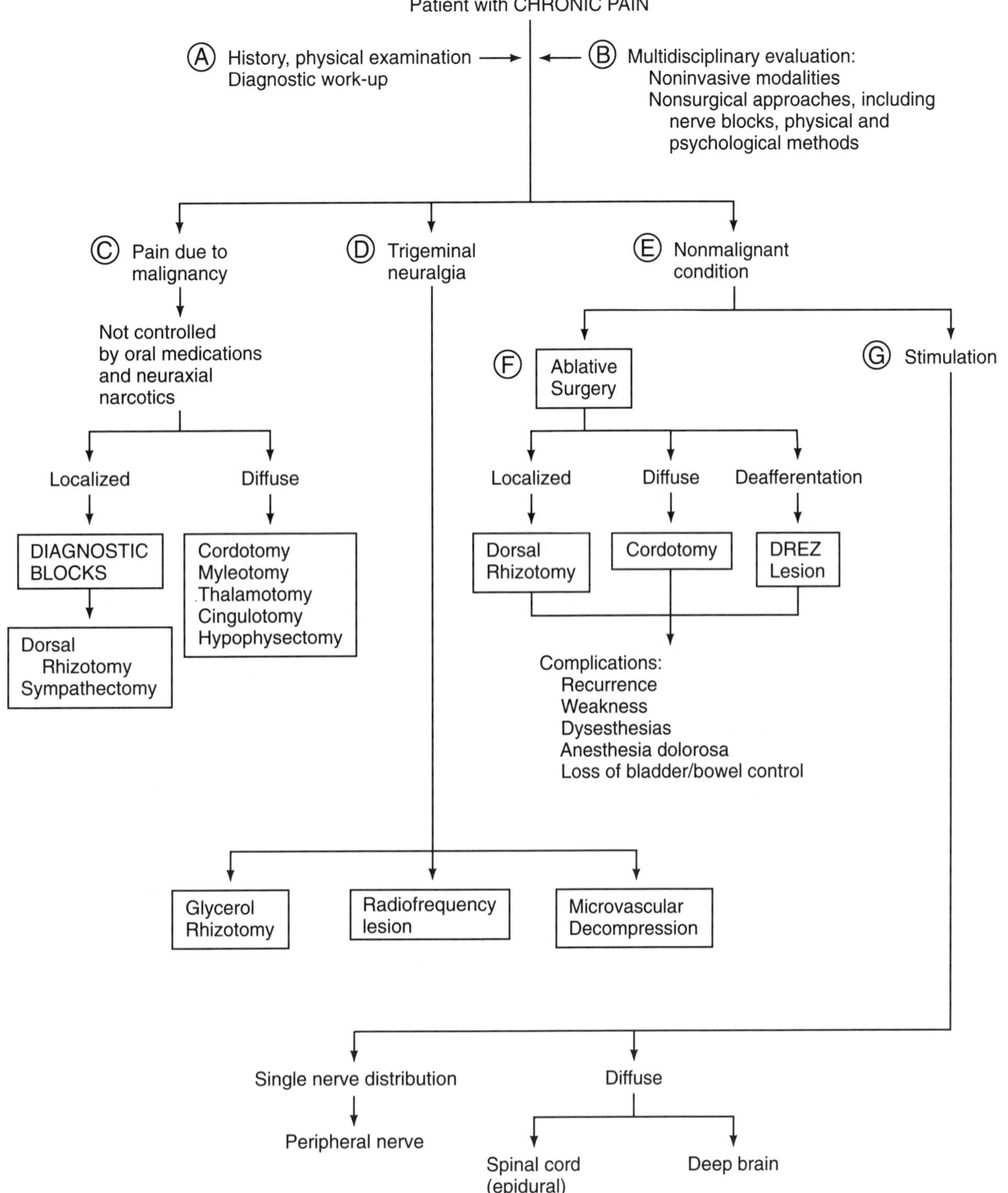

Patient with CHRONIC PAIN
(A) History, physical examination
Diagnostic work-up
(B) Multidisciplinary evaluation:
Noninvasive modalities
Nonsurgical approaches, including
nerve blocks, physical and
psychological methods
(C) Pain due to
malignancy
Not controlled
by oral medications
and neuraxial
narcotics
Localized
Diffuse
DIAGNOSTIC
BLOCKS
Dorsal
Rhizotomy
Sympathectomy
Cordotomy
Myleotomy
Thalamotomy
Cingulotomy
Hypophysectomy
(D) Trigeminal
neuralgia
Glycerol
Rhizotomy
Radiofrequency
lesion
Microvascular
Decompression
(E) Nonmalignant
condition
(F) Ablative
Surgery
Localized
Diffuse
Deafferentation
Dorsal
Rhizotomy
Cordotomy
DREZ
Lesion
Complications:
Recurrence
Weakness
Dysesthesias
Anesthesia dolorosa
Loss of bladder/bowel control
(G) Stimulation
Single nerve distribution
Peripheral nerve
Diffuse
Spinal cord
(epidural)
Deep brain

SPECIFIC BLOCKS

Contraindications to Regional Anesthesia
Peripheral Nerve Stimulators
Radiographic Contrast Media
Epidural Blockade
Subarachnoid Blockade
Stellate Ganglion Block
Thoracic Sympathetic Block
Celiac Plexus Block
Lumbar Sympathetic Block
Interpleural Analgesia
Intercostal Nerve Block
Somatic Paravertebral Nerve Root Block
Trigeminal Ganglion Blockade
Sphenopalatine Ganglion Block
Brachial Plexus Block
Spinal Accessory Nerve Block
Long Thoracic Nerve Block
Facet Joint Injection
Sacroiliac Joint Injection
Trigger Point Injection
Sciatic Nerve Block
Femoral Nerve Block
Lateral Femoral Cutaneous Nerve Block
Obturator Nerve Block
Tibial Nerve Block
Wrist Block
Ankle Block

CONTRAINDICATIONS TO REGIONAL ANESTHESIA

Robert Sprague, M.D.

The term *regional anesthesia* (RA) encompasses a wide variety of techniques, including spinal, epidural, caudal, Bier, and major nerve trunk blocks. Advantages and disadvantages to RA exist, but certain conditions are contraindications to performing any regional block. Medical conditions may also dictate against RA. Patients with severe lung disease, for example, may not tolerate a pneumothorax, and techniques of brachial block with the possibility of lung puncture, such as supraclavicular block, should not be used except by those with longstanding clinical experience.

A. Absolute contraindications to RA include localized infection; a dermatologic condition that precludes skin preparation; the existence of tumor at the injection site; patient refusal; a history of allergy to amide local anesthetics; the presence of severe hypovolemia; gross coagulation defects; increased intracranial pressure (spinal, caudal, epidural); and septicemia.

B. Relative contraindications include the inability to perform surgery adequately in the presence of a regional block. In certain diseases, such as aortic stenosis, the patient may not tolerate spinal, caudal, or epidural blockade. In addition, certain pathologic states such as ankylosing spondylitis, severe arthritis, and kyphoscoliosis may make it difficult to perform the block. Minor coagulation abnormalities, including the use of "minidose" heparin, and a difficult airway may also be contraindications in some patients. Pre-existing neurologic diseases such as multiple sclerosis or amyotrophic lateral sclerosis may be aggravated during spinal anesthesia. Finally, lack of skill on the part of the operator is also a relative contraindication to RA.

C. Block-specific contraindications also exist. A Bier block (IV regional block [IVRB]) should not be used in patients with sickle cell anemia or trait because the stasis and deoxygenation of blood left in the extremity during tourniquet inflation may lead to a sickling event. Prilocaine should not be used in doses >600 mg, because significant methemoglobinemia may result (Table 1). Bupivacaine is inappropriate for use in IVRB because of its cardiotoxic effects.

TABLE 1 Maximum Local Anesthetic Dosages

Drug	*Concentration (%)*	*Maximum Dosage (mg/kg adult)*
Procaine	1–2	10–14
Chloroprocaine	1–2	12–15
Tetracaine	0.1–0.25	2
Lidocaine	1–2	8–11
Mepivicaine	1–2	8–11
Bupivacaine	0.25–0.5	2.5–3.5
Etidocaine	0.5–1	4–5.5

References

Bridenbaugh PO, Greene NM. Spinal neural blockade. In: Cousins MJ, Bridenbaugh PO, eds. Neural blockade in clinical anesthesia and management of pain. 2nd ed. Philadelphia: JB Lippincott, 1988.

Covino BG, Lambert DH. Regional anesthesia. In: Barash PG, Cullen BF, Stoelting RK, eds. Clinical anesthesia. Philadelphia: JB Lippincott, 1989.

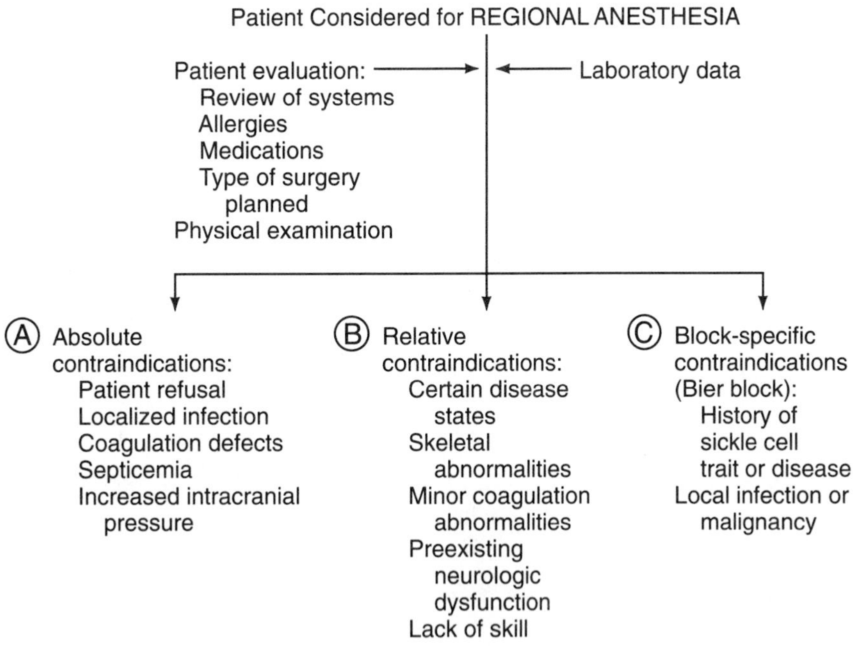

Patient Considered for REGIONAL ANESTHESIA

Patient evaluation: →
- Review of systems
- Allergies
- Medications
- Type of surgery planned

Physical examination

← Laboratory data

Ⓐ Absolute contraindications:
- Patient refusal
- Localized infection
- Coagulation defects
- Septicemia
- Increased intracranial pressure

Ⓑ Relative contraindications:
- Certain disease states
- Skeletal abnormalities
- Minor coagulation abnormalities
- Preexisting neurologic dysfunction
- Lack of skill

Ⓒ Block-specific contraindications (Bier block):
- History of sickle cell trait or disease
- Local infection or malignancy

PERIPHERAL NERVE STIMULATORS

Jay S. Ellis, Jr., M.D.

Peripheral nerve stimulators (PNSs) are a valuable aid in the performance of peripheral nerve blocks. Although most peripheral nerve blocks require only simple equipment and a sound knowledge of anatomy, the use of PNSs can more precisely identify the location of peripheral nerves, especially in the anesthetized or otherwise uncooperative patient. In addition, a PNS may reduce the chance of getting a paresthesia. Eliciting paresthesias increases the risk for neurologic complications from peripheral nerve blocks.

Whether the use of a PNS increases the success rate of peripheral nerve blocks is unclear. It does not increase the success of axillary blocks over the more traditional transarterial or paresthesia-seeking approaches, but other nerve blocks may be much easier to accomplish with its use. The obturator nerve, for example, is difficult to locate exactly, even if paresthesias are actively sought. With a PNS, the anesthetist can identify the obturator nerve by watching for muscular activity in the adductor muscles of the hip.

When choosing a PNS for neural blockade, make sure that the device has most, if not all, of the desirable features of PNSs listed in the review by Pither et al. As a minimum, the PNS must have a voltage range of 1 to 10 V and a display that shows the electrical current level over a range of 0.1 to 1.0 mA. Most commercially available PNS devices designed for neural blockade meet acceptable standards. Nerve stimulators designed for monitoring neuromuscular blockade do not deliver current in the low range of 0.1 to 1.0 mA.

Next, decide whether to use an insulated needle or the more common uninsulated type. The advantage of insulated needles is that the maximum current density appears at the tip of the needle, whereas the maximum current density of an uninsulated needle occurs proximal to the needle tip. This difference means that the maximum stimulation of a nerve by an uninsulated needle occurs once the tip of the needle is past the nerve. The knowledge of this difference allows the anesthetist to use the uninsulated needle effectively, allowing for the difference in current density. The advantages of the uninsulated needle are low cost and ready availability.

A. Prepare the patient for nerve block as usual.

B. Attach the anode (+) lead to the patient, and the cathode (−) lead to the needle. This step reduces the amount of current needed to stimulate the nerve.

C. When the needle approaches the expected location of the nerve, turn the nerve stimulator on to a current level of 5 mA or less. (If the muscle twitches increase and then diminish while advancing the needle, the needle has passed the nerve and needs to be redirected. Remember when using an uninsulated needle that the maximum current stimulation occurs once the needle tip has passed the nerve. Pull the needle back 1 to 2 mm to compensate for this difference.)

D. As the needle is advanced toward the nerve, the muscles supplied by the nerve begin to twitch (ignore local muscle contractions). Reduce the current while advancing the needle.

E. The goal of needle placement is to reach a point where muscle contractions are still maximal at a current setting <1.0 mA. A current level of 0.5 mA or less is ideal and indicates very precise localization of the nerve. Higher current requirements are a sign that needle position may not be optimal.

F. Once the point of minimal current stimulation is established, give a test dose of 2 ml of local anesthetic.

G. This test dose should abolish the muscle twitches; the remainder of the local anesthetic can then be administered. If the test dose fails to abolish the muscle twitches, reposition the needle so that, again, the minimum current needed to stimulate muscle twitches is 1.0 mA or less.

References

Bashein G, Ready LB, Haschke RH. Electrolocation: insulated versus noninsulated needles. Reg Anesth 1984; 9:31.

Goldberg ME, Gregg C, Larijani GE, et al. A comparison of three methods of axillary approach to brachial plexus blockade for upper extremity surgery. Anesthesiology 1987; 66:814.

Pither CE, Raj PP, Ford DJ. The use of peripheral nerve stimulators for regional anesthesia: a review of experimental characteristics: technique and clinical applications. Reg Anesth 1985; 10:49.

Selander D, Edshage S, Wolf T. Paresthesiae or no paresthesiae? nerve lesions after axillary blocks. Acta Anaesth Scand 1979; 23:27.

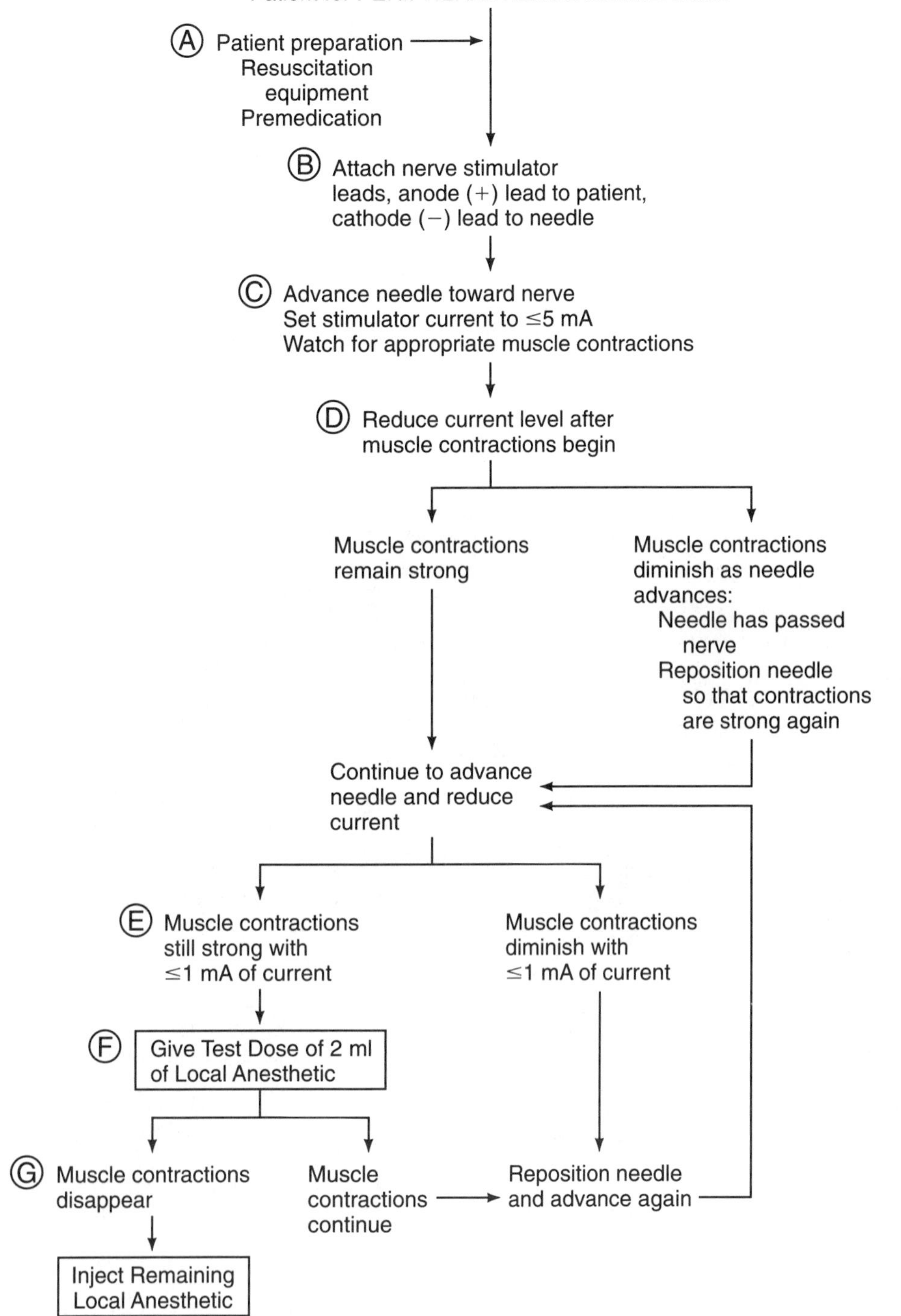
Patient for PERIPHERAL NERVE STIMULATION
Ⓐ Patient preparation
Resuscitation equipment
Premedication
Ⓑ Attach nerve stimulator leads, anode (+) lead to patient, cathode (−) lead to needle
Ⓒ Advance needle toward nerve
Set stimulator current to ≤5 mA
Watch for appropriate muscle contractions
Ⓓ Reduce current level after muscle contractions begin
Muscle contractions remain strong
Muscle contractions diminish as needle advances:
Needle has passed nerve
Reposition needle so that contractions are strong again
Continue to advance needle and reduce current
Ⓔ Muscle contractions still strong with ≤1 mA of current
Muscle contractions diminish with ≤1 mA of current
Ⓕ Give Test Dose of 2 ml of Local Anesthetic
Ⓖ Muscle contractions disappear
Muscle contractions continue
Reposition needle and advance again
Inject Remaining Local Anesthetic

RADIOGRAPHIC CONTRAST MEDIA

Scott D. Murtha, M.D.

Fluoroscopic assistance for nerve blocks has become an important tool in pain management. Correct placement of local anesthetics and neurolytic agents is imperative. Unfortunately, many use radiographic contrast media on a daily basis, yet know very little about their properties. Conventional agents, such as Hypaque, Renografin, and Conray are ionic tri-iodinated derivatives of benzoic acid and are water soluble and high in osmolarity. Two types of low osmolar contrast agents are available. These were developed in the hope of diminishing the number of reactions to contrast medium. The first is an ionic monoacidic dimer such as ioxaglate (Hexabrix). The second type consists of nonionic agents such as iopamidol (Isovue) and iohexol (Omnipaque). Low osmolar agents have less than half of the osmolarity of the conventional ionic contrast agents but still more than twice the osmolarity of plasma.

A. In general, conventional ionic contrast media are both technically acceptable and safe for most pain management procedures. They are not recommended for myelography or epidurography because of their neurotoxicity. Conventional media can induce epileptiform activity when applied to cortical tissue, probably as a result of the free salt-forming ions; however, their hyperosmolarity can affect CSF composition.

B. It is recommended that low osmolar contrast media be used selectively because of their high cost. They have proved less neurotoxic and less likely to produce arachnoiditis. Both iopamidol and iohexol are approved for intrathecal use and should also be used in epidurography or any procedure in which dural puncture is likely (e.g., selective nerve root blocks). Current recommendations emphasize limiting the intrathecal dose of iodine to less than 3 g in adult patients (10 ml of a 300-mg/ml agent). Injected intrathecally, these agents can cause headaches, nausea, vomiting, dizziness, or exacerbation of existing pain.

C. Low osmolar nonionic agents should also be employed in patients with a history of a reaction to contrast agents or at high risk for an anaphylactoid reaction (e.g., asthmatics or those with multiple food or medication allergies). Reactions to conventional ionic contrast agents are listed in Table 1. Reactions occur three to eight times less often with the newer nonionic agents. In particular, anaphylactoid reactions are fewer, although more case reports of fatal reactions to intravascular nonionic contrast media are surfacing in the radiology literature. Steroid prophylaxis should also be considered for any patient at high risk for an anaphylactoid reaction. Current prophylaxis recommendations are listed in Table 2.

TABLE 1 Incidence of Adverse Reactions to Ionic Contrast Agents

Reactions	*Number (%)*
Minor reactions: nausea, vomiting, limited urticaria, lightheadedness, mild dyspnea	1/20 (5%)
Intermediate reactions: extensive urticaria, dyspnea, bronchospasm, mild chest pain	1/100 (1%)
Severe reactions: laryngeal edema, severe angina, seizures, refractory hypotension	1/2000 (0.05%)
Cardiac arrest	1/6000 (0.017%)
Death	1/40,000 (0.0025%)

TABLE 2 Suggested Prophylaxis for Patients at Risk for an Anaphylactoid Reaction to Contrast Media

Steroids
Methylprednisolone: 32 mg po 12 hr and 1 hr before procedure
or
Prednisone: 20 mg po q6 hr × 3
or
Hydrocortisone: 100 mg IV q6 hr × 3

*Antihistamines**
Cimetidine: 300 mg PO or IV 1 hr before procedure *and*
Diphenhydramine: 50 mg PO or IV 1 hr before procedure

*If previous reaction was severe or had a respiratory component.

References

Cohan RH. Radiographic contrast media. In: Kadir S, ed. Current practice of interventional radiology. Philadelphia: BC Decker, 1991:14.

Curry NS, et al. Fatal reactions to intravenous non-ionic contrast material. Radiology 1991; 178:361.

Skucas J. Radiographic contrast agents. 2nd ed. Rockville: Aspen, 1989.

Slappendel R, et al. Spread of radiographic dye in the thoracic epidural space. Anaesthesia 1988; 43:939.

Sutton D. A textbook of radiology and imaging. 4th ed. New York: Churchill Livingstone, 1987.

Wang H, et al. Lumbar myelography with iohexol in outpatients: Prospective multicenter evaluation of safety. Radiology 1989; 173:239.

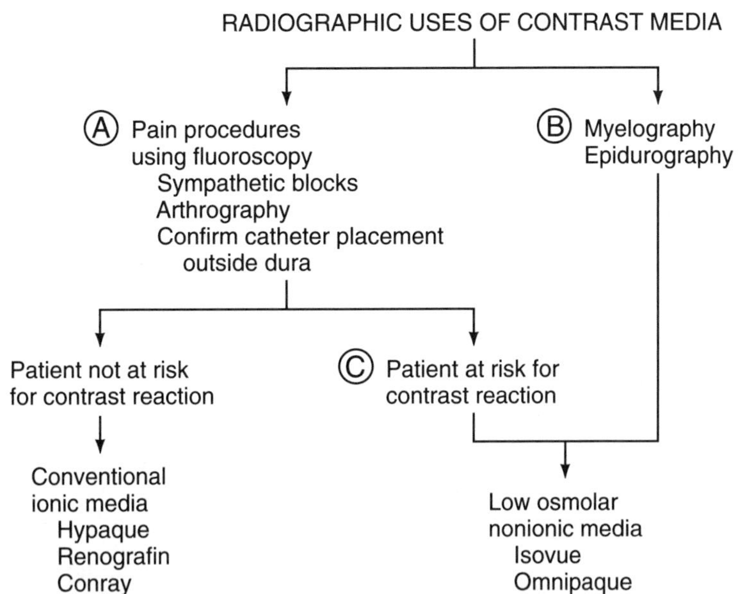
RADIOGRAPHIC USES OF CONTRAST MEDIA
Ⓐ Pain procedures
using fluoroscopy
Sympathetic blocks
Arthrography
Confirm catheter placement
outside dura
Ⓑ Myelography
Epidurography
Patient not at risk
for contrast reaction
Ⓒ Patient at risk for
contrast reaction
Conventional
ionic media
Hypaque
Renografin
Conray
Low osmolar
nonionic media
Isovue
Omnipaque

EPIDURAL BLOCKADE

Dale Solomon, M.D.

The epidural space is a potential space filled with fat, lymphatics, and vascular structures located between the ligamentum flavum and vertebral laminae posteriorly and the dura mater anteriorly. It extends from the foramen magnum to the sacral hiatus and can be entered with a needle anywhere along the length of its course. Drugs deposited in this space are taken up by adipose tissue and blood vessels so that significant systemic absorption occurs, but a portion of the drug diffuses through the dura mater or to adjacent nerve roots to affect neural transmission.

A. Epidural blockade can modulate the pain of both acute and chronic conditions of the neck, extremities, and torso. Candidates for the procedure should have no systemic infection, coagulopathy, or local inflammation near the proposed site of injection. The patient should have stable neurologic function and should consent to the procedure. Patients with a low circulating blood volume have an exaggerated hypotensive response when a sympathectomy is caused by local anesthetics. The epidural space may be difficult to locate in areas of previous spinal laminectomy.

B. Place epidurally administered drugs as close as possible to the nerve roots transmitting the pain impulses. For example, the thoracic epidural space may be entered for upper abdominal pain, the lumbar region for lower extremity pain, and the caudal epidural space, for pelvic pain. Use a midline or paramedian approach in the lumbar region, but a paramedian approach in the midthoracic region of the spine because of the severe caudad angulation of the spinous processes.

C. Any drug injected into the epidural space should have a record of safety when used in the epidural space and be preservative free. Local anesthetics, opiates, and various other drugs have been placed into the epidural space to modulate pain. Administer these drugs by intermittent bolus or continuous infusion. Local anesthetics provide the most intense analgesia but impair sympathetic nerve activity and can impair motor function. Opiates preserve motor and sympathetic nervous function, but may cause respiratory depression, itching, urinary retention, and nausea and vomiting. A combination of low concentrations of local anesthetic and opiate solutions has provided excellent analgesia with few side effects.

D. The dose and volume of solution to be injected depends on (1) clinical aspects of the patient, (2) the distance from the site of injection to the pertinent nerve roots, (3) the region of the spine being entered, and (4) the physicochemical properties of the drug being administered. For example, 20 to 30 cc of local anesthetic solution may be required to reach the T4 dermatome from the lumbar region, whereas 5 cc of the same solution in the thoracic region may spread over several dermatomal levels. Three to five mg of morphine in the lumbar region may be adequate for lower extremity pain, whereas 5 to 10 mg is needed to alleviate thoracic pain when injected from the same region of the spine.

E. Because of the risk for complications, resuscitation equipment and IV access must be present before proceeding with an epidural blockade. Scrub the skin over the spine with disinfectant while the patient is sitting or in the lateral decubitus position. Obtain cutaneous and subcutaneous anesthesia with local anesthetic, and pass an epidural needle to the ligamentum flavum. Advance the needle slowly until the epidural space is identified by the loss of resistance or hanging-drop technique. After a negative aspiration for CSF and blood, inject an appropriate test solution, usually 3 ml of 2% lidocaine with 1:200,000 epinephrine, through the needle to detect IV or subarachnoid placement of the needle. Check vital signs every 5 minutes. For short surgical procedures, inject the remainder of the local anesthetic solution through the needle, and then withdraw it. For longer procedures and for short- and long-term pain management, thread a catheter through the needle into the epidural space and secure to the skin in a sterile fashion. For long-term use, the catheter can be tunneled subcutaneously away from the site of insertion.

F. Complications of epidural blockade with local anesthetics include (1) hypotension caused by sympathetic blockade, (2) local anesthetic toxicity due to intravascular injection or uptake from the epidural space, and (3) motor paralysis and apnea caused by high epidural, subarachnoid, or subdural injection. Epidurally administered narcotics can cause respiratory depression, pruritus, nausea and vomiting, and urinary retention. Perform frequent inspection and redressing of long-term catheters to avoid infection. Epidural hematomas should be suspected with increasing back pain and progressing neurologic deficits. Accidental dural puncture may result in a spinal headache.

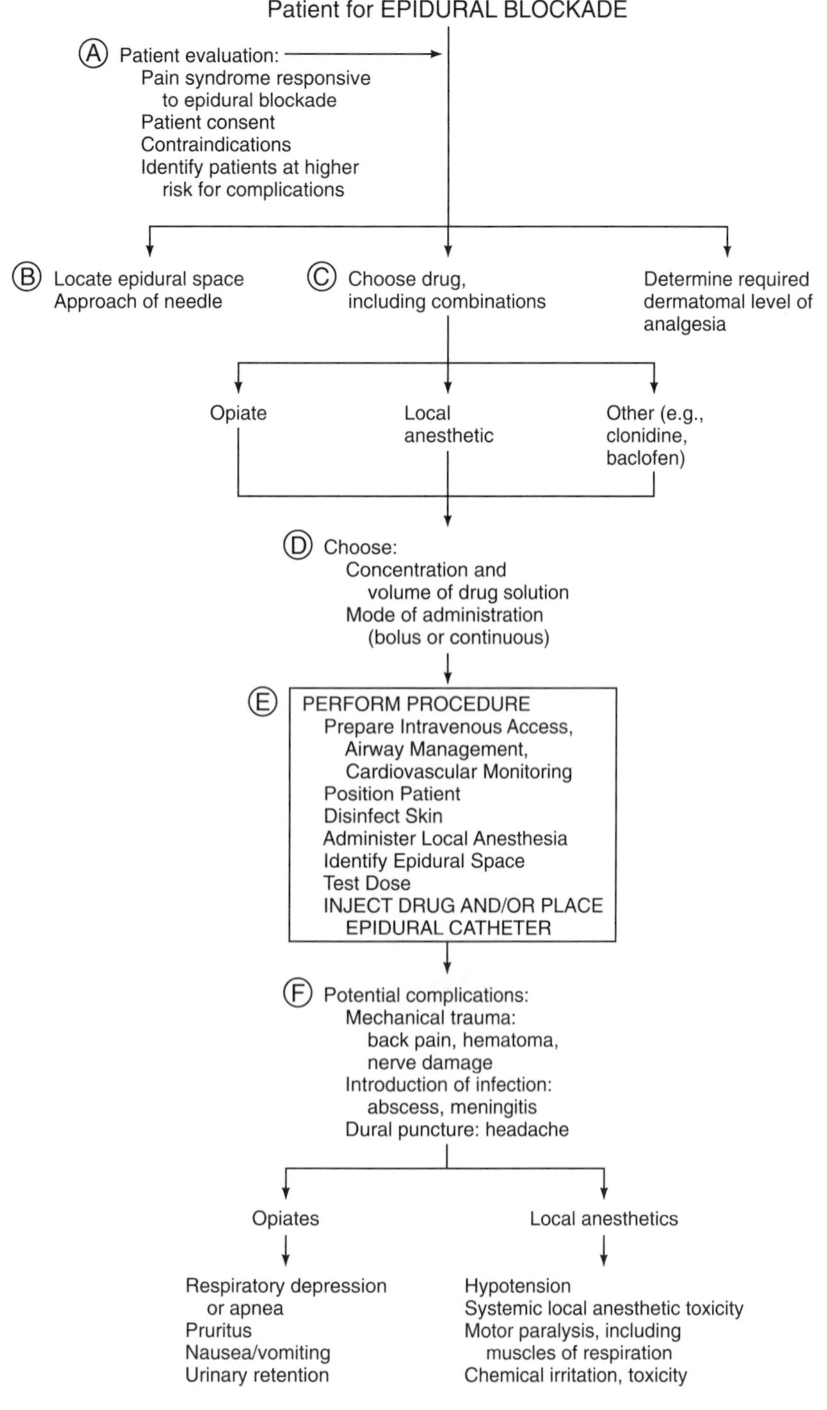

References

Bromage PR. Epidural analgesia. Philadelphia: WB Saunders, 1978:8.

Cousins MJ, Mather LE. Intrathecal and epidural administration of opioids. Anesthesiology 1984; 61:276.

Eisenach JC. Pain relief in obstetrics. In: Raj PP, ed. Practical management of pain. St Louis: Mosby–Year Biol, 1992:391.

Elliott RD. Continuous infusion epidural analgesia for obstetrics: bupivacaine versus bupivacaine-fentanyl mixture. Can J Anaesth 1991; 38:303.

Loeser JD, Cousins MJ. Contemporary pain management. Med J Aust 1990; 153:208.

Mulroy MF. Regional anesthesia. Boston: Little, Brown, 1989:93.

Raj SP, Pai U. Techniques of nerve blocking. Conduction blocks. In: Raj P, ed. Handbook of regional anesthesia. New York: Churchill Livingstone, 1985:237.

SUBARACHNOID BLOCKADE

Dale Solomon, M.D.

The subarachnoid space is contiguous with the intracranial CSF pathways and ends at the S2 spinal level in adults. Drugs injected into the CSF of the spine have a rapid action on exposed nerve membranes of the spinal cord and nerve roots. Subarachnoid blocks (SAB) are used to treat various acute and chronic pain syndromes, for diagnostic purposes, and to treat muscular spasms associated with cerebral, motor, or spinal cord dysfunction.

A. Candidates for SAB should consent to the procedure and have stable neurologic function, normal clotting function, no evidence of systemic sepsis, and no inflammation or infection over the proposed site of injection. Hypovolemic patients have an exaggerated hypotensive response to the sympathectomy caused by local anesthetics. Because of the risk for downward herniation of the brain, the dura must not be punctured when CSF pressure is elevated intracranially.

B. The subarachnoid space can be entered with a needle anywhere along its path, but to prevent injury to the spinal cord a site of entrance caudad to the conus medullaris (L1–2 in adults, L2–3 in infants) is normally chosen. In the lumbar area, use either a midline or paramedian approach to access the subarachnoid space through the interlaminar foramen. Because the spinous processes run nearly perpendicular to the long axis of the spine in this region, a spinal needle placed into the interspinous ligament is directed perpendicularly. Alternatively, the needle may be directed toward the midline from a position 1 cm lateral to the midline.

C. The choice and quantity of drug injected into the subarachnoid space are based on patient characteristics, the desired goal of the blockade, and the desired duration of the blockade. Any drug chosen should have a record of safety in the CSF and be preservative free. For short surgical procedures, lidocaine is most often chosen. For longer procedures, use either tetracaine or bupivacaine. Vasoconstrictors (usually epinephrine, 1:200,000) can intensify the analgesia and prolong the blockade of most local anesthetics. The local anesthetic can be diluted with water, saline, or dextrose to make the specific gravity of the final solution less, equal to, or greater than the specific gravity of CSF. In the case of hypobaric or hyperbaric solutions, some degree of control of the spread of the local anesthetic in the CSF can be attained by patient positioning. For isobaric solutions, the spread of the blockade is governed primarily by the number of milligrams of local anesthetic injected, rather than the volume.

D. The required dermatomal level of any blockade depends on the level of the spinal cord at which the afferent pain impulses insert. For example, a blockade of somatic pain afferents may be effected by a blockade of lower thoracic dermatomes during intra-abdominal surgery, but visceral pain passing through the celiac plexus and communicating fibers of the sympathetic chain requires a much higher level of blockade. Neurolytic agents can be placed into the subarachnoid space and directed toward the dorsal root ganglia while preserving motor tracts by using hypobaric or hyperbaric solutions.

E. Airway management devices must be at the bedside and there must be IV access before an SAB is instituted. Scrub the skin overlying the proposed site of entrance with disinfectant solution while the patient is in the sitting, lateral decubitus, or prone position. Obtain local anesthesia of the skin and subcutaneous area, and pass the needle toward the dura with the bevel oriented parallel to the long axis of the spine. As the dura is punctured, a distinct pop is often felt and CSF should return freely. Any red blood cells should quickly clear, and there should be no paresthesias before or during injection. After an injection of local anesthetic, the patient may be turned immediately or left in the same position while the block is set up. Take vital signs every 5 minutes after injection of the local anesthetic, and follow the spread of anesthesia closely. For short surgical procedures, local anesthetics can be injected in a "one-shot" technique. For longer procedures and chronic pain therapy, pass a catheter through the spinal needle and leave it in the subarachnoid space for intermittent or continuous injections of local anesthetic or opiates. The catheter may also be tunneled subcutaneously.

F. Potential complications of SAB with local anesthetics include (1) backache in up to 40% of patients, (2) hypotension caused by sympathectomy, (3) post–dural puncture headache, (4) nausea caused by unopposed vagal activity, (5) bradycardia from blockade of cardiac sympathetic fibers, (6) respiratory insufficiency due to hypotension or high motor blockade, (7) spinal cord or nerve root damage due to mechanical or chemical irritation, (8) chemical or bacterial meningitis, and (9) spinal and/or epidural hematoma and abscess. Subarachnoid opiates also cause the same complications as do epidural opiates (p 238).

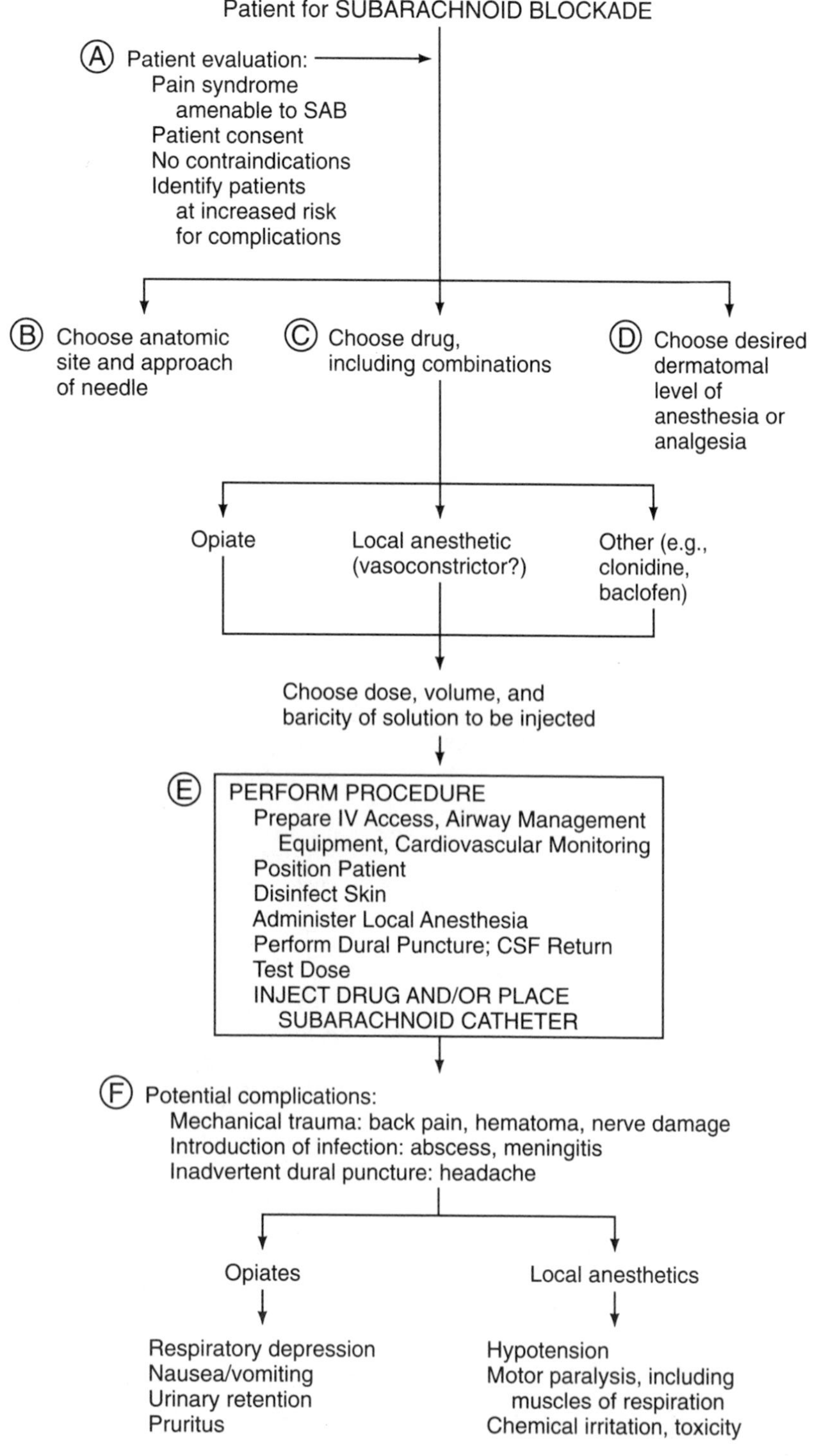

References

Albright AL, Cervi A, Singletary J. Intrathecal baclofen for spasticity in cerebral palsy. JAMA 1991; 265:1418.

Bonnet F, Brisson VB, Francois Y, et al. Effects of oral and subarachnoid clonidine on spinal anesthesia with bupivacaine. Reg Anesth 1990; 15:211.

Cousins MJ, Cherry DA, Gourlay GK. Acute and chronic pain: use of spinal opioids. In: Cousins MJ, Bridenbaugh PO, eds. Neural blockade in clinical anesthesia and management of pain. 2nd ed. Philadelphia: JB Lippincott, 1988:955.

Lee JA, Atkinson RS, Watt JM. Lumbar puncture and spinal analgesia: intradural and extradural. Edinburgh: Churchill Livingstone, 1985:60.

Mulroy MF. Regional anesthesia. Boston: Little, Brown, 1989:86.

Stienstra R, Greene NM. Factors affecting the subarachnoid spread of local anesthetic solutions. Reg Anesth 1991; 16:1.

STELLATE GANGLION BLOCK

Linda Tingle, M.D.

Sympathetic innervation of the head, neck, and upper extremity is by way of the cervical and upper thoracic sympathetic chain. The sympathetic chain lies at the anterolateral aspect of the vertebral body in the lower cervical region, and adjacent to the neck of the ribs in the thoracic region. The first thoracic and inferior cervical ganglion may be separate or fused to form the stellate ganglion.

The cervical sympathetic chain lies in the fascial space, limited by the fascia over the prevertebral muscles posteriorly and the carotid sheath anteriorly. The stellate ganglion is in front of the head of the first rib and transverse process of the seventh cervical vertebra. It lies posterior to the subclavian artery, at the origin of the vertebral artery. The dome of the pleura lies inferiorly, the scalene muscles lie laterally, and the vertebral column lies medially. Many of the complications of stellate ganglion block (SGB) are related to its proximity to important anatomic structures.

A. Indications include circulatory insufficiency of the arm (e.g., Raynaud's syndrome, arterial embolism, vasospasm) or pain from RSD, herpes zoster, or phantom limb. SGB has been beneficial for visual changes associated with quinine toxicity, sudden profound hearing loss, and Bell's palsy.

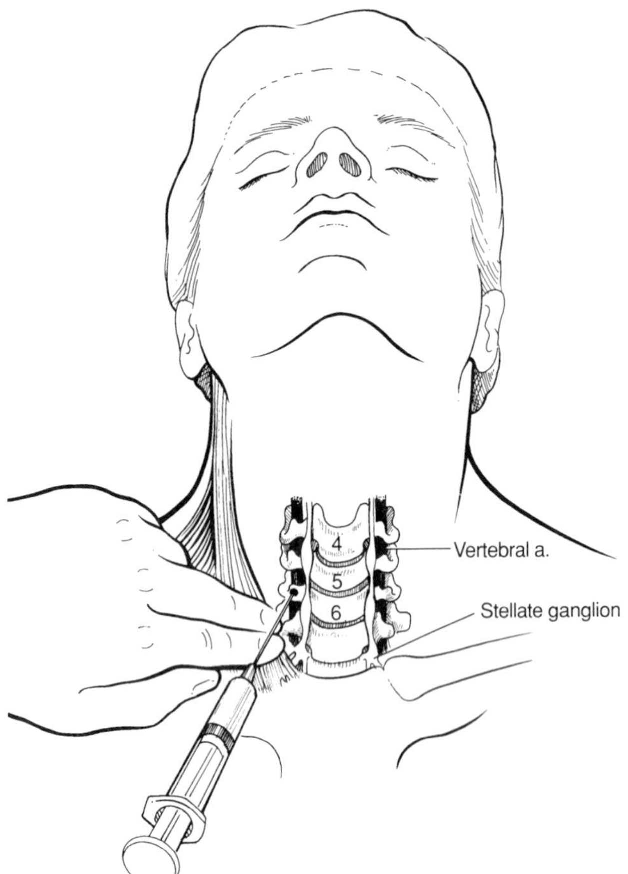

Figure 1 Placement of stellate ganglion block.

B. The paratracheal or anterior approach is the one most commonly used. The patient lies supine with the head slightly extended on a small pillow to stretch the esophagus away from the transverse process. The mouth slightly opened helps relax the neck muscles. The trachea and sternocleidomastoid (SCM) muscle are palpated. By retracting the SCM muscle laterally, the internal carotid artery and internal jugular vein are also pulled laterally. The most prominent cervical transverse process, C6 (Chassaignac's tubercle), lies at the level of the cricoid cartilage. This tubercle feels hard, like a marble. C6 is chosen as a landmark rather than C7, because C7 has no anterior tubercle to palpate, C7 is closer to the pleura, and the vertebral artery runs anterior to the transverse process of C7. Make a skin wheal over the C6 tubercle. Advance a 22-gauge, 1.5-inch needle until it contacts the transverse process medial to the tubercle, and then withdraw it 2 mm out of the prevertebral muscle. Perform an aspiration test and inject a test dose of 0.5 ml. Negative aspiration does not guarantee an extravascular injection. High resistance to injection may reflect subperiosteal injection. Significant but less resistance indicates that the needle is within the longus colli muscle. Radiating pain to the arm on injection indicates that a nerve root has been penetrated and the needle is too deep. Inject 10 to 20 ml of local anesthetic. Instruct the patient not to talk or swallow while the needle is in place, to avoid damage to adjacent structures in the neck. However, tell the patient to nonverbally communicate any abnormal sensation by raising the contralateral arm. When sympathetic block of the upper extremity is desired, the patient should sit up to facilitate the spread of local anesthetic caudad over the thoracic ganglion.

C. The presence of Horner's syndrome (ptosis, myosis, and enophthalmos) indicates a sympathetic block of the head but does not necessarily mean that the upper extremity has been blocked. Pre- and postblock temperatures taken on the distal hand indicate a sympathetic block that includes the upper extremity.

D. Common complications of SGB include temporary hoarseness (from recurrent laryngeal nerve block), hematoma, Horner's syndrome, and brachial plexus block. The phrenic nerve may be blocked, and for this reason it is prudent to block only one side at a time. Pneumothorax and epidural or subarachnoid injection can occur. Injection into the vertebral artery will result in loss of consciousness or generalized seizures. Brachial plexus block can create a diagnostic dilemma.

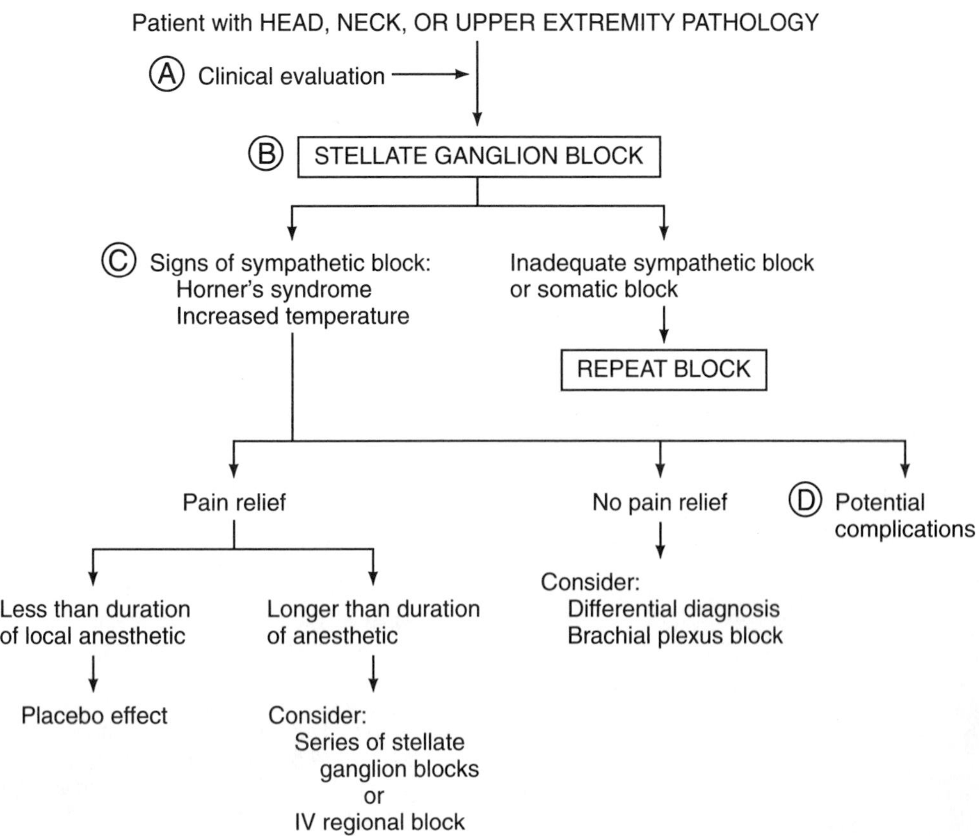

References

Ellis JS, Ramamurthy S. Seizure following stellate ganglion block after negative aspiration and test dose. Anesthesiology 1986; 64:533.

Lofstrom JB, Cousins MJ. Sympathetic neural blockade of upper and lower extremity. In: Cousins MJ, Bridenbaugh PO, eds. Neural blockade in clinical anesthesia and management of pain. 2nd ed. Philadelphia: JB Lippincott, 1987:461.

Milligan NS, Nash TP. Treatment of post-herpetic neuralgia. A review of 77 consecutive cases. Pain 1985; 23:381.

Thomas D. Forced acid diuresis and stellate ganglion block in the treatment of quinine poisoning. Anaesthesia 1984; 39:259.

THORACIC SYMPATHETIC BLOCK

Linda Tingle, M.D.

Of all the sympathetic blocks, thoracic sympathetic block has the most limited application and is most often reserved for permanent interruption of the sympathetic chain in a specific distribution of the arm or chest. Stellate ganglion block (SGB), used for sympathetic block of the upper extremity, can result in prolonged duration of undesirable side effects with the use of neurolytic agents. The less specific thoracic epidural block is often used for temporary blockade of the thoracic sympathetic chain.

The thoracic sympathetic chain lies posterolateral to the vertebral bodies and anterior to the neck of the ribs. In the thoracic region, the sympathetic chain is not separated from the somatic root by a muscle barrier as it is in the cervical and lumbar regions. The pleura is immediately lateral to the sympathetic chain.

A. Radiologic visualization is recommended to determine the relationship between the spinous process of one vertebrae and the lamina to be contacted at the cross-sectional plane.

B. Indications for blockade of thoracic sympathetic ganglia include reflex sympathetic dystrophy (RSD) in a thoracic distribution and hyperhidrosis. It is useful as a diagnostic tool for identifying specific nociceptive pathways. Blockade of the thoracic sympathetic chain is indicated in recent-onset herpes zoster, postherpetic neuralgia (PHN), chronic occlusive vascular disease, and intractable cardiac pain. It can be useful for intractable pain caused by aortic aneurysm (T2–T6), cancer of the upper two-thirds of the esophagus (T1–T8), and cancer of the viscera or chronic pancreatitis (lower two-thirds of the thoracic chain). A few patients have an anomalous sympathetic pathway known as Kuntz's nerve that bypasses the stellate ganglion. These patients may require thoracic sympathetic blockade to achieve blockade of the upper extremity.

C. The classic technique of blocking the thoracic ganglia involves positioning the patient prone with arms dangling off the table. Identify the spinous process of T2 or T3. Make a skin wheal 6 cm lateral to the spinous process and introduce a 10-cm needle in a parasagittal plane until it strikes the transverse process on the same side. Withdraw the needle 0.5 to 1 cm and angle it to pass just below the inferior edge of the rib. With the needle in a sagittal plane, contact the vertebral body about 1 cm deeper. Redirect the needle slightly to pass by the vertebral body. Inject radiopaque contrast media and verify the position in the postanterior and lateral planes with fluoroscopy. Aspirate, then inject 1.5 to 2 ml of a local anesthetic or neurolytic agent.

D. Bonica described the paralaminar technique, suggesting that it carried less risk of involving the somatic spinal nerve and of puncturing the dura. Position the patient in a lateral decubitus position with the spine flexed. Make a skin wheal 2 cm lateral to the spinous process. Advance an 8- to 10-cm, 22-gauge, short-beveled needle attached to a 2-ml glass syringe with a Luer-Lok containing saline until the lamina is contacted. Withdraw the needle until its point is in the subcutaneous tissue and the skin is moved 0.5 cm laterally. Advance the needle parallel to the first insertion. When advanced to the same depth as the lamina, the needletip contacts either the lateral edge of the lamina or the superior costotransverse ligament, which is lateral to the lateral edge of the lamina and just above the transverse process of the vertebrae below. The ligament is much less resistant than bone and more resistant than muscle. Advance the needle slowly while exerting continuous pressure on the syringe plunger. Sudden loss of resistance indicates that the bevel is anterior to the ligament. Then, advance the needle another 7 to 10 mm so that its bevel is in the same coronal plane as the anterior surface of the neck of the rib. Inject 1 ml saline to dislodge tissue in the needle. Aspirate in two planes, then inject 1 ml 0.5% bupivicaine as a test dose. If there are no signs of complications, inject 2 to 3 ml 0.25% bupivicaine or a neurolytic agent. This will block one ganglion and its upper interganglionic fibers. Repeat at subsequent lower levels.

E. Complications include somatic nerve block, pneumothorax, causalgia, nerve injury, puncture of the intercostal artery or vein, and epidural or intradural injection via insertion of the needle through an intervertebral foramen.

References

Bonica JJ. Neurolytic blockade and hypophysectomy. In: Bonica JJ, ed. The management of pain. Philadelphia: Lea & Febiger, 1990:2012.

Lofstrom JB, Cousins MJ. Sympathetic neural blockade of upper and lower extremity. In: Cousins MJ, Bridenbaugh PO, eds. Neural blockade in clinical anesthesia and management of pain. 2nd ed. Philadelphia: JB Lippincott, 1987:482.

Stanton-Hicks M. Sympathetic blocks. In: Raj PP. Practical management of pain. Chicago: Year Book, 1986:663.

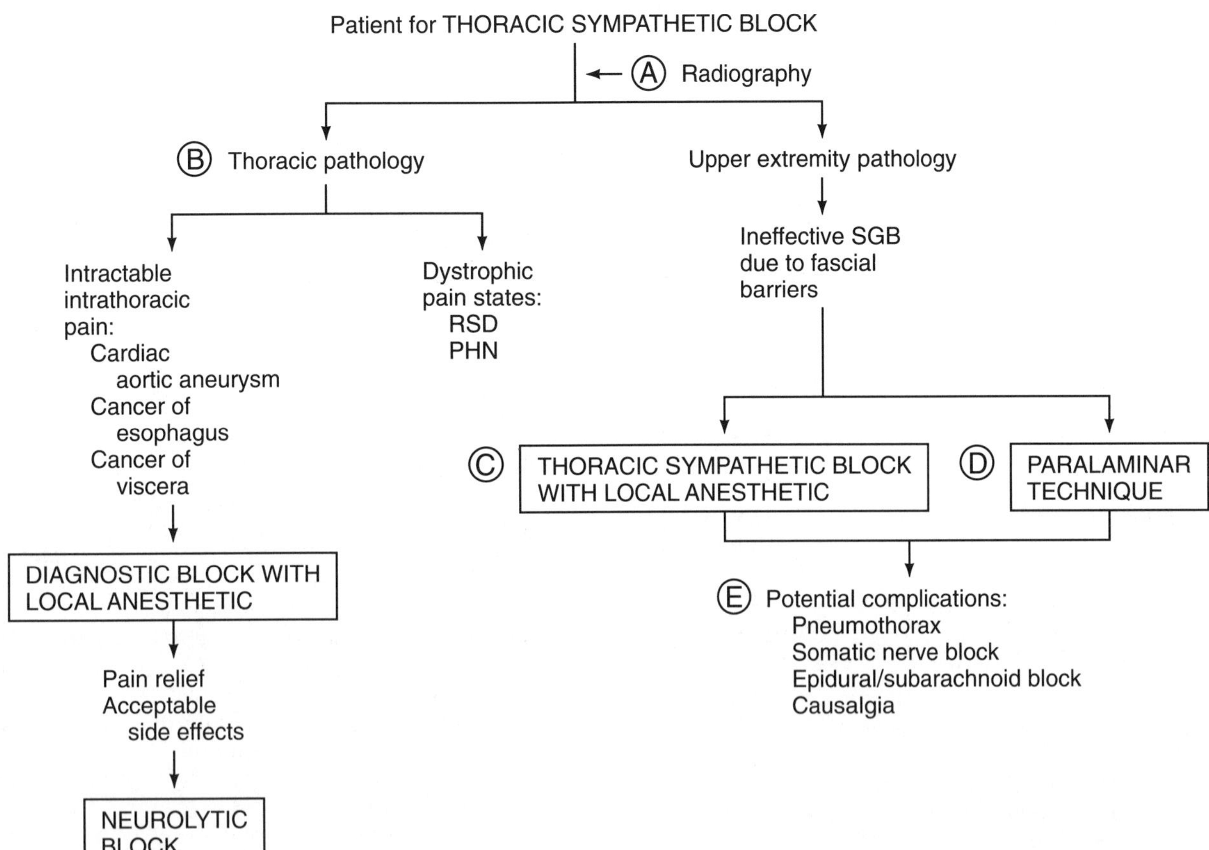

Patient for THORACIC SYMPATHETIC BLOCK
(A) Radiography
(B) Thoracic pathology
Upper extremity pathology
Intractable intrathoracic pain:
Cardiac
aortic aneurysm
Cancer of esophagus
Cancer of viscera
Dystrophic pain states:
RSD
PHN
Ineffective SGB due to fascial barriers
(C) THORACIC SYMPATHETIC BLOCK WITH LOCAL ANESTHETIC
(D) PARALAMINAR TECHNIQUE
DIAGNOSTIC BLOCK WITH LOCAL ANESTHETIC
(E) Potential complications:
Pneumothorax
Somatic nerve block
Epidural/subarachnoid block
Causalgia
Pain relief
Acceptable side effects
NEUROLYTIC BLOCK

CELIAC PLEXUS BLOCK

Linda Tingle, M.D.

The celiac ganglia lie midline in the prevertebral region of L1, anterior to the aorta, immediately above the pancreas, and in close approximation to the adrenals. The celiac plexus, composed of autonomic fibers and the celiac ganglia, surrounds the aorta and origin of the celiac and superior mesenteric arteries. The vena cava lies to the right and anteriorly. The kidneys lie laterally.

A. The indications for celiac plexus blockade (CPB) include assisting in the identification of abdominal visceral pain, treating acute pancreatitis, and treating chronic pancreatitis (controversial). It is mostly indicated for relief of intractable cancer pain from upper abdominal malignancies. CPB can also be used to provide anesthesia for abdominal procedures along with intercostal nerve blocks, and it may facilitate interventional radiologic procedures on the biliary tract.

B. It is useful to have an ECG display available and to obtain both sitting and supine blood pressure before the block, because hypotension may occur after the block and baseline values may aid in assessment. An IV catheter in place makes possible fluid boluses.

C. The classic posterolateral approach defined by Kappis and refined by Moore is the most practiced and proven route. Position the patient prone with a pillow under the abdomen and arms dangling down at the side. Identify the following landmarks and mark them on the skin: the lower edges of the twelfth ribs 7 to 8 cm lateral to the midline, and the inferior aspects of the T12 and L1 spinous processes. The points connected form a shallow isosceles triangle, the equal sides of which serve as directional guides for the two needles. Prepare the skin in a sterile fashion and place skin wheals at intersection points under the twelfth ribs. Angulate a 6-inch, 20-gauge spinal needle at 45 degrees from the horizontal plane of the patient's back and advance it toward the body of the first lumbar vertebrae until contact is made, usually at a depth of 6 to 9 cm. By grasping the needle at skin level, the operator can note the depth of the pass on subsequent insertions. Increase the angle to 60 degrees and readvance the needle meeting bone 2 to 3 cm deeper than the previous attempt. The needle is then "walked off" the lumbar body. Correct needle placement on the left can be confirmed by observation of needle pulsation transmitted from the aorta. The right side needle should be advanced in a similar fashion to a similar depth. Both needles should be 1 to 1.5 cm anterior to the anterior vertebral margin. CT or fluoroscopy in two planes can help confirm correct needle placement. After negative aspiration in four quadrants, an injection of 3 to 5 ml of a radiopaque contrast media provides confirmation of correct needle placement. Injection of local anesthetic should meet little resistance.

A single-needle technique with a transaortic approach has been described by Ischia and Feldstein, using the same landmarks as for the posterolateral approach. Advance the needle until a characteristic sense of aortic wall penetration occurs and free-flowing blood is aspirated. Advance the needle through the anterior wall of the aorta until either no blood is aspirated or a 5-ml loss of resistance syringe filled with saline meets an increased resistance to injection, indicative of aortic wall penetration, followed by a loss of resistance as the needle enters the periaortic space. A test dose of local anesthetic with epinephrine can then be injected.

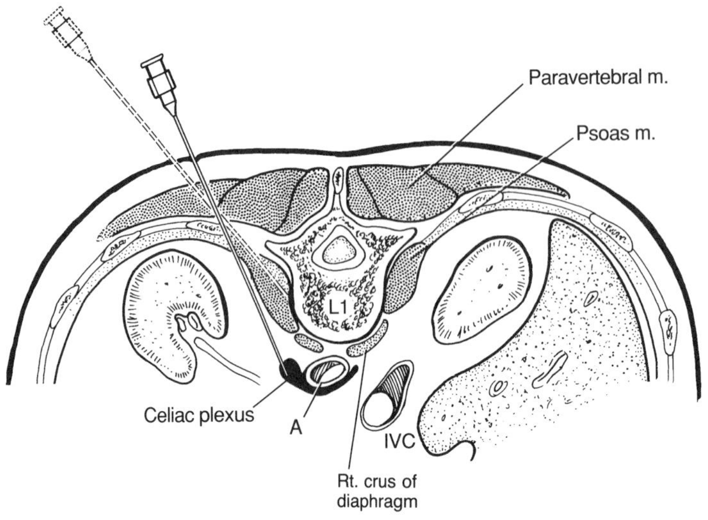

Figure 1 Placement of celiac plexus block. A = artery; IVC = inferior vena cava.

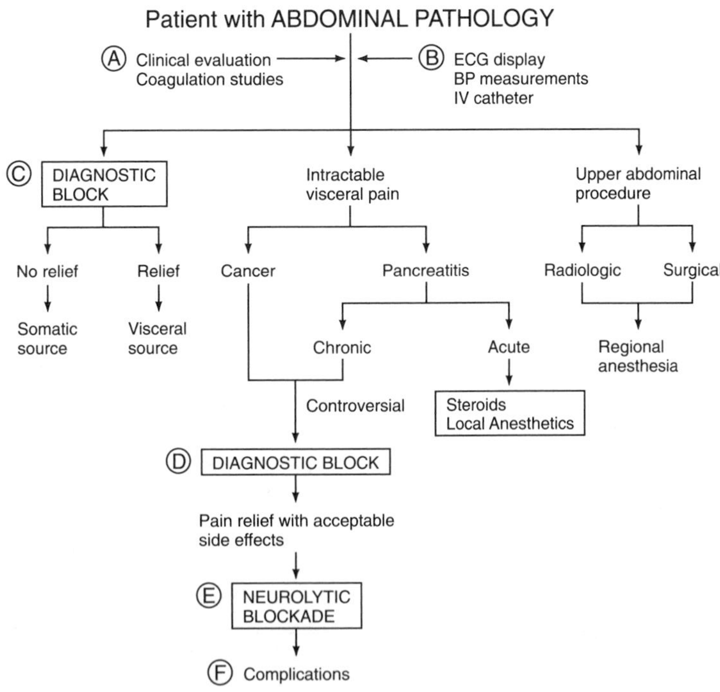

The splanchnic nerves can be blocked at the level of T12 in a similar fashion to the CPB. However, place the needle so that the tip is at the anterolateral border of the vertebral body. A smaller volume of local anesthetic is required, usually 3 to 5 ml. Complications are similar to those of the CPB, although postural hypotension may be less of a problem. The splanchnic nerve block usually does not result in a parasympathetic block of the abdomen. The risk of pneumothorax is higher than with a CPB.

D. Diagnostic blocks can be performed with 10 to 15 ml of lidocaine, 0.5 to 1% per side. Epinephrine (1:200,000) in the solution acts as a marker of intravascular injection; 10 to 15 ml of 0.25% bupivacaine or 0.1% tetracaine can be added to give longer pain relief.

E. Neurolytic blocks performed with 50 to 100% alcohol produce a deep visceral type pain initially, confirming needle placement. Addition of 20 to 25 ml of 1% lidocaine on each side attenuates this pain. Alcohol is not compatible with radiographic contrast media. Fifteen to 20 ml of 6% phenol may be added to contrast media, allowing fluoroscopic visualization during placement of the neurolytic agent. Neurolytic blocks are usually reserved for patients with intractable cancer pain, although there have been reports of successful management of chronic pancreatitis pain with CPB. The block may be performed at 2- to 6-month intervals if necessary.

F. Orthostatic hypotension related to sympathectomy usually disappears within 24 to 48 hours and is often ameliorated by preblock volume loading. Rarely, injury to other organs has resulted in pneumothorax, chylothorax, renal impairment, and paralysis due to injury to the artery of Adamkiewicz. Needle placement into the intervertebral disk and epidural and subarachnoid spaces, and unintentional transgression of the aorta and vena cava, have been reported. Incorrect placement of solution has resulted in paralysis, sexual dysfunction, and dysesthetic changes in the lower extremities secondary to spread of the solution to the lumbar plexus or centrally. For this reason, some clinicians prefer to perform neurolytic blocks only under radiographic guidance.

References

Bell SN, Cole R, Roberts-Thompson IC. Coeliac plexus block for control of pain in chronic pancreatitis. Br Med J 1980; 281:1604.

Brown DL, Moore DC. The use of neurolytic celiac plexus block for pancreatic cancer: Anatomy and technique. J Pain Symptom Management 1988; 3:206.

Cousins MJ, Bridenbaugh PO, eds. Neural blockade in clinical anesthesia and management of pain. 2nd ed. Philadelphia: JB Lippincott, 1988.

Feldstein GS, Waldman SD, Allen ML. Loss of resistance technique for transaortic celiac plexus block. Anesth Analg 1986; 65:1092.

Ischia S, Huzzani A, Ischia A, Faggian S. A new approach to the neurolytic block of the celiac plexus: The transaortic technique. Pain 1983; 16:333.

Kune GA, Cole R, Bell S. Observations on the relief of pancreatic pain. Med J Aust 1975; 2:789.

Moore PC. Regional block. A handbook for use in the clinical practice of medicine and surgery. 4th ed. Springfield, IL: Charles C Thomas, 1965:145.

Sprague R, Ramamurthy S. Celiac plexus block. In: Rogers MC, ed. Current practice in anesthesiology. 2nd ed. Philadelphia: BC Decker, 1992:442.

Stanton-Hicks M. Sympathetic blocks. In: Raj PP, ed. Practical management of pain. Chicago: Year Book Medical Publishers, 1986.

Verill P. Sympathetic ganglion lesions. In: Wall PD, Melzack R, eds. Textbook of pain. New York: Churchill Livingstone, 1989.

LUMBAR SYMPATHETIC BLOCK

Linda Tingle, M.D.

The lumbar sympathetic chain contains both preganglionic and postganglionic fibers that supply the pelvic viscera and vessels of the lower limbs as well as afferent sensory fibers. Nearly all the postganglionic fibers to the leg leave the sympathetic chain at or below L2. A small volume of local anesthetic deposited at the L2 level of the lumbar chain should block the sympathetic outflow to the lower extremity.

In cadaveric anatomic dissection, the ganglia are most frequently found at the level of the lower third of L2, at the L2-L3 interspace, and at the level of the upper third of L3 bilaterally. The needle tip is best placed at the lower third of L2 or upper third of L3 to avoid the lumbar arteries that cross the sympathetic chain at the middle third of the L2 and L3 vertebral body. The level of the disk should be avoided to avoid disk puncture.

The sympathetic chain is separated from the somatic roots by the psoas muscle and psoas fascia. The inferior vena cava lies anterior to the right sympathetic chain, and the aorta lies anterior and slightly medial to the left chain. The kidneys lie posterior from T11-L3 between two vertical lines 2.5 and 9.5 cm from the midline. The genitofemoral nerve arises from the first and second lumbar nerves and passes through the psoas to emerge near its medial border opposite L3 and L4.

A. Lumbar sympathetic block (LSB) may be used to diagnose and treat reflex sympathetic dystrophy of the lower extremities, circulatory insufficiency of the lower extremities, herpes zoster, postherpetic neuralgia of lumbar dermatomes, phantom limb pain, stump pain, and renal colic.

B. The classic approach (Mandel) has been simplified to a two-needle technique at L2 and L4. The patient is prone with arms off the side of the bed. The spinous processes of L1 and L4 are marked. L1 is level with the line between the two points where the lateral side of the erector spinae muscles meets the twelfth ribs; a line joining the posterosuperior iliac crests passes through the lower part of the spine at L4. Raise a subcutaneous wheal 8 to 10 cm lateral to the midpoint of the spinous processes of L2 and L4. Insert the needle lateral to the erector spinae muscles, with passage of the needle anterior to the muscle. This reduces patient discomfort and prevents needle movement with tensing of the muscle. Advance a 12-cm, 20-gauge needle with rubber marker until contact is made with the transverse process. The distance to the lateral side of the vertebral body is twice the distance from skin to transverse process. Reintroduce the needle and direct it slightly medial to pass between the two transverse processes, toward the lateral side of the vertebral body. Redirection of the needle allows it to slide off the vertebrae and reach the sympathetic chain. Place a second needle at L4, the depth being somewhat greater than at L2 owing to the lumbar lordosis at L4.

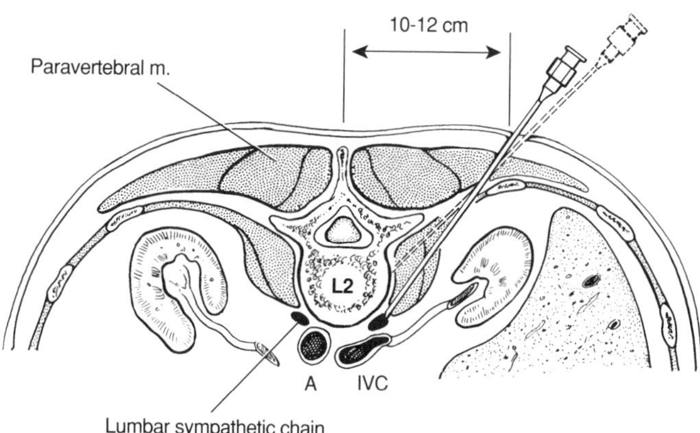

Figure 1 Placement of lumbar sympathetic block. A = artery; IVC = inferior vena cava.

C. The Reid technique is often preferred because it avoids the transverse process; is quicker, easier, and less painful to the patient; and gives virtual certainty of needle placement in the correct tissue plane. Positioning is the same. Locate the L2 and L4 spinous processes. Prepare the lumbar area and place the skin wheal 8 to 10 cm lateral to the superior part of the spinous process of the desired lumbar vertebrae. Advance a 12- to 15-cm, 20-gauge needle in an anteromedial direction approximately 45 degrees from the sagittal plane until the periosteum is contacted at a depth of 3 1/2 inches. Grasp the needle 2 cm from the skin and withdraw it until the tip is in the subcutaneous tissue; then redirect it more acutely, walking the needle off the anterolateral edge of the periosteum. Penetration of the psoas muscle should result in loss of resistance. Aspirate for blood or CSF, then inject 10 ml of 2% lidocaine. If no sensory or motor changes occur after 5 to 10 minutes and skin temperature is increasing, inject 10 ml of 0.5% bupivicaine. Attenuation of pain in the presence of increased temperature and absence of sensory block suggests, but does not guarantee, an autonomic cause. Continuous catheters are useful and may be placed at L2 and L4 with this technique. Radiographic guidance is an excellent tool in the proper placement of needles, particularly when small amounts of agent are used for a diagnostic or neurolytic block. Lateral and posteroanterior views confirm needletip position at the anterolateral edge of the vertical center of the vertebral body. Injection of contrast material into the psoas muscle produces characteristic longitudinal lines along the muscle bundles. Advancement of the needle produces tenting of the psoas muscle until the needle is advanced through the psoas fascia. This technique is a useful adjunct to correct needle placement. If a vessel has been entered by the needle, the contrast

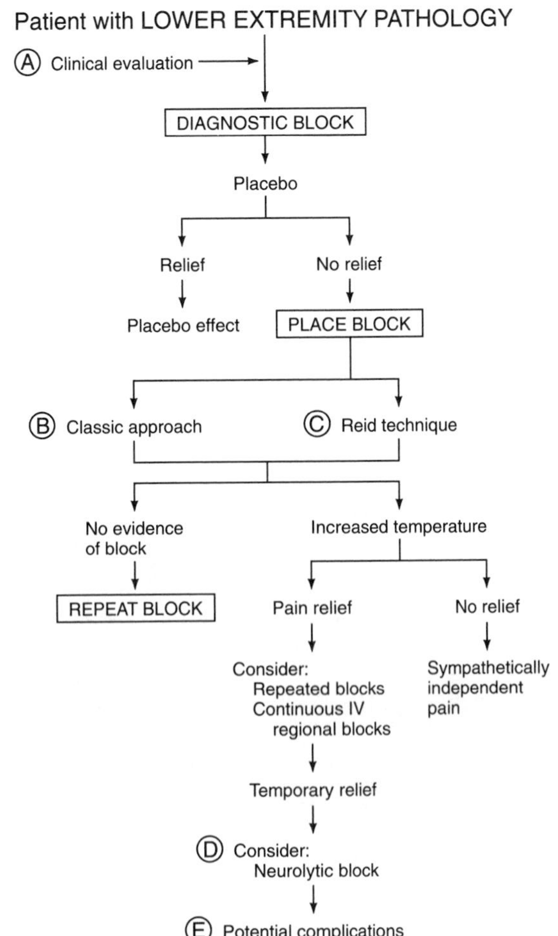

quickly vanishes as it is carried away. If the block is performed for therapeutic reasons with a relatively large volume of anesthetic, radiologic visualization is not necessary.

D. Neurolytic block may be considered in patients who respond favorably but temporarily to LSB with local anesthetics. Initially, an injection of 0.1 ml of contrast medium should reveal a sharp, almost vertical linear spread outlining the medial aspect of the psoas muscle. Inject a neurolytic agent such as phenol, mixed with a contrast agent, under fluoroscopic vision to confirm coverage of the sympathetic chain; as little as 2 to 4 ml of solution is adequate. Inject a small amount of saline (0.5 to 1 ml) before removal of the needle to prevent deposition of the neurolytic agent on somatic nerve roots during removal.

E. Complications include groin pain in L1-L2 distributions, which is thought to be secondary to genitofemoral neuralgia and may last 2 to 5 weeks. This may respond to transcutaneous electrical nerve stimulation. Other less common complications include subarachnoid puncture, lumbar somatic nerve block, perforation of the intervertebral disk, orthostatic hypotension, epidural spread of agent, bilateral block after attempted unilateral block, and renal trauma. Other complications noted after neurolytic block include difficulties with ejaculation after bilateral neurolytic block, and retroperitoneal hemorrhage associated with anticoagulation after neurolytic block.

References

Boas RA: Sympathetic blocks in clinical practice. Int Anesthesiol Clin 1978; 16:149.

Hatangdi VS, Boas RV. Lumbar sympathectomy: A single needle technique. Br J Anaesth 1985; 57:285.

Lofstrom JB, Cousins MJ. Sympathetic neural blockade of upper and lower extremity. In: Cousins MJ, Bridenbaugh PO, eds. Neural blockade in clinical anesthesia and management of pain. 2nd ed. Philadelphia: JB Lippincott, 1987.

Reid W, Watt JK, Gray TG. Phenol injection of the sympathetic chain. Br J Surg 1970; 57:45.

Sprague RS, Ramamurthy S. Identification of the anterior psoas sheath as a landmark for lumbar sympathetic block. Reg Anesth 1990; 15:253.

Stanton-Hicks M. Sympathetic blocks. In: Raj PP, ed. Practical management of pain. Chicago: Year Book Medical Publishers, 1988.

Umeda S, Arai T, Hantano Y, et al. Cadaver anatomic analysis of the best site for chemical lumbar sympathectomy. Anesth Analg 1987; 66:643.

Verrill P. Sympathetic ganglion lesions. In: Wall PD, Melzack R, eds. Textbook of pain. New York: Churchill Livingstone, 1989.

INTERPLEURAL ANALGESIA

Eric B. Lefever, M.D.

Interpleural analgesia is a relatively new technique for pain relief, first described by Reiestad in 1984. The technique provides unilateral blockade of multiple intercostal nerves by placement of local anesthetic solution into the potential space between the parietal and visceral pleura. The advantages of this technique include a single needle puncture for insertion, the ability to administer multiple doses of local anesthetic, and a low incidence of complications.

A. The technique is well suited to both acute and chronic pain control involving thoracic and upper abdominal regions. It has been used effectively after thoracotomy, cholecystectomy, unilateral breast surgery, and renal surgery. In this setting, it may significantly decrease the incidence of pulmonary complications. It has also been employed to relieve the pain of multiple rib fractures. Chronic pain states resulting from postherpetic neuralgia involving thoracic dermatomes, reflex sympathetic dystrophy of an upper extremity, and pancreatic carcinoma have been treated with good results.

B. Contraindications to the interpleural technique include lack of patient cooperation or consent, disorders of coagulation, localized infection or tumor at the insertion site, and sepsis. Pleural fibrosis or focal pleural thickening at the insertion site on recent chest radiography are relative contraindications, because it may be difficult to identify the interpleural space. Fluid within the interpleural space, from either hemothorax or pleural effusion, may dilute the local anesthetic to ineffective levels. Inflammatory processes involving the pleura may contribute to local anesthetic toxicity by speeding absorption from the pleural space.

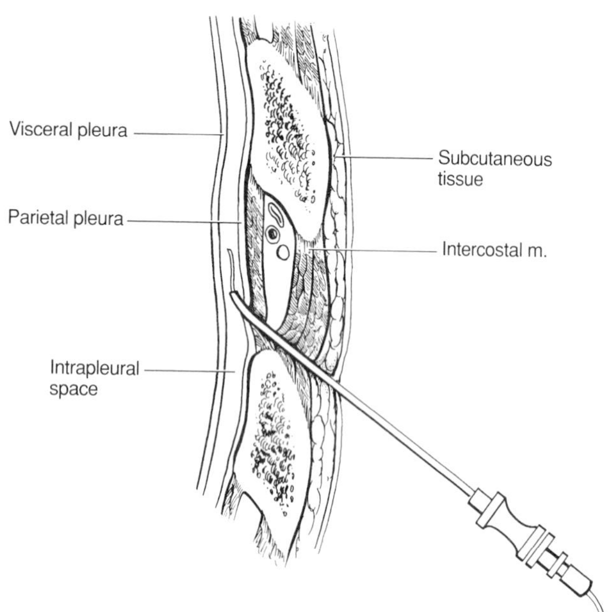

Figure 1 Administration of interpleural analgesia.

C. The interpleural catheter may be placed during spontaneous or controlled ventilation, although the latter may be associated with a higher incidence of complications. Place the patient laterally on the unaffected side and give appropriate sedation, skin preparation, and subcutaneous infiltration with local anesthetic. Insert a thin-walled Tuohy needle over the superior aspect of the fifth to eighth ribs, approximately 8 to 10 cm from the spine. Attach a well-lubricated glass syringe filled with air, and advance the needle in a medial direction at an angle of 30 to 40° to the skin. The interpleural space is identified by loss of resistance as the plunger of the syringe spontaneously drops because of the negative pressure in the pleural space. Remove the syringe from the needle, introduce a catheter 5 to 6 cm into the pleural space, and secure it with a sterile dressing.

D. Inject the interpleural catheter with local anesthetic after careful aspiration to prevent placement of the catheter into a blood vessel or the lung parenchyma. For intermittent dosing schedules, 20 to 30 ml of 0.25% bupivacaine with epinephrine (1:200,000) has been used. Continuous infusion techniques are also possible. Post-thoracotomy pain control may require clamping of the chest tubes for 15 minutes immediately after dosing the catheter.

E. There may be adverse effects related to systemic local anesthetic toxicity from direct intravascular injection, enhanced absorption in the setting of pleural inflammation, or inadvertent injection of a catheter into the vascular lung parenchyma. Pneumothorax is an obvious but uncommon complication. Air entrainment into the interpleural space should be prevented by occluding the needle as much as possible during catheter placement. In addition, spontaneous respiration with the patient instructed to exhale as the needle is advanced, or temporary holding of respirations if ventilation is controlled, may further decrease the incidence of pneumothorax. Unilateral phrenic nerve blockade and Horner's syndrome have been described but usually resolve without intervention.

References

Durrani Z, Winnie AP, Ikuta P. Interpleural catheter analgesia for pancreatic pain. Anesth Analg 1988; 67:479.

Reiestad F, Kvaleim L, McIlvaine WB, et al. Interpleural analgesia in the treatment of severe thoracic post-herpetic neuralgia. Reg Anesth 1990; 15:113.

Reiestad F, McIllvaine WB, Kvalheim L, et al. Interpleural

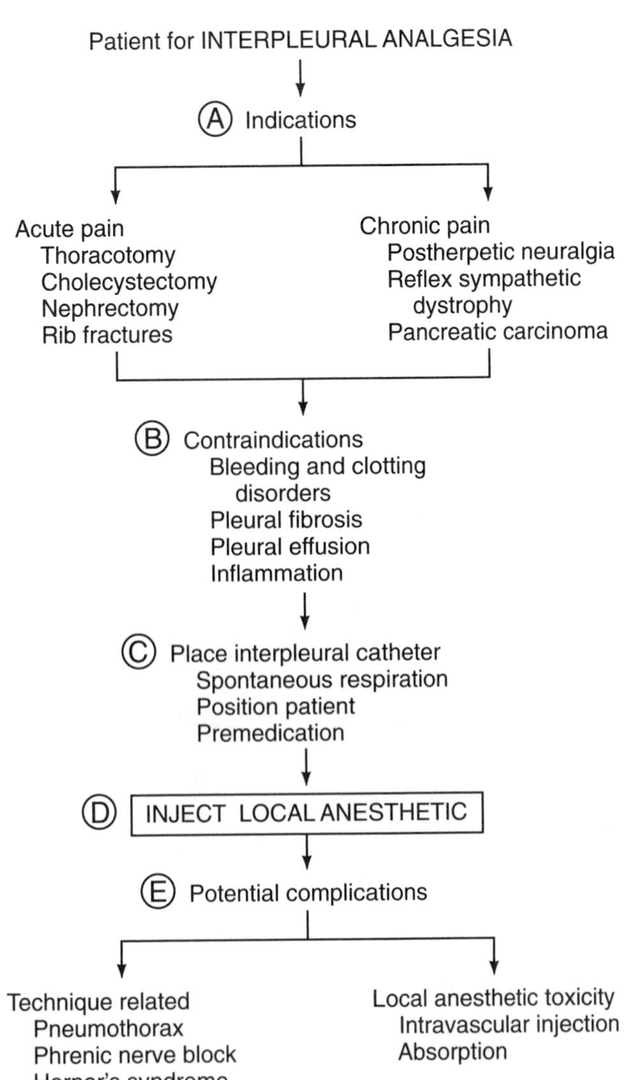

analgesia in treatment of upper extremity reflex sympathetic dystrophy. Anesth Analg 1989; 69:671.

Reiestad, F, Stromskag KE. Interpleural catheter in the management of postoperative pain. Reg Anesth 1986; 11:89.

Rocco A, Reiestad F, Gudman J, McKay W. Intrapleural administration of local anesthetics for pain relief in patients with multiple rib fractures. Reg Anesth 1987; 12:10.

INTERCOSTAL NERVE BLOCK

Jay S. Ellis, Jr., M.D.

Intercostal nerve blocks are a simple and effective method of providing analgesia for painful disorders of the chest and abdominal wall. Despite the benefits and simplicity of this technique, it is an underused method of pain control, for two reasons. First, practitioners have an exaggerated opinion of the risk associated with these blocks. Pneumothorax, the most feared complication, occurs in <1% of all patients. In addition, most pneumothoraces associated with intercostal nerve block are easily treated by aspiration of air, administration of supplemental oxygen, and close observation of the patient. Only those pneumothoraces that are symptomatic, resulting in severe dyspnea, and those under tension require tube thoracostomy and drainage. An additional, but less worrisome risk is local anesthetic (LA) toxicity. Blood levels of LA are higher after intercostal nerve block than after epidural, spinal, and other peripheral nerve blocks. However, toxicity is easily avoided by limiting the total dose of LA to a known, safe level and guarding against inadvertent IV administration by (1) aspirating for blood before injecting and removing the needle if blood is aspirated and (2) injecting the LA solution in increments ≦5 ml. Incremental injection protects the patient from serious toxic reactions if the LA is injected IV despite a negative aspiration for blood (a frustrating but well-described occurrence). The second reason for underuse of intercostal nerve blocks is that repeated injections of intercostal nerves are considered too labor intensive to be of value. True, even intercostal nerve blocks with 0.5% bupivacaine and epinephrine seldom last >12 hours. However, the analgesia associated with these blocks is usually superior to that achieved with parenteral narcotics, especially when used for rib fractures, subcostal incisional pain, or other unilateral chest and abdominal wall pain. In addition, intercostal nerve blocks are not associated with the sedation, nausea, and vomiting so common with narcotic administration. This makes them worth the extra effort, especially in high-risk patients.

There are also methods for reducing the work associated with repeat injections. A catheter can be placed in the intercostal space for repeat injections. There is some evidence that a single, large injection through an intercostal catheter spreads along the subpleural space to cover several intercostal nerves. It is also possible to place a catheter in the interpleural space, inject 20 ml of 0.5% bupivacaine, and obtain good analgesia over a large segment on one side of the chest and abdominal wall. If catheter techniques are impractical or ineffective, epidural analgesia with LA and/or epidural narcotics is a good alternative for pain control.

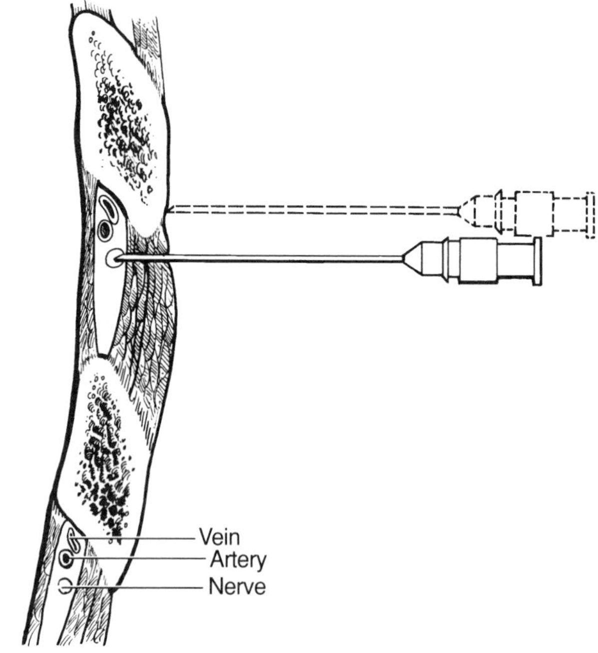

Figure 1 Placement of intercostal nerve block.

A. Select a patient with chest wall or abdominal pain. There should be no evidence of a coagulopathy or of a history of allergy to the class of LA to be used.

B. Place the patient in the prone position; the lateral position can be used if he or she cannot lie prone. In this case the injection point will lie along the midaxillary line. Injection at the midaxillary line may miss the lateral cutaneous branch of the intercostal nerve, but a volume of 5 ml usually ensures enough proximal spread of LA so that the lateral cutaneous branch is anesthetized before it leaves the intercostal groove.

C. Mark each of the ribs to be injected at the angle of the rib or along the midaxillary line, as appropriate. If the ribs are not easily palpable, alternative techniques (paravertebral somatic nerve block, epidural analgesia) may be necessary.

D. Prepare the injection sites with an appropriate antimicrobial solution. Place the index finger of your hand in the intercostal space and slide the skin up over the rib; this makes it easier to walk the needle off the rib later.

E. For the injection, use a 5-ml syringe filled with LA attached to a 22-gauge needle. Puncture the skin directly over the rib (this is the skin you previously slid up from the intercostal space). The long axis of the needle and syringe should have a slight cephalad tilt.

F. After contacting the rib, walk the needle off the inferior edge of the rib by withdrawing the needle into the subcutaneous tissue and allowing the skin to move back toward its usual position in the intercostal space. Do not walk off the rib by rotating the long axis of the syringe. Rotating the syringe will result in the needle pointing caudad, away from the intercostal groove and the nerve.

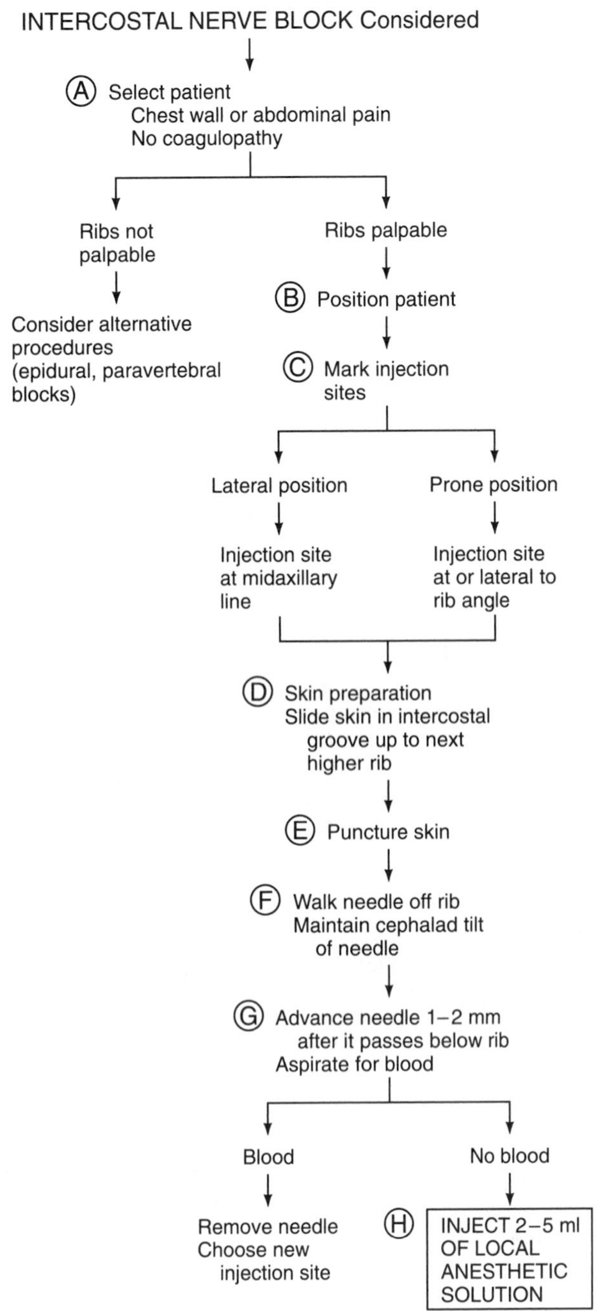

G. As the needle slips off the rib, advance the needle tip 1 to 2 mm. Take the hand used to palpate the rib and grab the needle at the hub. Use the hand on the syringe to aspirate for blood. After negative aspiration, inject 2 to 5 ml of LA. Some practitioners use a slight jiggling motion on the needle to improve spread of the LA and minimize the risk of intravascular injection.

H. Before repeating the injection at the next rib, it is best to use a new needle. Repeated contact with the rib can cause the needletip to bend into a barbed shape. If analgesia is incomplete, additional intercostal nerves may be blocked, or nerves blocked incompletely may require repeat injections. Of course, the total dose of LA must be within recognized safe levels.

References

Moore DC. Intercostal nerve block for postoperative somatic pain following surgery of thorax and upper abdomen. Br J Anaesth 1975; 47:284.

Murphy DF. Continuous intercostal nerve blockade: An anatomical study to elucidate its mode of action. Br J Anaesth 1984; 56:627.

Rauck RL. Techniques for postoperative pain control in 1990. Annual Refresher Course Lectures. Park Ridge, IL: American Society of Anesthesiologists, 1990.

Tucker GT, Moore DC, Bridenbaugh PO, et al. Systemic absorption of mepivacaine in commonly used regional block procedures. Anesthesiology 1972; 37:277.

SOMATIC PARAVERTEBRAL NERVE ROOT BLOCK

Jay S. Ellis, Jr., M.D.

Somatic paravertebral nerve blocks have a useful role in management of painful disorders involving the nerve roots. They are analogous to intercostal nerve blocks because they provide anesthesia in a dermatomal distribution. The more common indications for these blocks are patients needing intercostal blocks who do not have palpable ribs owing to obesity. Also, painful disorders of the groin or lower extremity that are in the distribution of one or more paravertebral nerve roots often respond to paravertebral nerve blocks. Any disorder that responds to intercostal nerve blocks can also be managed with paravertebral nerve blocks.

Complications usually occur from injection of local anesthetic into areas adjacent to the paravertebral space such as the epidural or subarachnoid space. Even if the needletip is outside the spinal canal, local anesthetic may spread along the dural cuff of a nerve root, with a resultant epidural or subarachnoid block. It is important to give a small dose of local anesthetic, no more than 2 to 3 ml, as a test dose. If there are no signs or symptoms of subarachnoid injection after 5 minutes, it is safe to inject the remaining volume of local anesthetic. In the thoracic region it is possible to puncture the parietal pleura and cause a pneumothorax. In the lumbar region it is conceivable that needles may puncture retroperitoneal organs such as the kidney or even the abdominal organs if the practitioner does not pay attention to anatomic detail.

The technique of paravertebral somatic nerve block is similar to that of intercostal nerve block. The transverse process of the vertebral body serves as the depth marker for the nerve roots. Precise location of the transverse process requires a sound knowledge of the relationship between the spinous processes of the vertebra and the corresponding transverse process. In the lumbar region a line drawn along the inferior edges of the right and left transverse process will intersect the spinous process of the same vertebra at its most cephalad point. In the thoracic region the spinous processes extend caudally as far as two vertebral levels, especially in the midthoracic region.

We will discuss the technique for lumbar nerve block and then describe the differences in the thoracic region.

A. Place the patient in the prone position.

B. Draw a line perpendicular to the axis of the spine, through the top of the spinous process.

C. Measure along the line 3 to 5 cm laterally from the spinous process and raise a skin wheal with local anesthetic at this spot. This point lies over the transverse process.

D. Using a 22-g, 10-cm needle, advance the needle through the point over the transverse process, keeping the needle perpendicular to the skin. The needle should contact the transverse process at a depth of 3 to 5 cm. Once the transverse process is found, note the depth of the needle.

E. Withdraw the needle, then redirect the needle to pass below the transverse process.

F. Aspirate for blood or CSF. If no fluid is present, inject 5 to 10 ml of local anesthetic. This volume will anesthetize the nerve root and possibly the next higher nerve root as it passes laterally. In the thoracic region it is more difficult to localize the transverse process accurately. The spinous processes slope more caudally, so it is best to consult an anatomic model before attempting the block. This ensures that the operator has a clear idea of the relationship between the spinous and transverse processes. If there is uncertainty about the depth of the thoracic transverse process, use the following alternative approach: Move 1 cm off the midline and advance the needle until it contacts the lamina of the thoracic vertebra. Again, note the depth of the needle. Withdraw the needle and walk off the lamina until the needle is 1 to 2 cm deeper than the last point at which it contacted the lamina. An injection of 10 ml of local anesthetic in this area usually anesthetizes the paravertebral nerve. It is essential to perform careful aspiration before injecting local anesthetic. Again, give a 2-ml test dose of local anesthetic and observe for signs of subarachnoid injection before injecting the full dose.

References

Bridenbaugh PO. Complications of local anesthetic neural blockade. In: Cousins MJ, Bridenbaugh PO, eds. Neural blockade in clinical anesthesia and management of pain. 2nd ed. Philadelphia: JB Lippincott, 1988:695.

Moore D. Regional block. 4th ed. Springfield, IL: Charles C Thomas, 1965.

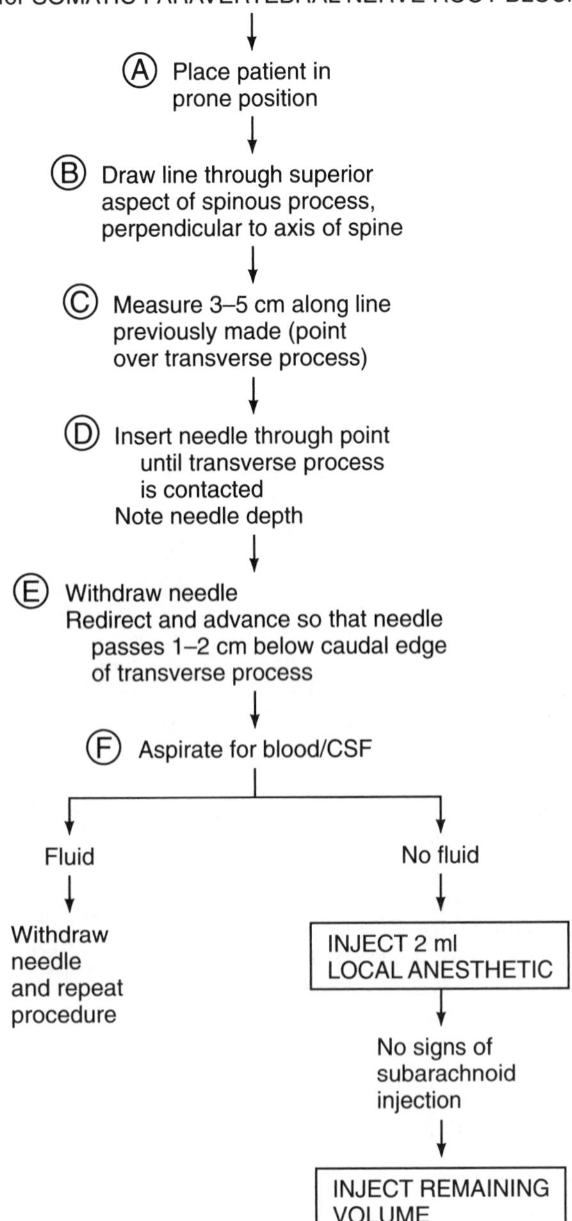
Patient for SOMATIC PARAVERTEBRAL NERVE ROOT BLOCK
(A) Place patient in prone position
(B) Draw line through superior aspect of spinous process, perpendicular to axis of spine
(C) Measure 3–5 cm along line previously made (point over transverse process)
(D) Insert needle through point until transverse process is contacted
Note needle depth
(E) Withdraw needle
Redirect and advance so that needle passes 1–2 cm below caudal edge of transverse process
(F) Aspirate for blood/CSF
Fluid
Withdraw needle and repeat procedure
No fluid
INJECT 2 ml LOCAL ANESTHETIC
No signs of subarachnoid injection
INJECT REMAINING VOLUME

TRIGEMINAL GANGLION BLOCKADE

David Vanos, M.D.

The trigeminal (or gasserian) ganglion gives rise to three major nerves or divisions, the ophthalmic (V1), maxillary (V2), and mandibular (V3), which provide the cutaneous sensation for the anterior half of the scalp, all of the face, the conjunctiva, the cornea, the iris, and the ciliary body. Other structures supplied are the lacrimal gland, deeper eye structures, skull, teeth, mandible, maxilla, tongue, muscles of mastication, falx cerebri, and tentorium cerebelli. Blockade of this ganglion has been useful for chronic pain conditions in the distributions noted above, when other pain management approaches have failed or proved impracticable (e.g., chronic cancer pain and trigeminal neuralgia). Currently, both diagnostic blocks with local anesthetic and therapeutic blocks with local and/or neurolytic agents are used.

The ganglion itself lies just inside the foramen ovale at the top of the petrous temporal bone at approximately the juncture between the middle and posterior cranial fossa. Its posterior two-thirds is enveloped by a fold of the dura matter called Meckel's cave, or cavum trigeminale. The medial boundary of the ganglion is the cavernous sinus where the carotid artery and the third, fourth, and sixth cranial nerves pass. Superior to the ganglion is the brain's inferior surface, the temporal lobe, and posteriorly is the brain stem.

A. Hartel's approach is the most popular. Introduce a 22-gauge, 8- to 10-cm needle under fluoroscopic guidance 1 cm lateral and posterior to the lateral corner of the mouth, and direct it cephalad and posteriorly to contact the inferior periosteum of the infratemporal fossa. Take care not to enter the oral cavity upon introduction of the needle, to avoid contamination of intracranial structures. A gloved finger introduced into the oral cavity can direct the needle appropriately. The anteroposterior plane of angulation should be parallel to that formed by the ipsilateral pupil and the skin insertion site. The lateral positioning should be such that the needletip transects the midpoint of the zygomatic arch. The needle can then be angled somewhat more posteriorly to enter the foramen ovale, noted usually by a mandibular nerve paresthesia. Advance the needle no more than 1 cm further; proper placement near the ganglion is confirmed by a first- or second-division paresthesia. Aspiration before injection of any substance is, of course, mandatory to avoid IV or subarachnoid spread. Mild sedation or analgesia with IV benzodiazepines and narcotics may be appropriate for this uncomfortable procedure. Nerve stimulators can help locate the sought-for structures when a paresthesia cannot be elicited.

B. Perform local anesthetic block first to assess the quality of pain relief with the block and to allow the patient to determine whether the resultant facial numbness is tolerable. Local anesthetics such as 1% lidocaine in small volumes, e.g., 0.25 mg at a time, can be used until analgesia occurs. If pain relief has been significant and the patient tolerates the side effects, a neurolytic block may be considered.

C. Neurolytics such as absolute alcohol, phenol, and glycerol have been used, but glycerol has the advantage of causing less interference with facial skin sensation. Alcohol blocks have such significant associated morbidity and mortality as almost to contraindicate their use, in view of the other agents available. Stender reported a 0.9% fatality rate with alcohol block of the trigeminal ganglion. Glycerol, 0.2 to 0.4 ml, has proved more efficacious. A total of 86% of patients were reported pain free initially, with a lower incidence of side effects than those from alcohol. Follow-up revealed a 31% recurrence rate over 1 to 6 years after use of glycerol.

D. Potential complications include hemorrhage, temporary or permanent cranial nerve dysfunction, Horner's syndrome, corneal ulcer, keratitis (secondary to corneal denervation and lack of tear formation), blindness, trophic disturbances (e.g., skin ulceration), anesthesia dolorosa, herpes simplex, delayed facial paralysis, dysphagia (ninth cranial nerve dysfunction), and osteomyelitis of the mandible.

E. Other methods of achieving neurolysis that have proved effective alternatives to chemical neurolysis include balloon compression and thermogangliolysis. Surgical rhizotomy is also very effective.

References

Hakanson S. Trigeminal neuralgia treated by the injection of glycerol into the trigeminal cistern. Neurosurgery 1981; 9:638.

Henderson WR. Trigeminal neuralgia: The pain and its treatment. Br Med J 1967; 1:7.

Loeser JD. Tic douloureux and atypical facial pain. In: Wall PD, Melzack R, eds. Textbook of pain. London, 1986, Churchill Livingstone, p 426.

Murphy TM. Somatic blockade of the head and neck. In: Cousins MJ, Bridenbaugh PO, eds. Neural blockade in clinical anesthesia and management of pain. Philadelphia: JB Lippincott, 1988:536, 541, 726, 1066.

Sweet WH, Wepsic JG. Controlled thermocoagulation of the trigeminal ganglion and rootlets for a differential destruction of pain fibers. I. Trigeminal neuralgia. J Neurosurg 1974; 39:143.

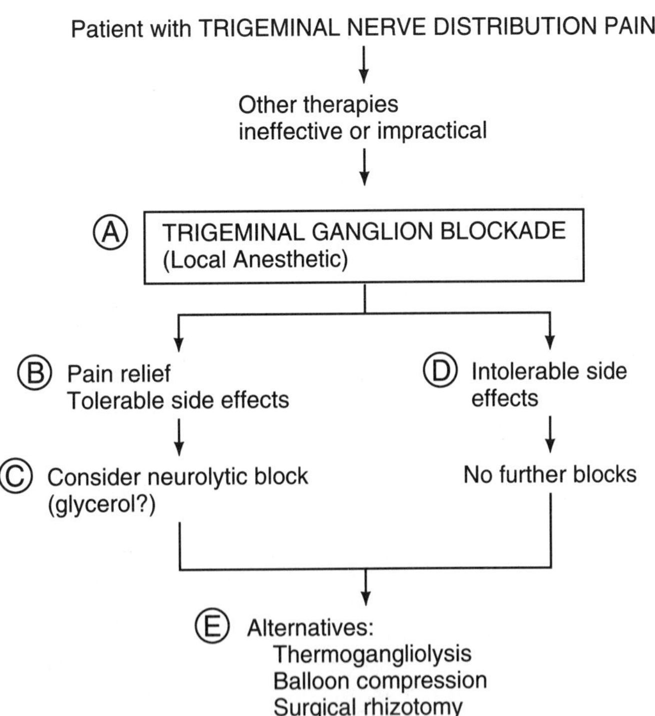
Patient with TRIGEMINAL NERVE DISTRIBUTION PAIN
Other therapies
ineffective or impractical
Ⓐ TRIGEMINAL GANGLION BLOCKADE
(Local Anesthetic)
Ⓑ Pain relief
Tolerable side effects
Ⓒ Consider neurolytic block
(glycerol?)
Ⓓ Intolerable side
effects
No further blocks
Ⓔ Alternatives:
Thermogangliolysis
Balloon compression
Surgical rhizotomy

SPHENOPALATINE GANGLION BLOCK

Jeffery T. Summers, M.D.
Emil J. Menk, M.D.

Anesthetization of the sphenopalatine ganglia (SPG) for the successful treatment of a painful condition was first described by Sluder in 1903, when he anesthetized the SPG for the treatment of a headache. Since then SPG block has been used to treat headaches, eye pain, sinus pain, mouth pain, earache, abdominal pain, asthma, angina pectoris, low back pain, diarrhea, trigger points, and numerous other conditions. Although many of these applications were described decades ago in case reports and "personal series," numerous successes reported by respected clinicians suggest the use of SPG blocks in cases of refractory pain.

The neural connections of the SPG are extensive and probably affect many areas of the CNS. The SPG themselves are composed of three types of nerve fibers: sensory, sympathetic, and motor. The sensory fibers provide connections with the trigeminal nerve via its maxillary branch. The sympathetic fibers link with the facial nerve (to the posterior scalp, neck, and external ear), the internal carotid artery plexus, and the superior cervical sympathetic ganglion via the great deep petrosal nerve. The motor fibers have parasympathetic (visceral motor) connections. The SPG also connects directly to the ventral horn of the spinal cord, and to the neurohumoral axis via a connection to the anterior lobe of the pituitary gland. These multiple and varied nerve connections could account for many of the otherwise seemingly unrelated reported "uses" of SPG block.

A. Conduct a full diagnostic work-up for the condition encountered and anatomic area involved.

B. Other painful conditions in this anatomic area have reportedly been successfully treated by SPG block, but are beyond the scope of this chapter. Many of these other uses have been described in case reports involving only one or two patients. For a description of these additional uses of SPG block, see the article by Byrd and Byrd.

C. Conservative treatment should include the usual and customary treatment for the given condition suspected. SPG block is typically used to treat the pain associated with a given condition and is usually not the cause of the pain itself. You may choose to consider SPG blocks for pain control while appropriate measures to treat the source of the condition are being initiated, however. Be sure to consider endpoints other than the elimination of pain for successful treatment of the condition; otherwise, pain control secondary to nerve blocks might be misinterpreted as resolution of the condition.

D. The SPG are located in the lateral walls of the pterygopalatine fossa, which makes them accessible to anesthetization via a topical "nasal" route. This approach is generally preferred because of its technical ease and relative lack of significant side effects. To perform, advance a cotton-tipped applicator soaked with local anesthetic through the nares and direct it along the inferior turbinate downward and posteriorly until the posterior wall of the nasopharynx is encountered. This procedure can then be repeated on the opposite side. An effective block can usually be produced if the applicators are left in place for about 10 minutes, and the procedure repeated. If the condition is acute, one to two blocks should provide noticeable improvement. If the condition is chronic, daily blocks (1 to 2 per day) for up to 2 to 3 weeks may be necessary to determine a response. Ganglion neurolysis can be considered if the SPG blocks provide consistent but only temporary relief.

E. Reported side effects include twitching of the nasal alae, lacrimation, sneezing, and mild intranasal discomfort—usually described as a deep "pressure" sensation. More significant side effects related to trauma of the intranasal structures can be avoided by not forcing the applicators when there is substantial resistance to their advancement.

References

Amster JL. Sphenopalatine ganglion block for relief of painful vascular and muscular spasm with special reference to lumbosacral pain. NY State J Med 1948; 48:2475.

Berger JJ, Pyles ST, Saga-Rumley SA. Does topical anesthesia of the sphenopalatine ganglion with cocaine or lidocaine relieve low back pain? Anesth Analg 1986; 65:700.

Byrd H, Byrd W. Sphenopalatine phenomena: present status of knowledge. Arch Intern Med 1930; 46:1026.

Murphy TM. Somatic blockade of head and neck. In: Cousins MJ, Bridenbaugh PO, eds. Neural blockade in clinical anesthesia and management of pain. 2nd ed. Philadelphia: JB Lippincott, 1988:543.

Reder M. Sphenopalatine ganglion block in treatment of acute and chronic pain. In: Hendler NH, Long DM, Wise TN, eds. Diagnosis and treatment of chronic pain. Boston: John Wright, 1982:104.

Ruskin AP. Sphenopalatine (nasal) remote effects including "psychosomatic" symptoms, rage reaction, pain and spasm. Arch Phys Med Rehabil. 1979; 60:353.

Ruskin SL. Herpes zoster oticus relieved by sphenopalatine ganglion treatment. Laryngoscope 1925; 35:301.

Ruskin SL. Neurologic aspects of nasal sinus infections, headaches and systemic disturbances of nasal ganglion origin. Arch Otolaryngol 1929; 10:337.

Sluder G. Nasal neurology, headaches and eye disorders. St Louis: CV Mosby, 1927.

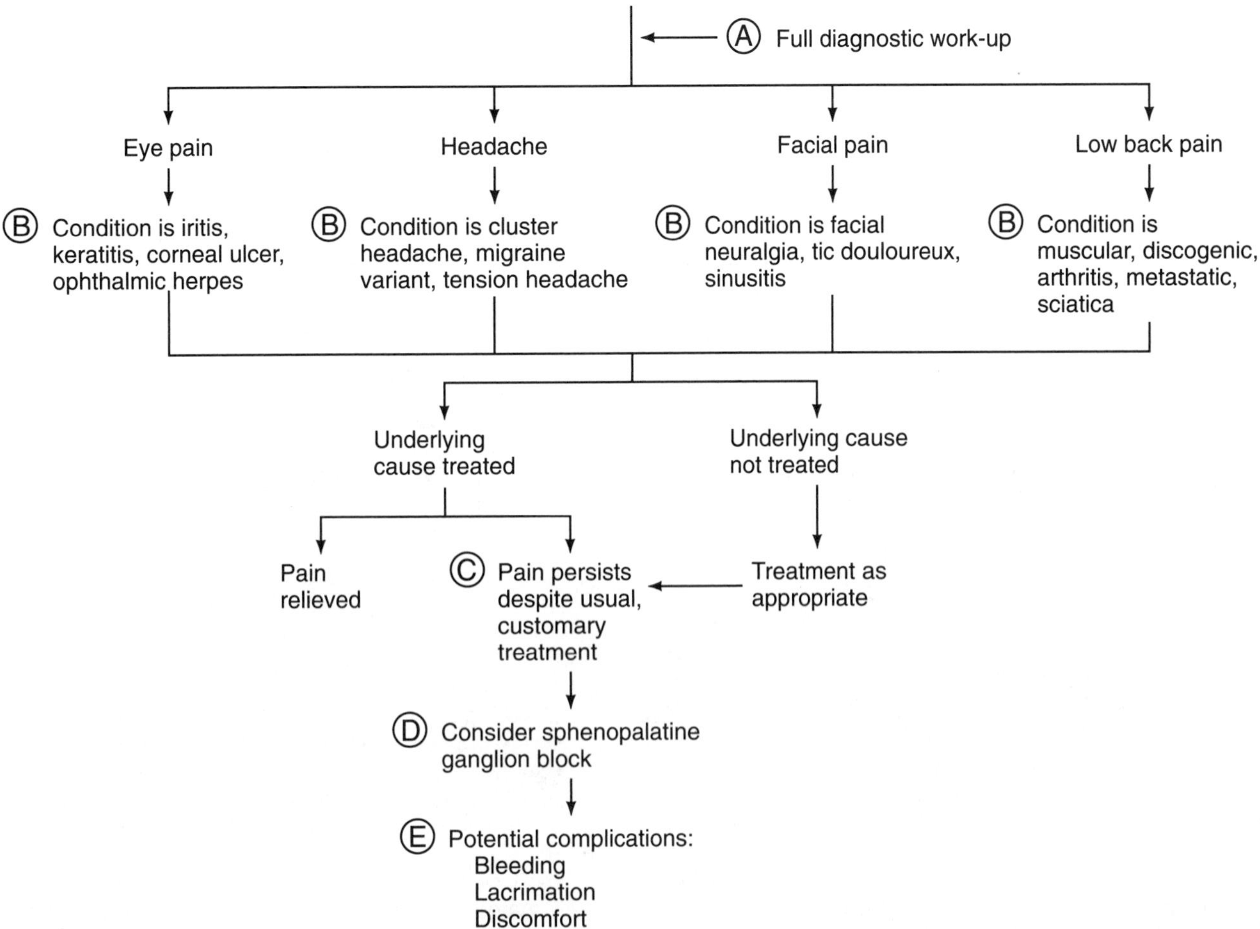
Patient considered for SPHENOPALATINE GANGLION BLOCK
(A) Full diagnostic work-up
Eye pain
Headache
Facial pain
Low back pain
(B) Condition is iritis, keratitis, corneal ulcer, ophthalmic herpes
(B) Condition is cluster headache, migraine variant, tension headache
(B) Condition is facial neuralgia, tic douloureux, sinusitis
(B) Condition is muscular, discogenic, arthritis, metastatic, sciatica
Underlying cause treated
Underlying cause not treated
Pain relieved
(C) Pain persists despite usual, customary treatment
Treatment as appropriate
(D) Consider sphenopalatine ganglion block
(E) Potential complications:
Bleeding
Lacrimation
Discomfort

BRACHIAL PLEXUS BLOCK

Rosemary Hickey, M.D.

Anesthesia for upper extremity and shoulder procedures can be provided by various brachial plexus block techniques. Advantages include less disturbance of general body physiology, prevention of reflex responses to pain (blocks afferent impulse transmission from the site of CNS surgery), less risk for pulmonary aspiration, and the ability to provide postoperative analgesia.

A. Contraindications include bleeding and clotting abnormalities, infection or tumor at the block site, and patient refusal. Pre-existing neurologic deficits in the extremity to be blocked dissuade some anesthesiologists from using regional anesthesia because of medicolegal concerns. However, brachial plexus blocks can be done in these patients if the deficits are carefully documented preoperatively.

B. Premedicate the patient to allay anxiety, raise the seizure threshold, and reduce pain that may occur with needle placement. Do not oversedate the patient so that cooperation is not possible or CNS signs of local anesthetic toxicity could be missed.

C. Choose the type of brachial plexus block based on the area of the upper extremity or shoulder to be blocked as well as your expertise with that particular technique. Interscalene block (ISB) is best for shoulder and proximal upper extremity procedures, but it may not block the C8 and T1 distribution (ulnar, medial brachial, and antebrachial cutaneous nerves). Subclavian perivascular block (SPB) and supraclavicular block (SCB) are the most effective for procedures involving the mid portion of the upper extremity, and axillary block (AB) is the most effective for surgery on the distal forearm, hand, and wrist.

D. To perform an ISB, place the patient in the supine position with the head turned opposite to the side being injected. Identify the lateral margin of the clavicular head of the sternocleidomastoid muscle at the level of C6 (determined by noting the level of the cricoid cartilage). Roll the index and middle finger of the palpating hand laterally across the anterior scalene muscle until the interscalene groove, between the anterior and middle scalene muscles, is palpated. Insert a 22-gauge 4 cm regional block needle (short bevel) in a direction perpendicular to the skin in all planes with a slight caudad direction to avoid vertebral artery, epidural, or subarachnoid injection.

E. For an SPB, position the patient and identify the interscalene groove at the level of C6, as described for ISB. Follow the interscalene groove as far inferiorly (toward the clavicle) as it can be easily palpated. Insert a 22-gauge regional block needle in the groove in a caudad direction. If you reach the subclavian artery, reinsert the needle in a more dorsal plane.

F. To perform SCB, position the patient as for an ISB or SPB. Introduce a 22-gauge regional block needle through the skin 0.5 cm above the midpoint of the clavicle and advance the needle until the first rib is encountered. Walk the needle along the first rib from the lateral border of the anterior scalene muscle to the anterior border of the middle scalene muscle.

G. For an AB, place the patient in the supine position with the arm abducted 90° and the forearm flexed 90°. Identify the axillary artery pulse and follow the pulse as far proximally as possible, ideally to the point where the pulse disappears under the pectoralis major muscle. Keeping the index finger of the palpating hand on the pulse, advance a 22-gauge regional block needle toward the apex of the axilla, approaching the neurovascular bundle at a 10° to 20° angle.

H. To confirm correct needle placement before injecting the local anesthetic, various endpoints may be chosen. For an ISB, elicit a paresthesia below the level of the shoulder. Alternatively, obtain muscle contractions of the arm or hand with a nerve stimulator, attaching the ground electrode to an ECG pad placed on the opposite shoulder and the other electrode to the regional block needle. When performing an SPB, use paresthesias to the hand or arm or muscle contractions elicited with a nerve stimulator to identify correct needle placement. For an SCB, attempt to elicit paresthesias in four to five different locations on the arm and inject local anesthetic with each paresthesia. When an AB is performed, locate the final needle position by (1) identifying the fascial click, indicating penetration of the brachial plexus sheath; (2) eliciting a paresthesia; (3) using a nerve stimulator to obtain muscle contractions of the arm or hand; or (4) injecting transarterially by advancing the needle through the posterior wall of the axillary artery. Inject a total of 30 ml of local anesthetic for an ISB or SPB, 40 ml for an SCB, and 40 to 50 ml for an AB. Keep total dosage below the maximum recommended safe limits and adjust dosages for children. With each of the techniques, obtain anesthesia for tourniquet placement (T2 block) by injecting local anesthetic (3 to 5 ml) subcutaneously over the axillary artery pulse.

I. When brachial plexus blocks are performed above the clavicle, phrenic nerve block, pneumothorax, Horner's syndrome, and recurrent laryngeal nerve block may result. With an ISB, advancement into the vertebral artery, epidural, or subarachnoid space may occur if a slightly caudad needle direction is not maintained. Avoid intravascular injection by carefully aspirating before making a local anesthetic injection.

References

Ramamurthy S. Anesthesia. In: Green DP, ed. Operative hand surgery. New York: Churchill Livingstone, 1982.

Winnie AP. Plexus anesthesia. Vol 1. Philadelphia: WB Saunders, 1990.

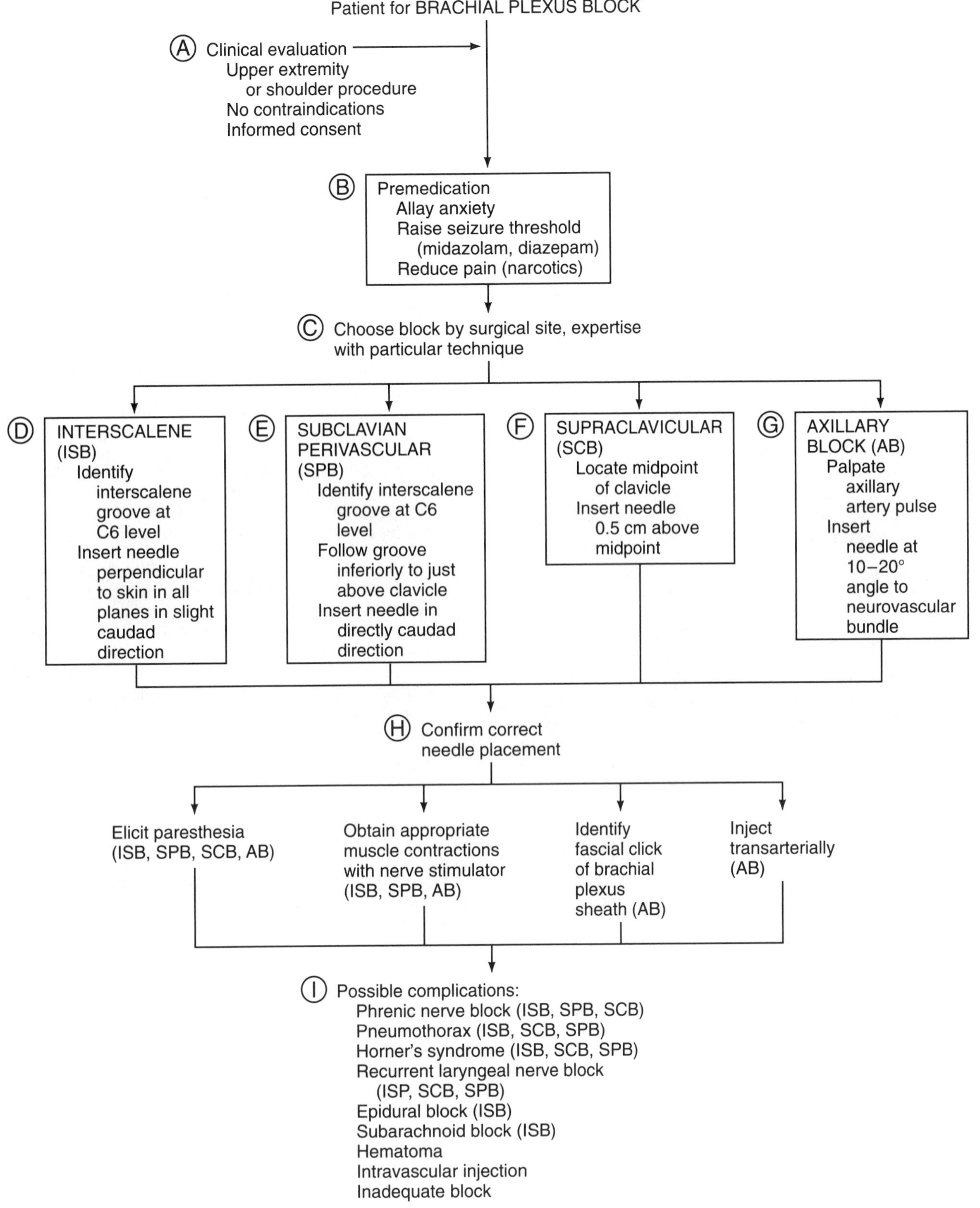
Patient for BRACHIAL PLEXUS BLOCK
(A) Clinical evaluation
Upper extremity or shoulder procedure
No contraindications
Informed consent
(B) Premedication
Allay anxiety
Raise seizure threshold (midazolam, diazepam)
Reduce pain (narcotics)
(C) Choose block by surgical site, expertise with particular technique
(D) INTERSCALENE (ISB)
Identify interscalene groove at C6 level
Insert needle perpendicular to skin in all planes in slight caudad direction
(E) SUBCLAVIAN PERIVASCULAR (SPB)
Identify interscalene groove at C6 level
Follow groove inferiorly to just above clavicle
Insert needle in directly caudad direction
(F) SUPRACLAVICULAR (SCB)
Locate midpoint of clavicle
Insert needle 0.5 cm above midpoint
(G) AXILLARY BLOCK (AB)
Palpate axillary artery pulse
Insert needle at 10–20° angle to neurovascular bundle
(H) Confirm correct needle placement
Elicit paresthesia (ISB, SPB, SCB, AB)
Obtain appropriate muscle contractions with nerve stimulator (ISB, SPB, AB)
Identify fascial click of brachial plexus sheath (AB)
Inject transarterially (AB)
(I) Possible complications:
Phrenic nerve block (ISB, SPB, SCB)
Pneumothorax (ISB, SCB, SPB)
Horner's syndrome (ISB, SCB, SPB)
Recurrent laryngeal nerve block (ISP, SCB, SPB)
Epidural block (ISB)
Subarachnoid block (ISB)
Hematoma
Intravascular injection
Inadequate block

SPINAL ACCESSORY NERVE BLOCK

Tara L. Chronister, M.D.

The spinal accessory nerve (SAN), or 11th cranial nerve, arises from rootlets of the first five cervical segments of the spinal cord. These rootlets join and then ascend through the subarachnoid space to enter the cranium through the foramen magnum. After joining its cranial portion, the nerve exits the cranium through the jugular foramen in a position that is usually anterior to the internal jugular vein. The cranial portion separates to join the vagus nerve. The nerve then pierces the sternocleidomastoid muscle (SCM), passing through the substance of the muscle and exiting at the border of the muscle's superior and middle thirds. At this point it crosses under the fascial covering of the posterior triangle of the neck to reach the trapezius 5 cm above the clavicle. The SAN can be blocked anywhere along its course.

A. One of the few indications to block the SAN is to treat pain associated with acute or chronic torticollis (p 90), to deal with the presence of multiple trapezius trigger points, or to manage spasm of the trapezius muscle.

B. This block can also be used as an adjunct to other regional procedures such as a cervical plexus block for carotid surgery or an interscalene block of the brachial plexus for shoulder surgery. An interscalene block provides adequate analgesia for shoulder surgery, but motor function of the trapezius is maintained, allowing patients to interfere with the surgical procedure by shrugging the shoulders. By means of an SAN block, the trapezius is paralyzed and surgery is facilitated. Blocking of this nerve also increases patient comfort owing to a decreased need for retraction and decreased "pull" when the head is turned to one side for prolonged periods.

C. Several techniques have been described for blocking the SAN in different positions along its course. Use of a nerve stimulator to locate the nerve increases accuracy. Proximal blocks have been associated with hoarseness secondary to subsequent block of the vagus or development of Horner's syndrome due to block of the sympathetic chain. Ramamurthy described a technique for blocking the SAN as it lies within the SCM that eliminates the above risk.

D. With the patient in the supine position, elevation of the head allows identification of the posterior border of the SCM. Deposit 5 to 10 ml local anesthetic (LA) in the belly of the SCM 2 cm below the tip of the mastoid process, using a 23-g, 2.5-cm needle. The LA agent chosen for the block should depend on the clinical situation. Use of 1 or 2% mepivacaine, 0.5 or 0.75% bupivacaine, and 1 or 2% chloroprocaine have all been described. Neurolytic blockade can be accomplished with 3 ml of 3 to 6% phenol or 50% alcohol.

E. A successful block is confirmed by absence of contraction of the SCM when the patient turns the head to the contralateral side, and weakness of the trapezius during attempts to shrug the shoulders.

F. Side effects include difficulty elevating the arm above 90 degrees, slight difficulty turning the head to the opposite side, and numbness behind the ear secondary to block of the lesser occipital nerve, all of which resolve with resolution of the block. Depending on the technique used, the SAN may be inadvertently blocked with superficial cervical plexus block, and vice versa.

References

Murphy TM, Raj PP, Stanton-Hicks M. In: Raj PP, ed. Practical management of pain. Chicago: Year Book, 1986:601.

Ramamurthy S, Akkineni SR, Winnie AP. A simple technic for block of the spinal accessory nerve. Anesth Analg 1978; 57:591.

Woodburne RT. Essentials of human anatomy. New York: Oxford University Press, 1983:50.

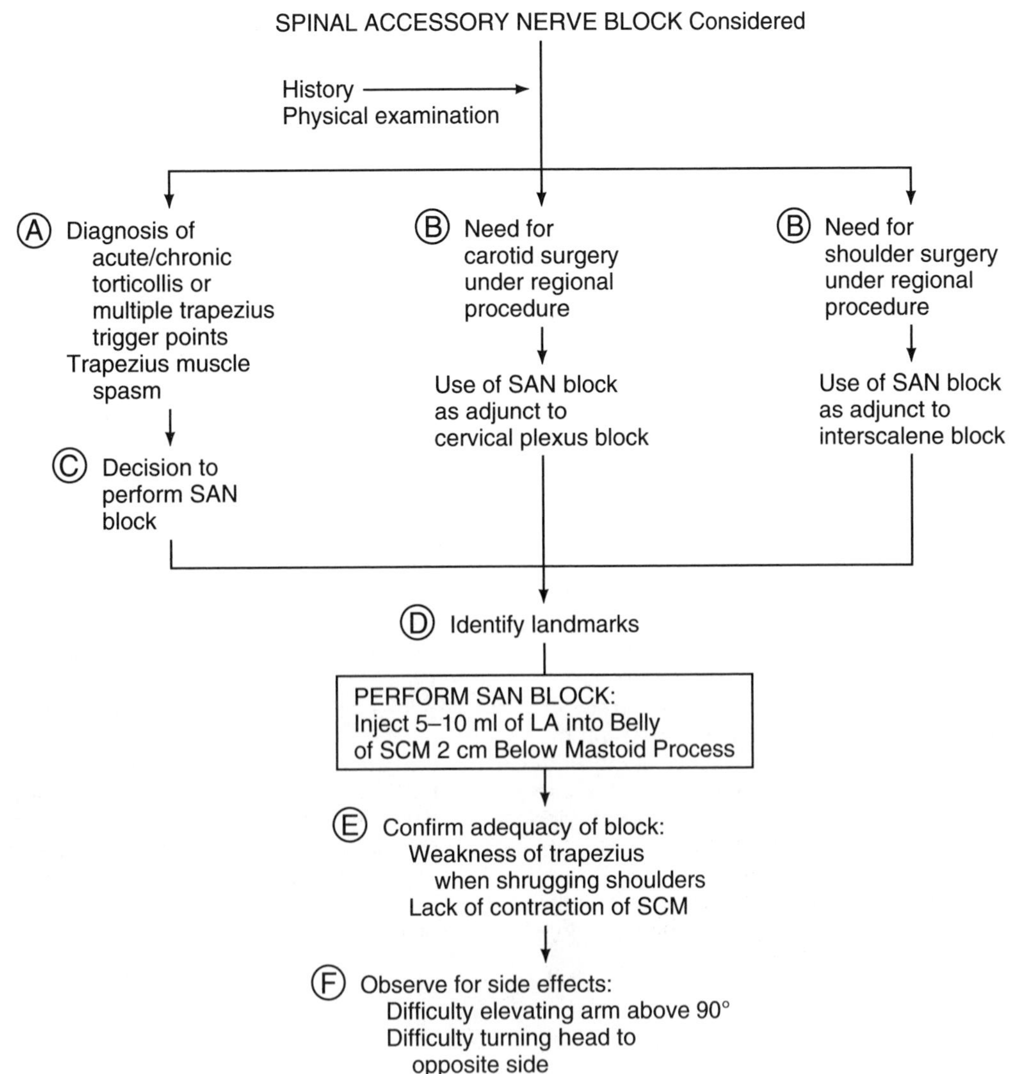

SPINAL ACCESSORY NERVE BLOCK Considered
History
Physical examination
(A) Diagnosis of acute/chronic torticollis or multiple trapezius trigger points
Trapezius muscle spasm
(B) Need for carotid surgery under regional procedure
(B) Need for shoulder surgery under regional procedure
Use of SAN block as adjunct to cervical plexus block
Use of SAN block as adjunct to interscalene block
(C) Decision to perform SAN block
(D) Identify landmarks
PERFORM SAN BLOCK: Inject 5–10 ml of LA into Belly of SCM 2 cm Below Mastoid Process
(E) Confirm adequacy of block:
Weakness of trapezius when shrugging shoulders
Lack of contraction of SCM
(F) Observe for side effects:
Difficulty elevating arm above 90°
Difficulty turning head to opposite side
Numbness behind ear

LONG THORACIC NERVE BLOCK

Rosemary Hickey, M.D.

Pain originating from spasm of the serratus anterior muscle may result in pain in the lateral chest wall under the axilla. This spasm may be relieved by blocking the long thoracic nerve, which arises from the anterior branches of the C5, C6, and C7 nerve roots and provides the motor innervation of the serratus anterior muscle.

A. Before performing the block, take a careful history to exclude other causes of chest wall pain. On physical examination, test the strength of the serratus anterior muscle by noting the presence of scapular "winging," which is accentuated when the arm is pressed against a wall and an attempt is made to push the body away from the wall. A chest film is taken before the block to confirm the absence of rib fractures.

B. To perform the block, place the patient in the supine position without a pillow and instruct him or her to raise the head to facilitate palpation of the sternocleidomastoid muscle (SCM) by making it more prominent. After palpating the posterior border of the SCM with the index finger, instruct the patient to lower the head and relax the neck muscles. Identify the anterior scalene muscle, the interscalene groove, and the middle scalene muscle by rolling the index and middle fingers of the palpating hand laterally from the SCM. Insert a 22-gauge, 3-cm regional block needle (short bevel) attached to a nerve stimulator into the middle scalene muscle in a direction that parallels the long axis of the middle scalene muscle (Fig. 1). Enter the muscle just above the level of C6, which is determined by noting the level of the cricoid cartilage. Expose the lateral chest wall over the serratus anterior muscle to observe muscle contractions, and have an assistant identify contractions induced with the nerve stimulator by placing his or her hand over the area of the muscle. Maintain the final needle position at the point where maximal contraction of the serratus anterior muscle occurs. After negative aspiration, inject 5 ml of local anesthetic solution (0.5% bupivacaine).

C. To evaluate the motor effect of the block, check the strength of the serratus anterior muscle after the block. When muscle function is impaired, the vertebral border of the scapula protrudes dorsomedially, producing scapular "winging"; the shoulder droops; and the arm cannot be abducted beyond 90 degrees. If EMG is available, use it to document that the block has interrupted innervation of the serratus anterior muscle. Teach the patient gentle stretching exercises to try and prevent return of the spasm. If no pain relief is obtained, consider repeating the block or evaluate other possible origins of pain.

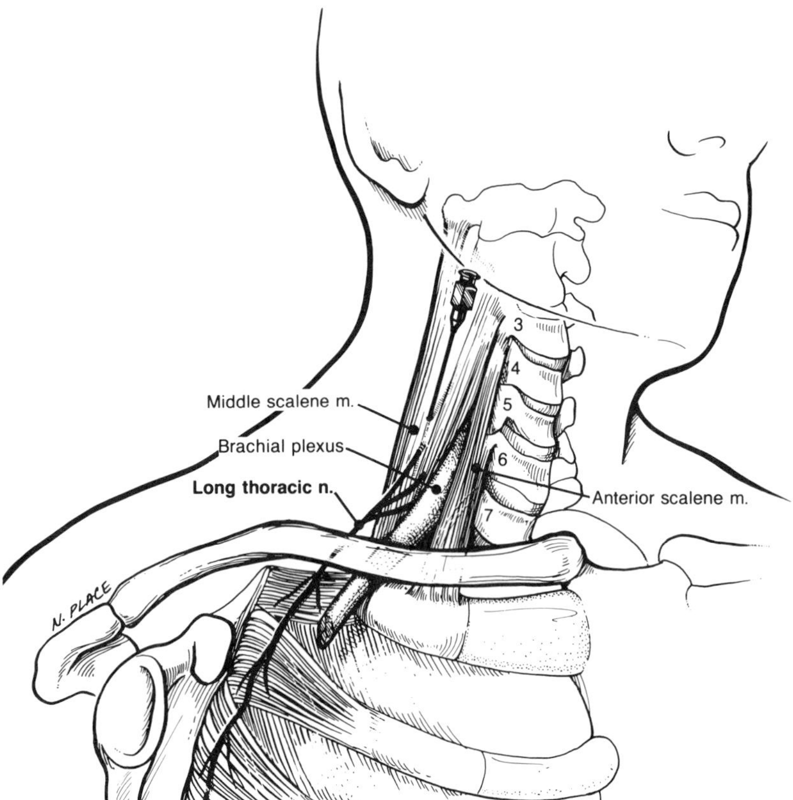

Figure 1 The long thoracic nerve, which innervates the serratus anterior muscle, is blocked as it pierces the middle scalene muscle. (From Ramamurthy S, Hickey R, Maytorena A, et al. Long thoracic nerve block. Anesth Analg 1990; 71:197–199; with permission.)

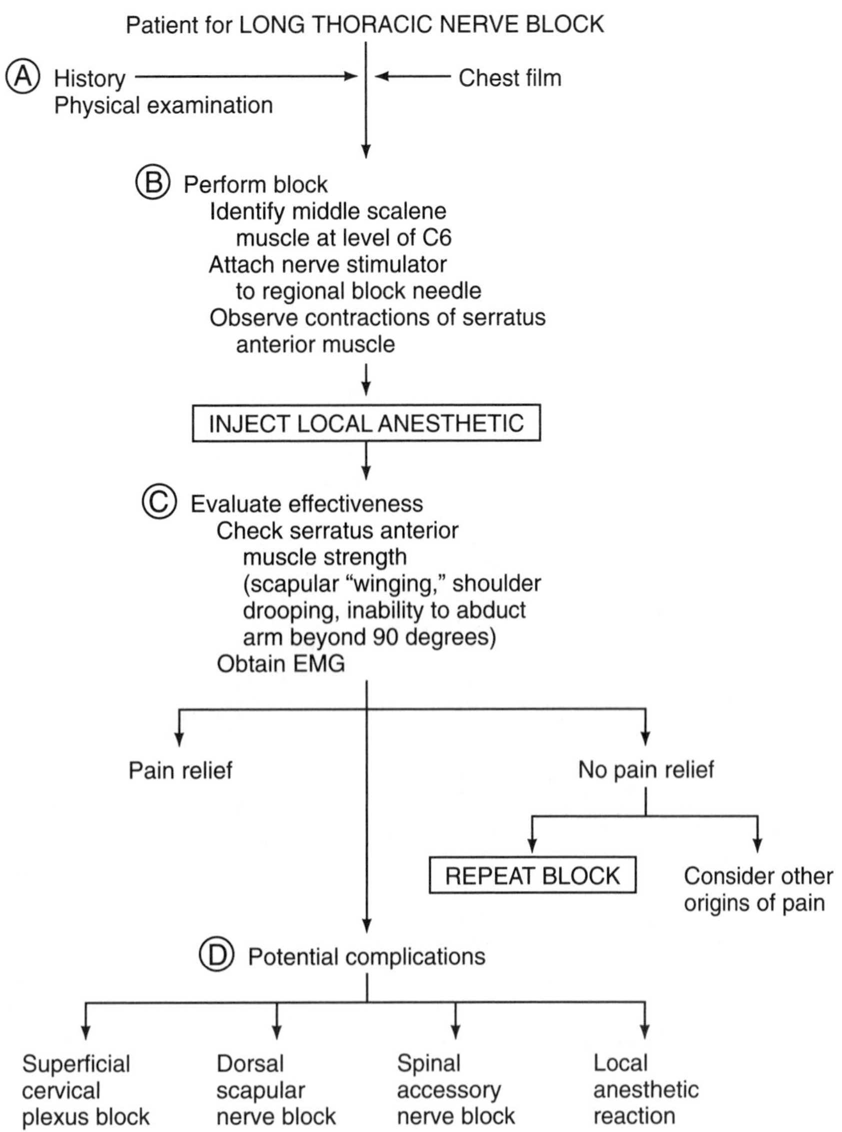

D. Potential complications include block of adjacent nerves such as the superficial cervical plexus, the dorsal scapular nerve (innervator of the rhomboids and levator scapulae), and the spinal accessory nerve (innervator of the SCM and trapezius). As with any other regional anesthetic, a local anesthetic reaction is possible, and precautions should be taken to minimize this possibility (aspiration before injection, limiting the total dose of local anesthetic, and use of appropriate monitoring equipment).

References

Martin JT. Postoperative isolated dysfunction of the long thoracic nerve: A rare entity of uncertain etiology. Anesth Analg 1989; 69:614.

Ramamurthy S, Hickey R, Maytorena A, et al. Long thoracic nerve block. Anesth Analg 1990; 71:197.

FACET JOINT INJECTION

Emil J. Menk, M.D.

Injection of the facet joint with local anesthetic solution remains the only way of definitively diagnosing facet joint syndrome. Injection of the facet joint with steroids may also be one of the most useful therapeutic interventions available. Should denervation techniques be justified, cryoanalgesia, radiofrequency neurolysis, and chemical neurolysis have all been proven effective. Signs and symptoms are described in the chapter "Facet Joint Syndrome" (p 140).

A. The performance of a diagnostic facet joint block has also been described in the "Facet Joint Syndrome" chapter. For obvious reasons I strongly recommend the use of fluoroscopy during a diagnostic procedure. Accurate needle location can be confirmed and recorded by making a radiograph of an arthrogram produced by injecting 0.5 ml of contrast medium. The diagnosis is confirmed if 1 ml of a local anesthetic solution (0.5% bupivacaine) injected into the facet joint is associated with significant improvement in symptoms.

B. Steroids in moderate doses (e.g., 40 mg methylprednisolone acetate) have been combined with local anesthetic solutions to produce prolonged relief of symptoms. There is a dearth of appropriate prospective, double-blind studies, but clinical reports have described widely varying success rates. Differences in study protocols, diagnostic criteria, and success-versus-failure criteria make overall assessments of the published results impossible. In my experience, steroids have proved very effective in selected patients.

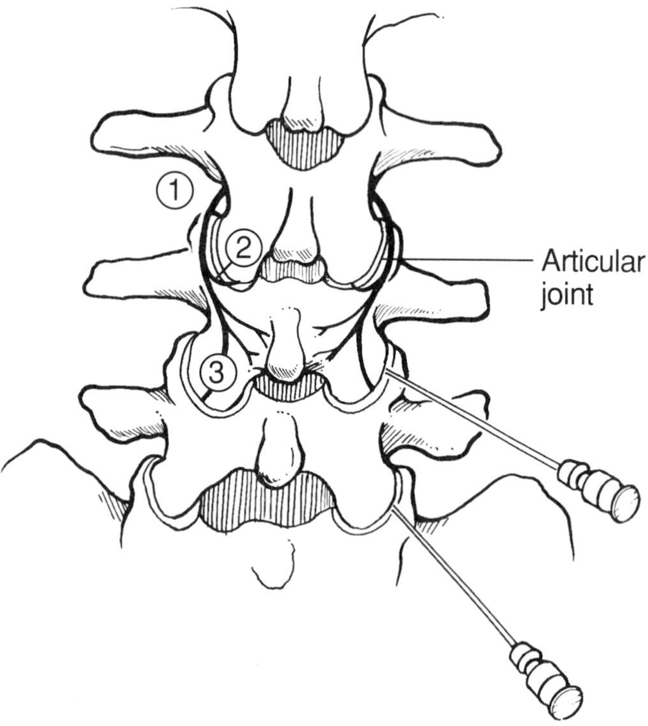

Figure 1 Facet joint injection. Facet innervation: 1, medial branch of dorsal branch of spinal nerve; 2, inferior articular branch of medial branch; 3, superior articular branch of medial branch.

C. If therapeutic blocks with steroids are successful acutely yet fail to produce satisfactory results for more than about 30 days, denervation techniques may be warranted. Although inherently more risky, they have proved effective and safe in experienced hands. Each facet joint receives sensory innervation from two medial branches of the lumbar dorsal rami. For effective analgesia the medial branches of the nerves must be blocked both above and below each joint selected. The block is commonly performed lateral to the facet process at the junction of the superior edge of the transverse process and the dorsal lumbar process of the spinal arch. Diagnostic nerve blocks using local anesthetics should be performed before considering neurolytic blocks. As with any denervation block, whether using cryoanalgesia, radiofrequency, or phenol, accurate placement should be evaluated by electrically stimulating the nerve before denervation. This should help identify nearby motor nerves. Interestingly, the denervation techniques normally are not permanent. Regeneration of the nerve accompanied by resumption of symptoms usually occurs after about 6 months, at which time the blocks may be repeated.

D. Repeated therapeutic injections may be more prudent in many patients who routinely receive more than 30 days' benefit from the initial series of injections. Regardless of the approach taken, therapy should be combined with NSAIDs and an exercise program.

E. Although complications are rare in experienced hands, they may include intravascular injection, epidural injection, subdural injection, rupture of the facet joint capsule, sensory/motor nerve block, and infection. Appropriate precautions must always be taken during a sensory or therapeutic block. Denervation techniques also include the risks of prolonged sensory/motor nerve blocks or neuritis.

References

Boas RA. Facet joint injections. In: Stanton-Hicks M, Boas R, eds. Chronic low back pain. New York: Raven Press, 1982:207.

Bogduk N. Back pain: Zygapophysial blocks and epidural steroids. In: Cousins MJ, Bridenbaugh PO, eds. Neural blockade in clinical anesthesia and management of pain. 2nd ed. Philadelphia: JB Lippincott, 1988:935.

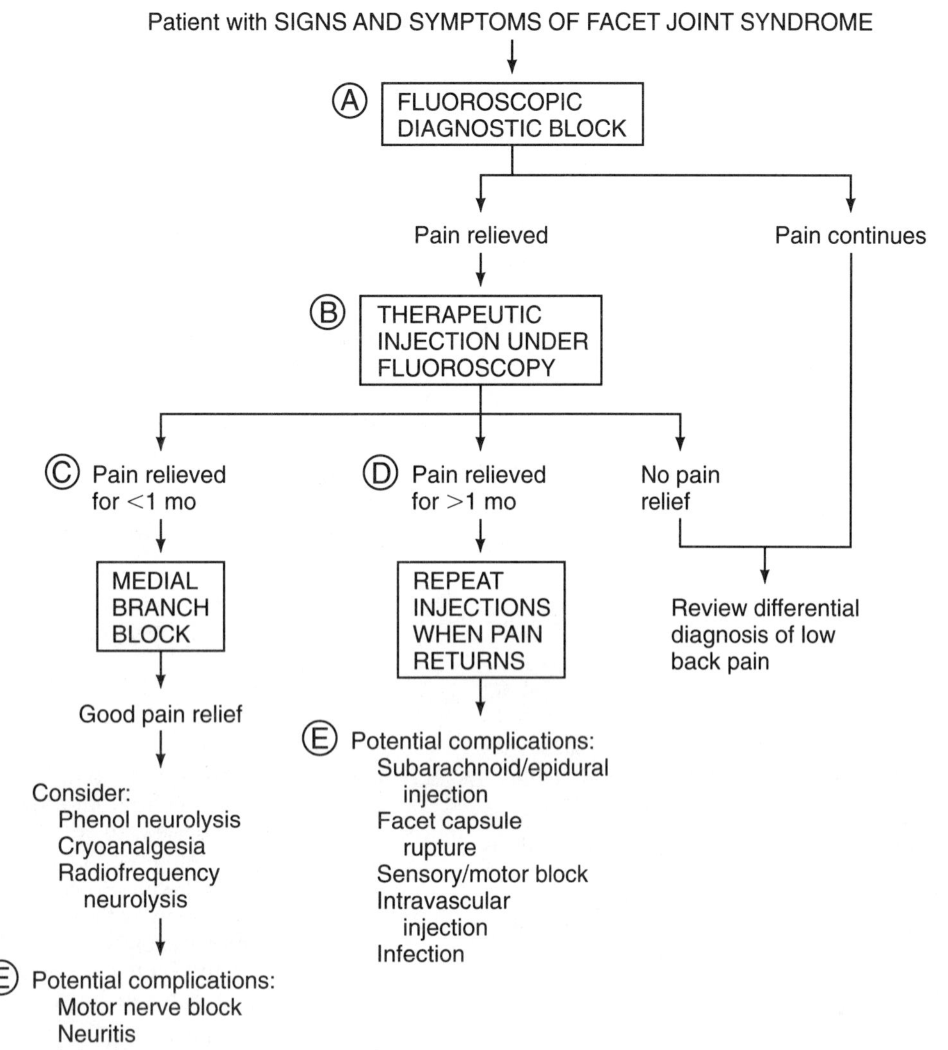
Patient with SIGNS AND SYMPTOMS OF FACET JOINT SYNDROME
(A) FLUOROSCOPIC DIAGNOSTIC BLOCK
Pain relieved
Pain continues
(B) THERAPEUTIC INJECTION UNDER FLUOROSCOPY
(C) Pain relieved for <1 mo
(D) Pain relieved for >1 mo
No pain relief
MEDIAL BRANCH BLOCK
REPEAT INJECTIONS WHEN PAIN RETURNS
Review differential diagnosis of low back pain
Good pain relief
(E) Potential complications:
Subarachnoid/epidural injection
Facet capsule rupture
Sensory/motor block
Intravascular injection
Infection
Consider:
Phenol neurolysis
Cryoanalgesia
Radiofrequency neurolysis
(E) Potential complications:
Motor nerve block
Neuritis
Infection

SACROILIAC JOINT INJECTION

Timothy Castro, Jr., M.D.

Inflammation in the sacroiliac joint can be a major source of low back pain, with symptoms occurring either unilaterally or bilaterally. It is rarely associated with neurologic deficits, but radiating pain into the posterior thigh is very common. A patient presenting with low back pain should have a good physical examination of the sacroiliac joint before potentially unfruitful radiographic studies are undertaken. Physical therapy of the sacroiliac joint remains the mainstay of treatment; however, injection into or near the sacroiliac joint with plain local anesthetic can serve as a useful diagnostic tool as well as be therapeutic to the patient. Virtually all patients with low back pain accompanied with no neurologic deficit should be examined for sacroiliac joint pathology.

A. Acute causes usually result from mechanical changes such as trauma or changes in posture or gait.

B. Chronic causes can include inflammatory bowel disease, rheumatologic diseases, persistent stress to the joint, or osteoarthritis. Early morning stiffness with localized tenderness may be a common complaint.

C. Take a careful history to rule out pyogenic sources of sacroiliac joint inflammation. The gut as well as intravenous drug abuse can seed the joint with bacteria. Although a physical examination may demonstrate inflammation of the joint, direct treatment to the primary source of the disease rather than to alleviation of the symptom.

D. Localized tenderness over the posterior inferior iliac spine is the best indicator of sacroiliac joint disease. The examiner can also use both thumbs to forcibly direct the anterior superior iliac spine to the midline while the patient is supine. If the patient complains of pain near the sacroiliac joint, joint pathology should be suspected.

E. Although there are many tests for stressing the sacroiliac joint, none is as reliable as palpation for localized tenderness over the joint.

F. An equivocal examination can result in patients whose low back pain has multiple causes. These patients may present with generalized tenderness as well as tenderness over the sacroiliac joint. A plain film can reveal joint pathology in many instances.

G. If the plain films are normal and the cause of the back pain cannot be determined, perform a CT scan or bone scan to evaluate sacroiliac joint pathology. Both of these tests are more sensitive than plain radiography, although the severity of the structural changes may not correlate with the patients' symptoms.

H. An injection with local anesthetic into the paraspinous muscle and ligaments over the sacroiliac joint can be an invaluable diagnostic tool to confirm physical or radiological findings. A patient with minor symptoms may not warrant such a diagnostic block, however. If the block yields partial relief or if sacroiliac joint pathology is strongly suspected, a direct injection into the joint with the aid of fluoroscopy may prove beneficial.

I. Once the diagnosis is established, physical therapy includes massage, exercise, and joint manipulation.

J. Usually, minor symptoms can be easily managed with NSAIDs.

K. An injection of steroids and local anesthetics into the paraspinous muscles and joint ligaments often allows the patient to benefit from physical therapy. The injection can be done with about 5 to 10 ml of a dilute local anesthetic with about 25 mg of triamcinolone or 40 mg of methylprednisolone. If joint penetration is desired, confirmation with 1 ml of renografin-60 is helpful. The block can be repeated in 1 or 2 weeks depending on the patient's symptoms and the total amount of steroids recently used.

L. If diagnostic and therapeutic measures do not aid the patient, other sources of the low back pain should be considered. The work-up may include a psychological evaluation to explore the possibility of secondary gain or contributing psychological factors.

References

Boyle AC. Discussion of the clinical and radiological aspects of sacro-iliac disease. Proc R Soc Med 1957; 50:847.

DonTigny RL. Anterior dysfunction of the sacroiliac joint as a major factor in the etiology of idiopathic low back pain syndrome. Phys Ther 1990; 70:250.

Fewins HE, Whitehouse GH, Bucknall RC. Role of computed tomography in the evaluation of suspected sacroiliac joint disease. J R Soc Med 1990; 83:430.

Guyot DR, Manoli A, Kling GA. Pyogenic sacroilitis in i.v. drug users. AJR 1987; 146:1209.

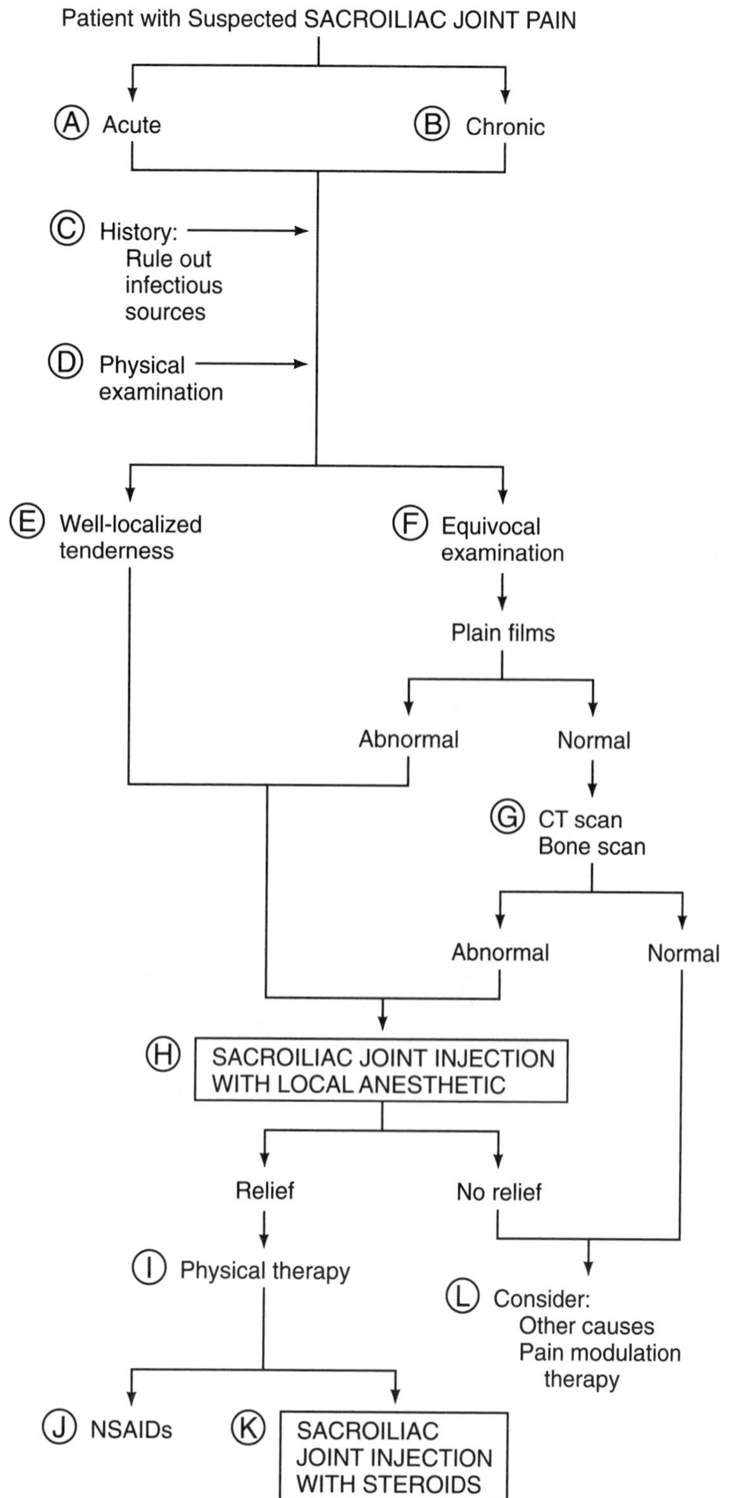

Patient with Suspected SACROILIAC JOINT PAIN
(A) Acute
(B) Chronic
(C) History:
Rule out
infectious
sources
(D) Physical
examination
(E) Well-localized
tenderness
(F) Equivocal
examination
Plain films
Abnormal
Normal
(G) CT scan
Bone scan
Abnormal
Normal
(H) SACROILIAC JOINT INJECTION
WITH LOCAL ANESTHETIC
Relief
No relief
(I) Physical therapy
(L) Consider:
Other causes
Pain modulation
therapy
(J) NSAIDs
(K) SACROILIAC
JOINT INJECTION
WITH STEROIDS

TRIGGER POINT INJECTION

Robert D. Culling, D.O.

Patients with myofascial pain have hyperirritable trigger points (TPs) within a taut band of muscle or its associated fascia. Palpation of a TP produces a characteristic local and referred pain pattern response. Trigger point injections (TPIs) interrupt the pain cycle to allow muscle stretching and range of motion exercises.

A. Identify TPs; active TPs reproduce the pain pattern when palpated. Mark the sites with a skin pencil. Clean the skin with an antiseptic solution before injection.

B. A 22- to 25-gauge 2-5-cm needle is attached to a 10-ml Luer-Lok syringe. Palpate the TP again and place the needle directly into the taut muscle band. The needle placement should aggravate the pain and tenderness in the referred pain region, which helps to confirm correct placement into the TP.

C. Dry needling, saline, sterile water, steroids, and local anesthetics have all proved effective. Local anesthetics reduce the local discomfort associated with the injection. 2 to 5 ml of lidocaine or bupivacaine may be used. Correct placement is confirmed if the injection results in pain relief. If relief is not obtained, it is likely that the TP was not injected; it should be relocated and the injection repeated.

D. Several TPs can be treated, but the total amount of local anesthetic should be kept below toxic levels. If the patient becomes pale, diaphoretic, or faint, stop the injection.

Reference

Travell JG, Simons DG. Myofascial pain and dysfunction. The trigger point manual. Baltimore: Williams & Wilkins, 1983.

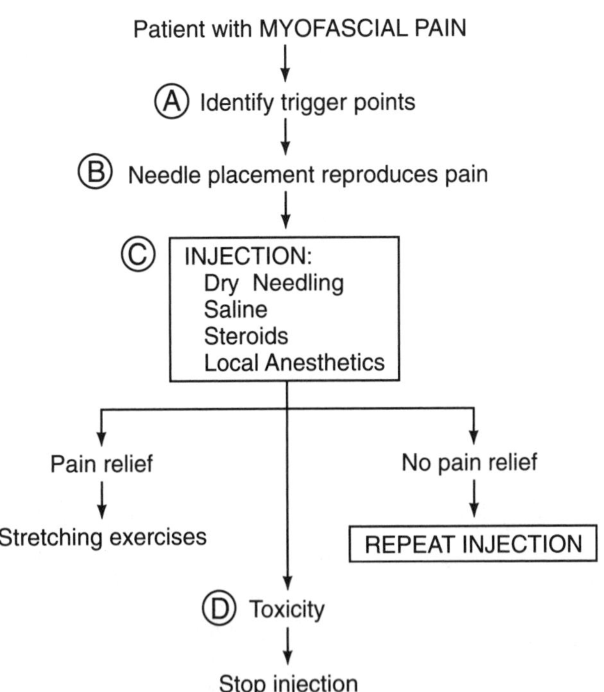
Patient with MYOFASCIAL PAIN
A Identify trigger points
B Needle placement reproduces pain
C INJECTION:
Dry Needling
Saline
Steroids
Local Anesthetics
Pain relief
Stretching exercises
No pain relief
REPEAT INJECTION
D Toxicity
Stop injection

SCIATIC NERVE BLOCK

Mary Ann Gurkowski, M.D.

The sciatic nerve (SN) is the largest nerve in the body. It can be blocked at the sciatic notch or at the level of the ischial tuberosity and greater trochanter. Anterior, posterior, and lateral approaches have been described. The SN consists of two major trunks, the lateral trunk (L4-S2), which makes up the common peroneal nerve, and the medial trunk (L4-S3), which forms the tibial nerve.

A. The indications for sciatic nerve block (SNB) include the need for repair of malleolar fractures and tendons in the foot and ankle. The SNB alone provides anesthesia for the sole of the foot and all but the medial area of the dorsum, which is supplied by the saphenous branch of the femoral nerve. Combined with the three-in-one block, complete blockade of the entire lower extremity can be achieved. SNB can be of great value in minimizing the pain from a fractured tibia during transport.

B. Contraindications include local skin infection, hematoma, osteomyelitis of the femur, coagulopathy, and patient refusal. Relative contraindications include organic nervous system disorders. The disadvantages include the need for large volumes of local anesthetics, the need to elicit paresthesia or muscle contraction with a nerve stimulator to confirm correct needle placement, and the need to be combined with other nerve blocks.

C. The SN travels anterior to the sacrum and exits the pelvis posteriorly through the greater sciatic notch, anterior to the piriformis muscle and between the ischial tuberosity and the greater trochanter of the femur. It runs behind the femur and divides into the common peroneal and tibial nerves at the superior aspect of the popliteal fossa.

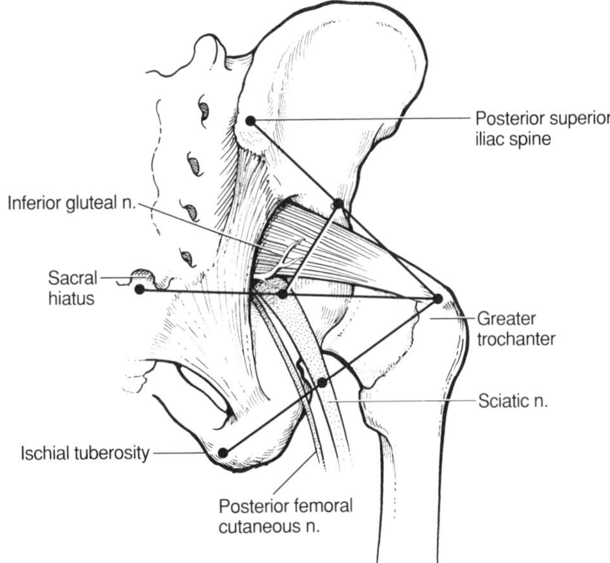

Figure 1 Placement of sciatic nerve block.

D. The classic posterior approach blocks the SN at the greater sciatic notch. At this level, the posterior femoral cutaneous nerve (PFCN) and pudendal nerve (PN) are blocked as well. Place the patient in lateral Sims' position with the side to be blocked uppermost. The upper knee is bent and the patient's back rotated slightly forward. A perpendicular line is dropped from the midpoint of a line drawn between the posterior superior iliac spine and the top of the greater trocanter. Insert the needle 3 to 4 cm caudad on this line. Advance a 3 1/2 inch, 22-gauge spinal needle until paresthesia or muscle contraction occurs in the distribution of the SN. If bone is contacted, the needle is walked off medially or superiorly. Inject 15 to 20 ml of local anesthetic. A modified posterior approach can be performed with the patient in either the lateral or prone position. Draw a line connecting the ischial tuberosity and the greater trochanter, and insert the needle at the midpoint. Paresthesia or muscle contraction again is used to confirm correct placement.

E. The supine sciatic block described by Winnie has the advantage of not requiring the patient to be turned. Movement of the leg, however, may be painful in patients with trauma. The hip is flexed, and landmarks and needle insertion site are the same as in the modified posterior approach (see D).

F. The anterior approach is helpful when movement of the lower extremity is painful. Sedation is important because this approach can be uncomfortable. The PFCN may not be blocked with this technique. Draw a line along the inguinal ligament joining the anterior superior iliac spine and the pubic tubercle. Divide the line into three equal parts and draw a perpendicular line from the junction of the medial and middle third. Draw a parallel line to the original line, beginning at the top of the greater trochanter. Insert the needle at the junction of the parallel and perpendicular lines. Advance a 6-inch, 22-gauge spinal needle until it contacts the bone, usually the lesser trochanter. Redirect the needle medially and posteriorly until a paresthesia is obtained. Inject 15 to 20 ml of local anesthetic after negative aspiration.

G. The lateral approach has the advantage of requiring no patient movement and may be better tolerated than the anterior approach. Care must be exercised when using a nerve stimulator. Contractions may be obtained in the thigh, leading the anesthesiologist into misplacing the local anesthetic. Contraction should be elicited in the calf muscles or anterior compartment muscles before injecting the local anesthetic. Insert a

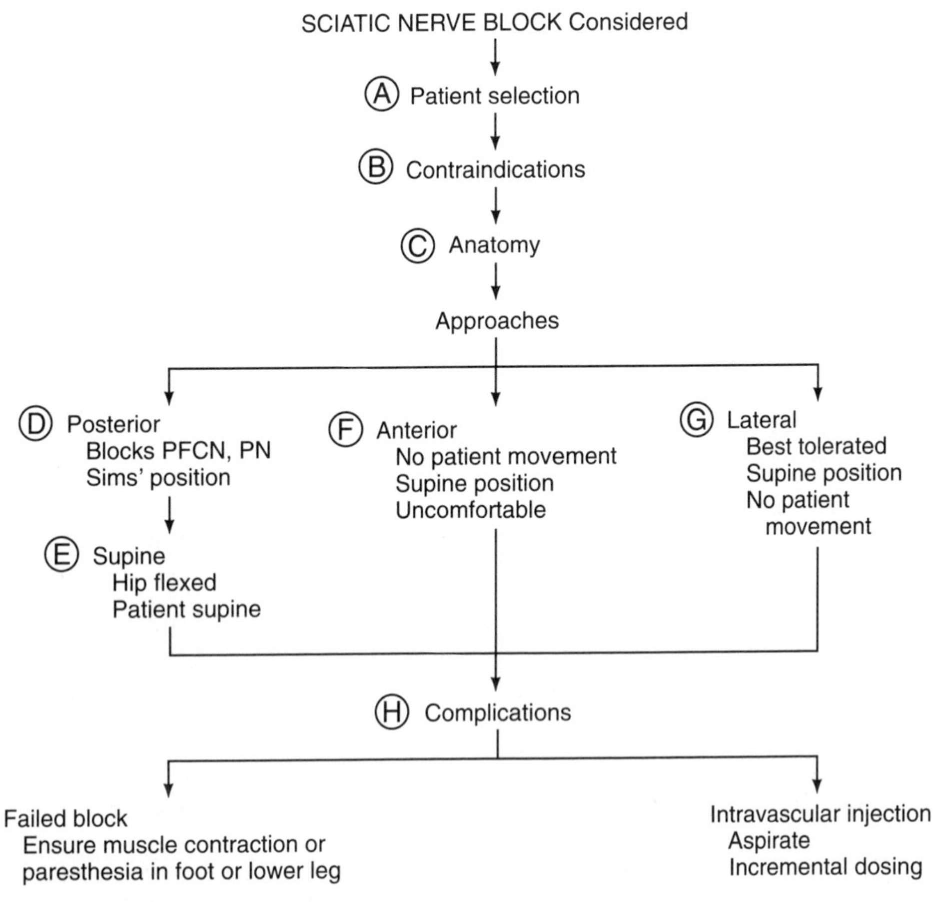

6-inch, 22-gauge needle 3 cm distal to the maximal lateral prominence of the greater trochanter, close to its posterior margin, until bone is contacted. Redirect the needle posteriorly and medially until paresthesia or contraction of calf or anterior compartment muscles is elicited. Inject 15 to 20 ml of local anesthetic.

H. The primary complications of this block include unintentional intravascular injection and failure to block the nerve. Intravascular injection is unlikely if a test dose is given initially and local anesthetic is injected incrementally with aspiration before each injection. A failed block most commonly occurs when the injection is performed without eliciting a paresthesia or muscle contraction of the foot or lower leg.

References

Dalens B, Tanquy A, Vanneuville G. Sciatic nerve blocks in children: Comparison of the posterior, anterior, and lateral approaches in 180 pediatric patients. Anesth Analg 1990; 70:131.

Guardini R, Waldron BA, Wallace WA. Sciatic nerve block: A new lateral approach. Acta Anaesthesiol Scand 1985; 29:515.

Magora F, Pessachovitch B, Shoham I. Sciatic nerve block by the anterior approach for operations on the lower extremity. Br J Anaesth 1974; 46:121.

Winnie AP, Ramamurthy S, Durrani Z, Radonjic R. Plexus blocks for lower extremity surgery. Anesthesiol Rev 1974; 1:11.

FEMORAL NERVE BLOCK

Alfonso Maytorena, M.D.

Femoral nerve block (FNB) is easy to perform as long as the anatomy is understood. The nerve arises from the L2–L4 nerve roots and runs between the psoas major and iliacus muscles. It passes beneath the inguinal ligament lateral to the femoral artery to enter the thigh. The nerve is deep to both the fascia lata and fascia iliaca, whereas the artery is only deep to the fascia lata. The nerve can be blocked individually or in conjunction with the lateral femoral cutaneous and obturator nerves, employing the 3-in-1 technique described by Winnie and colleagues.

A. FNB is most commonly used to control severe post-traumatic or postoperative pain. In early management of a fractured femoral shaft, it relieves muscle spasm and provides immediate analgesia. It can also be used as a diagnostic procedure in patients with chronic, severe anterior thigh pain.

B. The patient lies supine and a line is drawn joining the anterosuperior iliac spine and the pubic tubercle. The midpoint usually overlies the femoral artery. After skin preparation, raise a skin wheal 1 cm lateral to the junction of the femoral artery and inguinal ligament. Advance the needle cephalad at an angle of 30 degrees. Loss of resistance is felt twice when a short-beveled needle is used. A paresthesia or muscle contraction at the knee occurs when a nerve simulator is used. After a negative aspiration for blood, inject 8 to 10 ml of local anesthetic. A femoral nerve block provides sensory block of the anteromedial thigh, the medial aspect of the leg, and the proximal foot. There is loss of extension of the knee and some loss of flexion at the hip joint.

C. The 3-in-1 block described by Winnie requires only slight modifications. The point of entry is 1 cm lateral and 1 cm below the inguinal ligament. Introduce the needle cephalad and parallel to the artery. Inject 30 ml of local anesthetic into the sheath while obstructing the sheath distal to the point of injection. The local anesthetic flows proximally within the sheath, diffusing toward the paravertebral region and blocking the femoral, lateral femoral cutaneous, and obturator nerves. When combined with the sciatic nerve block (p 272), it provides analgesia of the entire lower extremity.

D. A continuous catheter may be introduced during the above technique, although an angle of 60 degrees may allow easier threading of the catheter. Thread the catheter approximately 3 cm into the sheath. This provides prolonged analgesia. Local anesthetics can be infused, usually 5 to 10 ml/hr.

E. Complications include unintentinal intra-arterial or IV injection, nerve injury, and subsequent dysesthesia, hematoma, or infection.

References

Berry FR. Analgesia in patients with fractures of neck of femur. Anesthesia 1979; 37:577.

Brands E, Callahan VL. Continuous lumbar plexus block. Analgesia for femoral neck fractures. Anaesth Intensive Care 1978; 6:265.

Cousins MJ, Bridenbaugh PO. Neural blockade in clinical anesthesia and management of pain. 2nd ed. Philadelphia: JB Lippincott, 1988.

Rosenblatt RM. Continuous femoral anesthesia for lower extremity surgery. Reg Anesth 1980; 4:2.

Winnie AP, Ramamurthy S, Durrani Z. The inguinal paravascular technique of lumbar plexus anesthesia: "The 3-in-1 block." Anesth Analg 1973; 52:989.

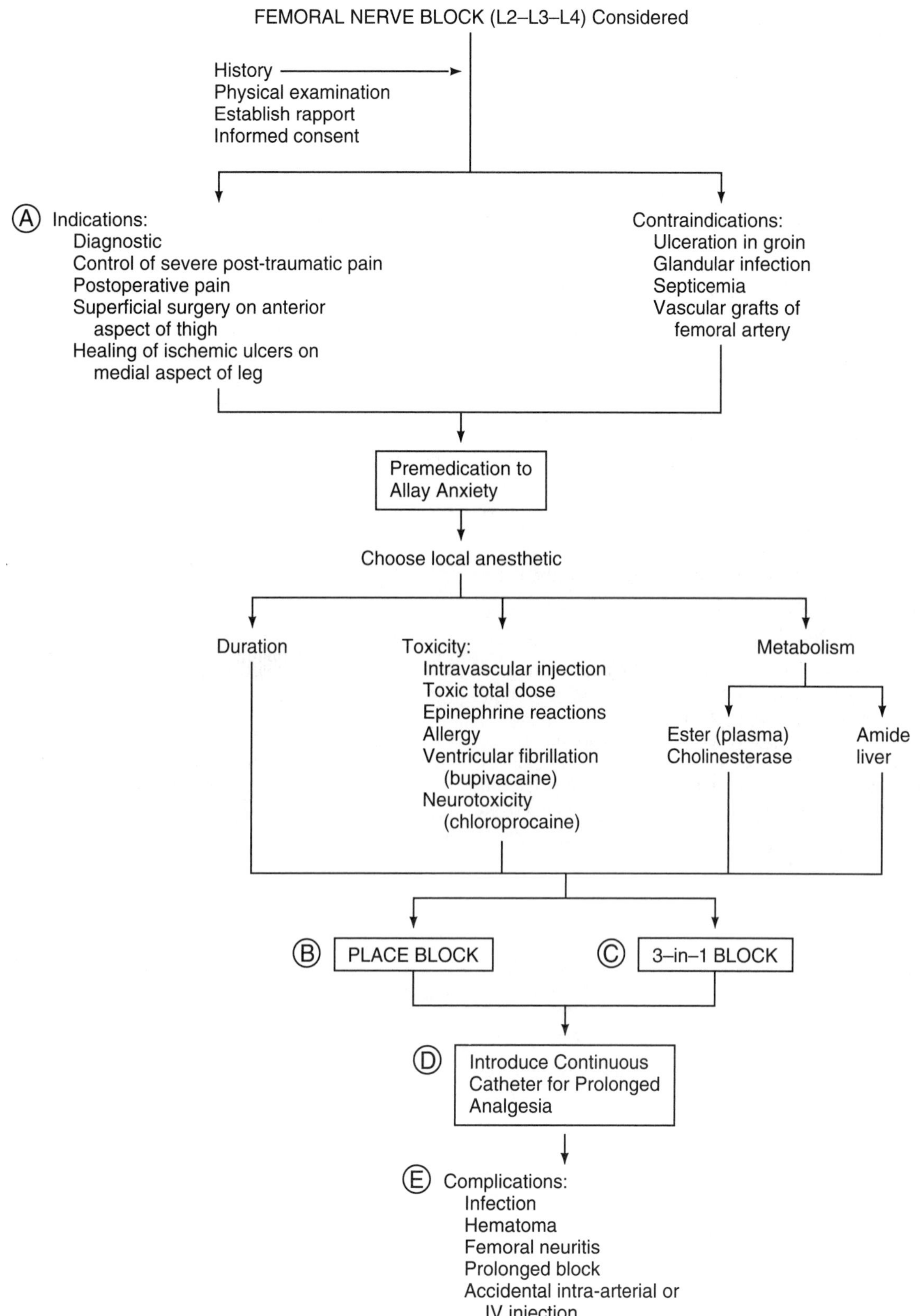

FEMORAL NERVE BLOCK (L2–L3–L4) Considered
History
Physical examination
Establish rapport
Informed consent
(A) Indications:
Diagnostic
Control of severe post-traumatic pain
Postoperative pain
Superficial surgery on anterior aspect of thigh
Healing of ischemic ulcers on medial aspect of leg
Contraindications:
Ulceration in groin
Glandular infection
Septicemia
Vascular grafts of femoral artery
Premedication to Allay Anxiety
Choose local anesthetic
Duration
Toxicity:
Intravascular injection
Toxic total dose
Epinephrine reactions
Allergy
Ventricular fibrillation (bupivacaine)
Neurotoxicity (chloroprocaine)
Metabolism
Ester (plasma) Cholinesterase
Amide liver
(B) PLACE BLOCK
(C) 3–in–1 BLOCK
(D) Introduce Continuous Catheter for Prolonged Analgesia
(E) Complications:
Infection
Hematoma
Femoral neuritis
Prolonged block
Accidental intra-arterial or IV injection

LATERAL FEMORAL CUTANEOUS NERVE BLOCK

Alfonso Maytorena, M.D.

The lateral femoral cutaneous nerve (LFCN) arises from the L2–L3 nerve roots and emerges at the lateral border of the psoas muscle at a level lower than the ilioinguinal nerve. It passes obliquely under the iliac fascia and across the iliac muscle to enter the thigh deep to the inguinal ligament at a point approximately 1 to 2 cm medial to the anterosuperior iliac spine. It supplies the skin of the anterolateral thigh to the knee and the skin of the lateral aspect of the buttock below the greater trochanter and upper two-thirds of the lateral side of the thigh.

A. The indications for LFCN block include acute pain settings involving the anatomic distribution, e.g., providing anesthesia for skin graft harvests. It is commonly used as a supplement to femoral and sciatic nerve blocks for knee operations, and to provide analgesia for tourniquet pain. It is also useful as a diagnostic block in patients with chronic anterolateral thigh pain, to rule out meralgia paresthetica.

B. Contraindications include local infection, septicemia, and patient refusal.

C. The patient is placed supine with the thigh in neutral position. Landmarks are the anterior superior iliac spine and the inguinal ligament. After skin preparation, a wheal is produced 1.5 cm caudad to the anterosuperior iliac spine. Introduce a 5-cm, 22- or 25-gauge short-beveled needle upward and lateral, and advance it until a paresthesia is obtained. If periosteum is contacted, withdraw the needle and redirect it in a line parallel to the inguinal ligament until a paresthesia is obtained. Inject 5 to 8 ml of local anesthetic. The superior approach requires placement of the needle just medial to the anterosuperior iliac spine in a vertical direction. An initial loss of resistance can be felt as the needle passes through the external oblique aponeurosis. A second loss of resistance is felt as the needle exits the internal oblique muscle. The needle now lies within the fascial canal that contains the nerve, and local anesthetic can be injected.

D. Complications are rare. Transient neuropathy may occur in cases of accidental nerve damage.

References

Bonica JJ. The management of pain. Vol II. 2nd ed. Philadelphia: Lea & Febiger, 1990.

Cousins MJ, Bridenbaugh PO. Neural blockade in clinical anesthesia and management of pain. Philadelphia: JB Lippincott, 1988.

Pansky B. Review of gross anatomy. 6th ed. New York: Macmillan, 1989.

Winnie AP, Ramamurthy S, Durrani Z. The inguinal paravascular technique of lumbar plexus anesthesia: The "3-in-1 block." Anesth Analg 1973; 52:989.

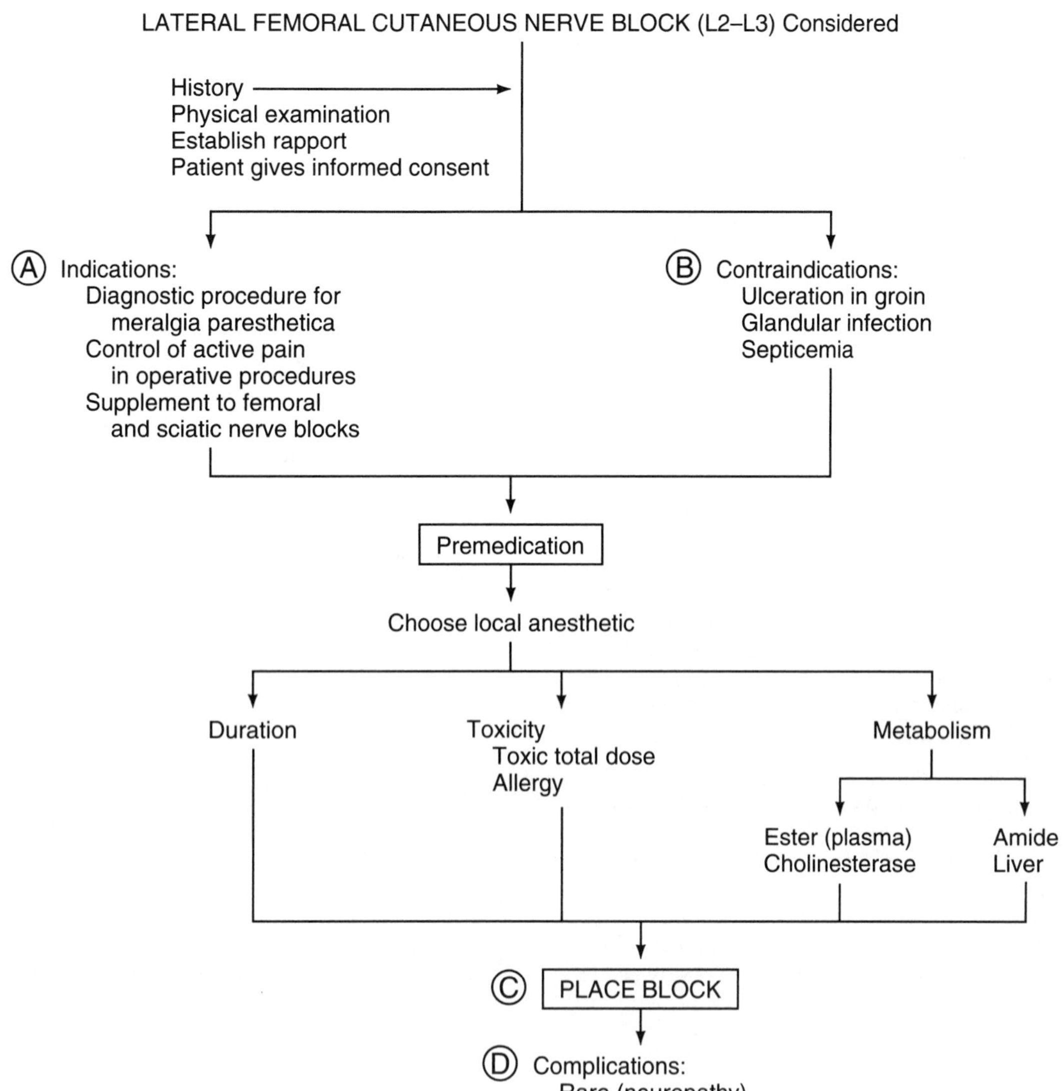
LATERAL FEMORAL CUTANEOUS NERVE BLOCK (L2–L3) Considered
History
Physical examination
Establish rapport
Patient gives informed consent
(A) Indications:
Diagnostic procedure for meralgia paresthetica
Control of active pain in operative procedures
Supplement to femoral and sciatic nerve blocks
(B) Contraindications:
Ulceration in groin
Glandular infection
Septicemia
Premedication
Choose local anesthetic
Duration
Toxicity
Toxic total dose
Allergy
Metabolism
Ester (plasma) Cholinesterase
Amide Liver
(C) PLACE BLOCK
(D) Complications:
Rare (neuropathy)

OBTURATOR NERVE BLOCK

Alfonso Maytorena, M.D.

Obturator nerve block (ONB) can be used as a diagnostic or prognostic procedure. The obturator nerve arises from the L2–L4 nerve roots. The nerve is covered anteriorly by the external iliac vessels, passing downward into the pelvis. It travels with the obturator vessels along the obturator groove and passes through the obturator foramen into the thigh. It divides into posterior and anterior branches as it passes through the obturator canal. The anterior branch supplies the hip joint, anterior adductor muscles, and skin of the lower inner thigh. The posterior branch innervates the deep adductor muscles and frequently the knee joint. The obturator nerve provides little to no cutaneous innervation to the leg.

A. ONB can be used in diagnosing hip pain and in relieving adductor spasm of the hip in individuals with spasticity from spinal cord injury. It is also necessary to provide complete analgesia for surgery above or on the knee, when combined with sciatic, femoral and lateral femoral cutaneous nerve blocks.

B. The nerve is difficult to find because of its deep location. The patient is supine and the leg is placed in slight abduction. Palpate the pubic tubercle and raise a skin wheal 1 to 2 cm below and 1 to 2 cm lateral to the tubercle. Introduce a 7- to 8-cm needle in a slightly medial direction until the inferior pubic ramus is contacted. Withdraw the needle and redirect it 45 degrees cephalad to identify the superior bony portion of the canal. Withdraw the needle and direct it slightly laterally and inferiorly 2 to 3 cm deeper into the obturator canal. Needle placement into the obturator canal is confirmed either by fluoroscopy or by nerve stimulator with adductor movement. After negative aspiration, inject 10 to 15 ml of local anesthetic.

C. The 3-in-1 block with the femoral nerve approach can be used to provide blockade of the femoral, lateral femoral cutaneous, and obturator nerves with a single injection.

D. Complications are nearly identical to those of the femoral nerve block (p 274). Hematoma, dysesthesias, and intravascular injection are possible.

References

Bonica JJ. The management of pain. Vol II. 2nd ed. Philadelphia: Lea & Febiger, 1990.

Cousins MJ, Bridenbaugh PO. Neural blockade in clinical anesthesia and management of pain. 2nd ed. Philadelphia: JB Lippincott, 1988.

Pansky B. Review of gross anatomy. 6th ed. New York: Macmillan, 1989.

Winnie AP, Ramamurthy S, Durrani Z. The inguinal paravascular technique of lumbar plexus anesthesia: The "3-in-1 block." Anesth Analg 1973; 52:989.

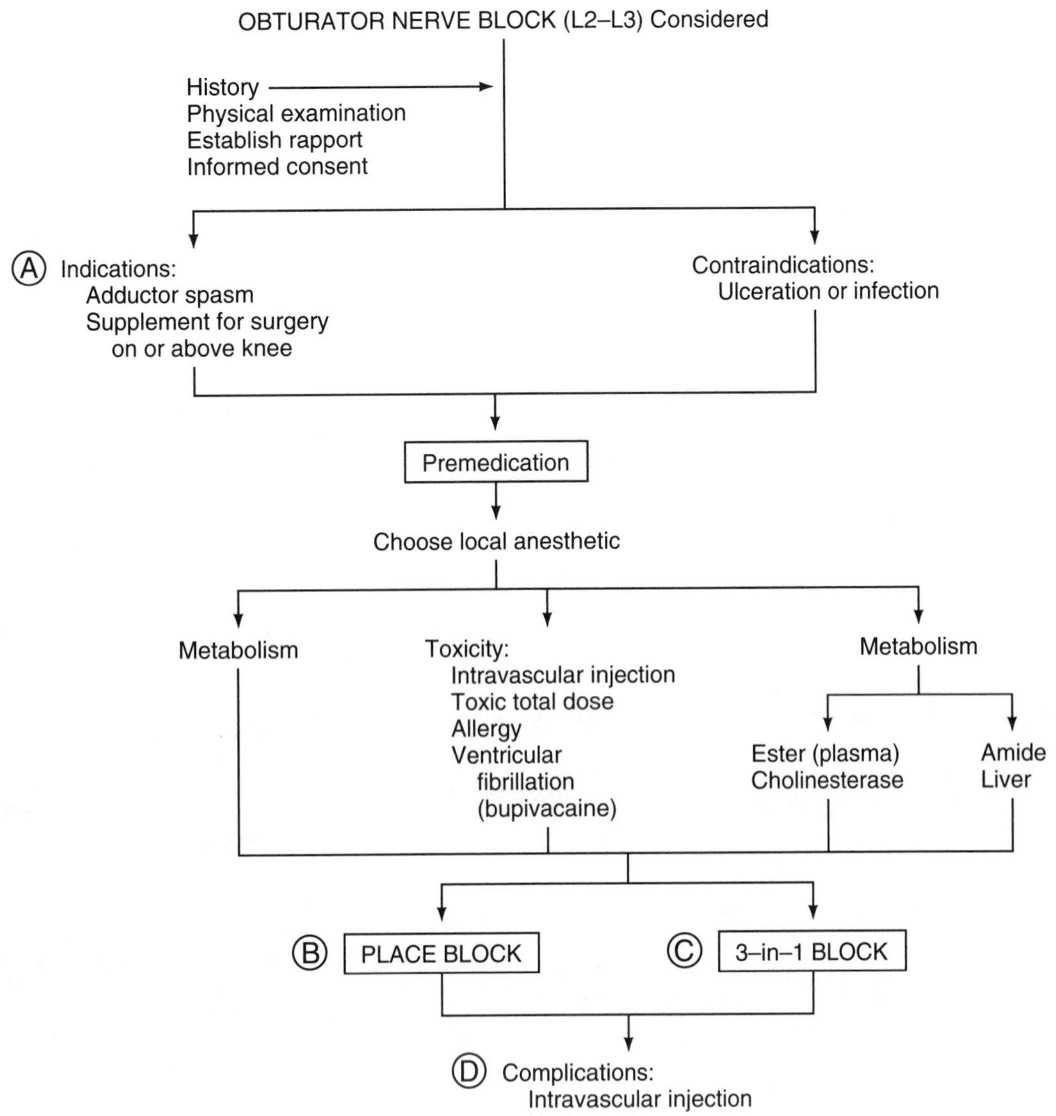
OBTURATOR NERVE BLOCK (L2–L3) Considered
History
Physical examination
Establish rapport
Informed consent
(A) Indications:
Adductor spasm
Supplement for surgery
on or above knee
Contraindications:
Ulceration or infection
Premedication
Choose local anesthetic
Metabolism
Toxicity:
Intravascular injection
Toxic total dose
Allergy
Ventricular
fibrillation
(bupivacaine)
Metabolism
Ester (plasma)
Cholinesterase
Amide
Liver
(B) PLACE BLOCK
(C) 3–in–1 BLOCK
(D) Complications:
Intravascular injection
Hematoma

TIBIAL NERVE BLOCK

Alfonso Maytorena, M.D.

The tibial nerve is the largest of the two branches of the sciatic nerve and lies medial to the common peroneal nerve. It arises at the most cephalad aspect of the popliteal fossa and provides both a muscular branch to the back of the leg and cutaneous branches to the back of the leg, knee joint, and popliteal fossa. It innervates the gastrocnemius, soleus, semimembranosus, semitendinosus, and popliteus muscles and the long head of the biceps muscles. It provides some sensation to the knee joint itself. The tibial nerve can be blocked either at its origin in the popliteal fossa or at the ankle as it lies behind the posterior tibial artery. The popliteal fossa is filled with fat, which means that the local anesthetic must be deposited as close as possible to the nerve. This can be achieved by use of a nerve stimulator (p 50).

A. Before performing a tibial nerve block, complete a careful history and physical examination. Perform a complete neurologic examination to document any preexisting neurologic deficits. After informed consent has been obtained, the patient may receive a premedication to relieve anxiety and aid in making the block more comfortable.

B. The indications for tibial nerve block include surgery in the lower leg and foot, the need for pain relief postoperatively, or chronic pain conditions (such as reflex sympathetic dystrophy) involving the foot. A tibial nerve block may also be useful in supplementing an incomplete epidural or sciatic nerve block.

C. Contraindications to a tibial nerve block include patient refusal, documented allergy to amide local anesthetics, and infection involving the popliteal fossa. Patients with bleeding and clotting abnormalities probably should not receive a nerve block.

D. The patient is usually placed either prone or in the lateral decubitus position with the knee extended. The landmarks to be identified include the medial and lateral epicondyles of the femur, the medial and lateral heads of the gastrocnemius muscle, and the lateral long head of the biceps femoris and the superimposed tendons of the semimembranosus and semitendinosus muscle medially. Make the injection above the midpoint of a line drawn connecting the femoral epicondyles above the knee joint. Advance the needle approximately 1.5 to 3.0 cm vertically to the skin until a paresthesia is elicited in the distal leg or sole of the foot. A nerve stimulator should elicit visible plantar flexion of the foot. The popliteal artery lies deep to the nerve and can serve as an additional landmark. Inject 5 to 10 ml of a local anesthetic solution close to the nerve; this should be adequate to block the tibial nerve.

E. Tibial nerve blocks have proved both effective and safe. Complications include intravascular injection and hematoma.

References

Bonica JJ, Buckley FP. Regional anesthesia with local anesthetics. In: Bonica JJ, ed. The management of pain. Vol II. 2nd ed. Philadelphia: Lea & Febiger, 1990:1883.

Bridenbaugh PO. The lower extremity: Somatic blockade. In: Cousins MJ, Bridenbaugh PO, eds. Neural blockade in clinical anesthesia and management of pain. 2nd ed. Philadelphia: JB Lippincott, 1988.

Kofoed H. Peripheral nerve blocks at the knee and ankle in operations for common foot disorders. Clin Orthop 1982; 168:97.

Panksy B. Review of gross anatomy. 6th ed. New York: Macmillan, 1989.

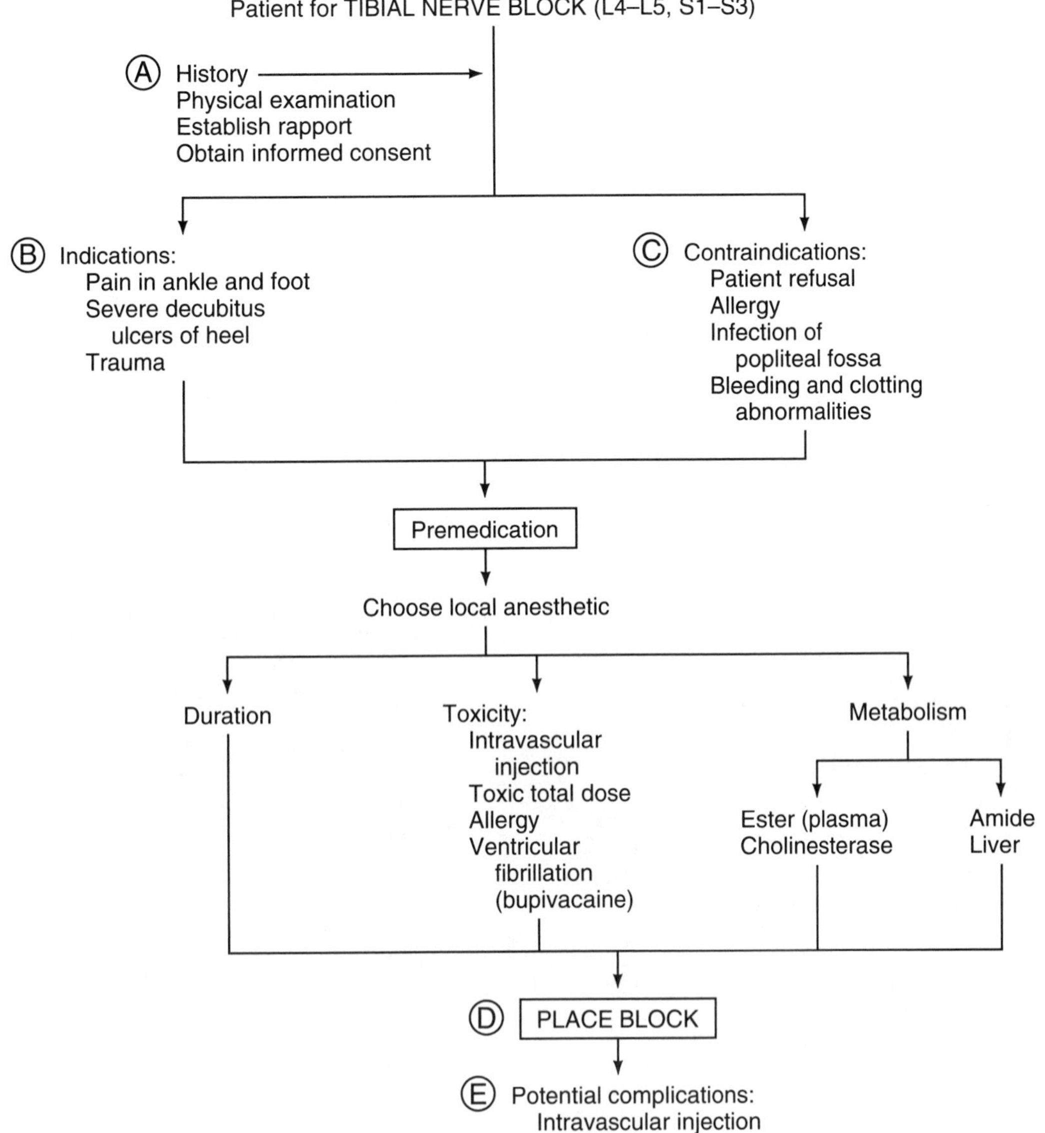
Patient for TIBIAL NERVE BLOCK (L4–L5, S1–S3)
Ⓐ History
Physical examination
Establish rapport
Obtain informed consent
Ⓑ Indications:
Pain in ankle and foot
Severe decubitus ulcers of heel
Trauma
Ⓒ Contraindications:
Patient refusal
Allergy
Infection of popliteal fossa
Bleeding and clotting abnormalities
Premedication
Choose local anesthetic
Duration
Toxicity:
Intravascular injection
Toxic total dose
Allergy
Ventricular fibrillation (bupivacaine)
Metabolism
Ester (plasma) Cholinesterase
Amide Liver
Ⓓ PLACE BLOCK
Ⓔ Potential complications:
Intravascular injection
Hematoma

WRIST BLOCK

Douglas E. Chapman, M.D.

A wrist block consists of individual blockade of the median, ulnar, and cutaneous branches of the radial nerves at the level of the metacarpal bones. These blocks are quick, technically easy, relatively safe, and tolerated well without patient sedation.

A. The primary indications for wrist block are intraoperative anesthesia and postoperative analgesia. The block is useful for minor procedures such as closed reduction of hand fractures and dislocations and for excision of lesions in the area of innervation. Wrist blocks are used as supplements to incomplete brachial plexus blocks. This is commonly seen when an interscalene block provides inadequate anesthesia in the ulnar nerve distribution. Blocking the median, ulnar, and radial nerves at the wrist rather than the elbow is easier and more reliable and precludes occasional ulnar neuritis caused by injection into a constricted compartment at the elbow. The incomplete hand anesthesia that results, and a lack of anesthesia under a tourniquet site, limit the use of wrist block in surgery.

B. Contraindications include cellulitis, osteomyelitis, bleeding diathesis, and patient refusal. Relative contraindications are preexisting neural deficit and probable high blood levels of local anesthetic from previous injections (inadequate brachial plexus block). Use of wrist block in chronic pain syndromes is limited, since most syndromes involve more than just the hand. Injections into painful sites are poorly tolerated and there are other simple ways to provide sympathectomy.

C. At the wrist the radial nerve is very superficial and provides only sensory innervation to the skin. Radial nerve innervation of the bone, joints, and muscles in the hand is provided by the superior interosseus nerve, which branches from the radial nerve near the elbow. The radial nerve lies lateral to the tendon of the brachioradialis and terminates at the level of the carpal bones in multiple inconsistent branches.

D. The patient should be supine with arm abducted. The point of entry is just lateral to the radial artery at the level of the ulnar styloid process (the proximal skin crease of the wrist). Advance a 25-gauge needle subcutaneously across the dorsal surface of the wrist toward the styloid process of the ulna. Deposit a ring of local anesthetic from the radial artery to the extensor carpi radialis tendon. Use 5 ml of 1% lidocaine or the equivalent.

E. The median nerve becomes superficial just before reaching the wrist. At the proximal skin crease it is located between the tendons of the palmaris longus and the flexor carpi radialis. It lies deep to the flexor retinaculum, but seldom deeper than 1.0 cm below the skin surface. At the level of the wrist the median nerve innervates both deep and superficial tissues in the hand.

F. The patient should be supine with arm abducted and supinated. The point of entry is at the proximal skin crease of the wrist between the tendons of the palmaris longus tendon and the flexor carpi radialis. If the palmaris longus tendon is absent, enter 1 cm ulnar to the flexor carpi radialis. Needle advancement should be 0.5 to 1.0 cm deep and perpendicular to the skin. Paresthesia may occur but need not be sought; an excellent block will result without it. A "fan" distribution of anesthetic in a cross-sectional plane will help ensure a good outcome. Subcutaneous deposition of 1 ml of local anesthetic on needle removal will block the palmar cutaneous branch. Infuse 3 to 5 ml of 1% lidocaine or the equivalent through a 25-gauge needle.

G. At the wrist the ulnar nerve lies just dorsal and radial to the flexor carpi ulnaris tendon. It is ulnar to the ulnar artery and deep to the flexor retinaculum. It innervates both deep and superficial tissues in the hand.

H. The patient should be supine with arm abducted and supinated. The point of entry is at the proximal skin crease of the wrist just radial to the flexor carpi ulnaris. Aspirate while advancing a 25-gauge needle vertically (in a dorsal direction) 1 to 2 cm deep. Paresthesia is not required. If none are elicited, proceed until the periosteum is reached. Inject 5 ml of 1% lidocaine or the equivalent while withdrawing the needle. Dorsal cutaneous branch can be blocked with subcutaneous infiltration across the ulnar half of the dorsum of the wrist.

I. Systemic toxicity of local anesthetics can result from unintended intravascular injection and additive systemic absorption from previously placed brachial plexus or elbow blocks. Bleeding and hematoma formation are unlikely and usually of little consequence. Other complications include infection of the skin or bone, failure to block the nerve, an allergic reaction to the anesthetic, and neuritis after the injection. Use of a 25-gauge needle may reduce the incidence of neuritis. Separating the needle from the syringe by flexible tubing can help provide better needle control and better fixation if paresthesias occur.

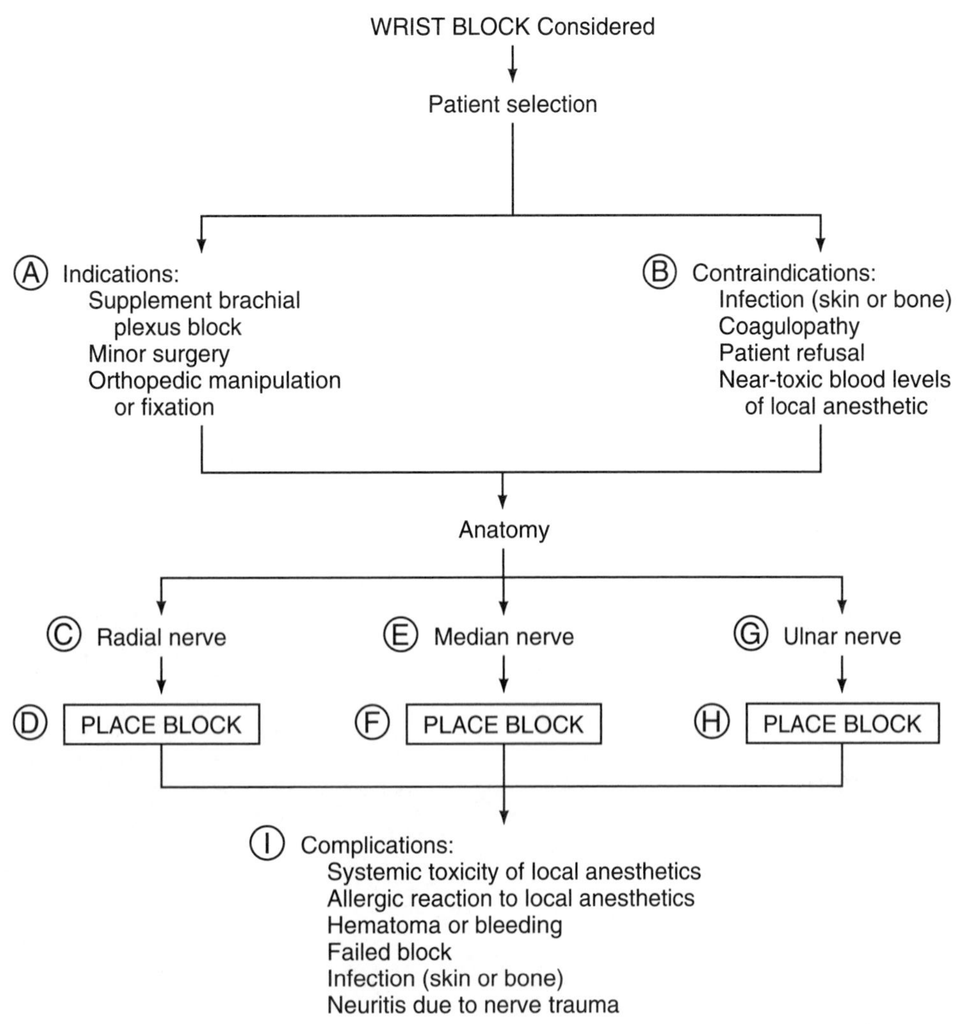

References

Adriani J. Labat's regional anesthesia: Techniques and clinical applications. St Louis: Warren H. Green, 1985:289.

Bridenbaugh L. The upper extremity: Somatic blockade. In: Cousins M, Bridenbaugh PO, eds. Neural blockade in clinical anesthesia and management of pain. 2nd ed. Philadelphia: JB Lippincott, 1988:406.

Covic D. Block of the peripheral nerves in the area of the wrist. In: Hoerster W, ed. Regional anesthesia. 2nd ed. St Louis: CV Mosby, 1990:94.

Scott D. Nerve blocks at the wrist. In: Techniques of regional anesthesia. Norwalk: Appleton & Lange, 1989:112.

ANKLE BLOCK

Douglas E. Chapman, M.D.

Ankle block consists of individual blockade of the tibial, deep peroneal, sural, saphenous, and superficial peroneal nerves near the level of the malleoli. These blocks are quick, technically easy, relatively safe, and well tolerated without patient sedation.

A. The primary indications for ankle block are intraoperative anesthesia and postoperative analgesia. The block is useful for a variety of surgical procedures and lends itself to day surgery patients. It is indicated for foot surgery when attempted central neural blockade is inadequate or when central blockade is contraindicated. Blockade of the tibial and deep peroneal nerves provides complete anesthesia to the bones, tendons, and joints of the foot. All five nerves carry innervation to the skin, but only these two supply the deeper structures. Blockade of both nerves is required for most surgical procedures.

B. Contraindications include cellulitis, osteomyelitis, bleeding diathesis, and patient refusal. Relative contraindications are preexisting neural deficit and probable high blood levels of local anesthetic (LA) from previous injections (inadequate epidural block). The use of ankle block in chronic pain syndromes is limited, since most such syndromes involve more than just the foot. Injections into painful sites are poorly tolerated and there are other simple ways to provide sympathectomy.

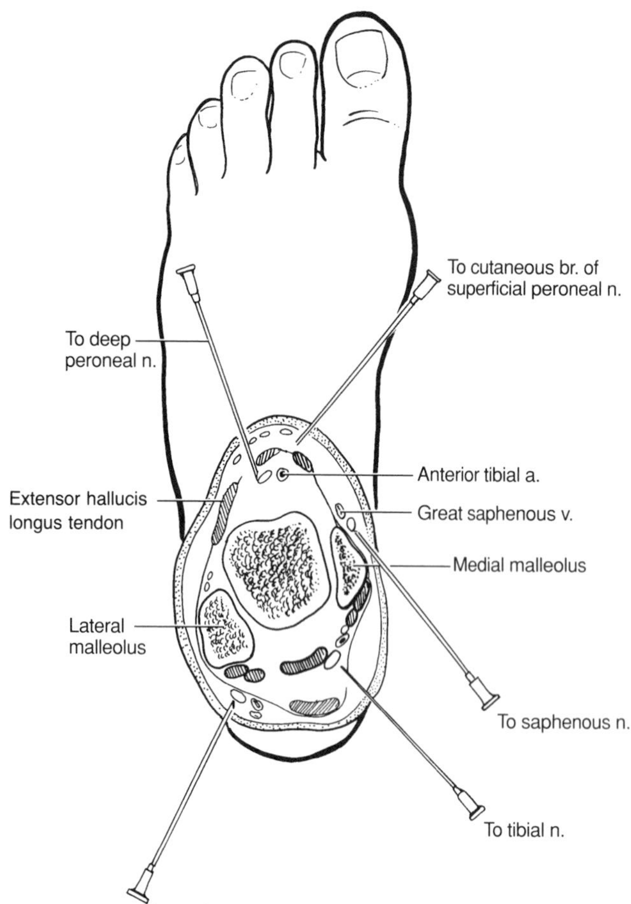

Figure 1 Placement of ankle block.

C. The deep peroneal nerve reaches the ankle beside the anterior tibial artery. As it emerges from under the extensor retinaculum, it lies just lateral to the dorsalis pedis artery. The nerve primarily innervates deep structures. A small area of skin at the dorsal surface of the great toe and second toe is supplied by the nerve.

D. Place the patient supine with hip and knee flexed and the foot flat on the table. Palpate the dorsalis pedis artery lateral to the extensor hallucis longus and anterior tibial muscles at a level just superior to the malleolus. Advance a 25-gauge needle perpendicular to the skin just lateral to the artery down to the tibial periosteum. Infuse 3 to 5 ml of 1 to 2% lidocaine or equivalent within 1 cm of the bone. If the anatomy is easily identified, the LA can be infused just lateral or deep to the artery. Use of epinephrine can safely prolong the block.

E. The tibial nerve lies beside the tibial artery just posterior to the medial malleolus between the Achilles and flexor digitorum longus tendons. It supplies deep structures as well as cutaneous innervation to most of the heel and the extensor surface of the foot and toes.

F. Place the patient supine with the thigh externally rotated, or prone with a pillow under the ankle. The point of insertion is just posterior to the posterior tibial artery above the level of the medial malleolus. Advance a 25-gauge needle to the periosteum while aspirating. Infuse 3 to 5 ml of 1 to 2% lidocaine or equivalent within 1 cm of the bone. If unable to palpate the artery, enter just above the medial malleolus at the medial margin of the Achilles tendon. Epinephrine can safely prolong the block.

G. The saphenous, sural, and superficial peroneal nerves are subcutaneous at the level of the malleolus. Branching is abundant and inconsistent and there may be overlap in innervation. These nerves innervate only cutaneous structures. Branches of the sural nerve lie between the Achilles tendon and lateral malleolus; they innervate the heel and lateral surface of the foot to the small toe. The saphenous nerve becomes subcutaneous at the knee, lying next to the saphenous vein between the medial malleolus and the anterior edge of the tibia. It supplies the skin over the medial malleolus but sometimes extends its coverage to the midfoot. The superficial peroneal nerve becomes subcutaneous at the distal third of the fibula. It has multiple branches between the tibia anteriorly and the

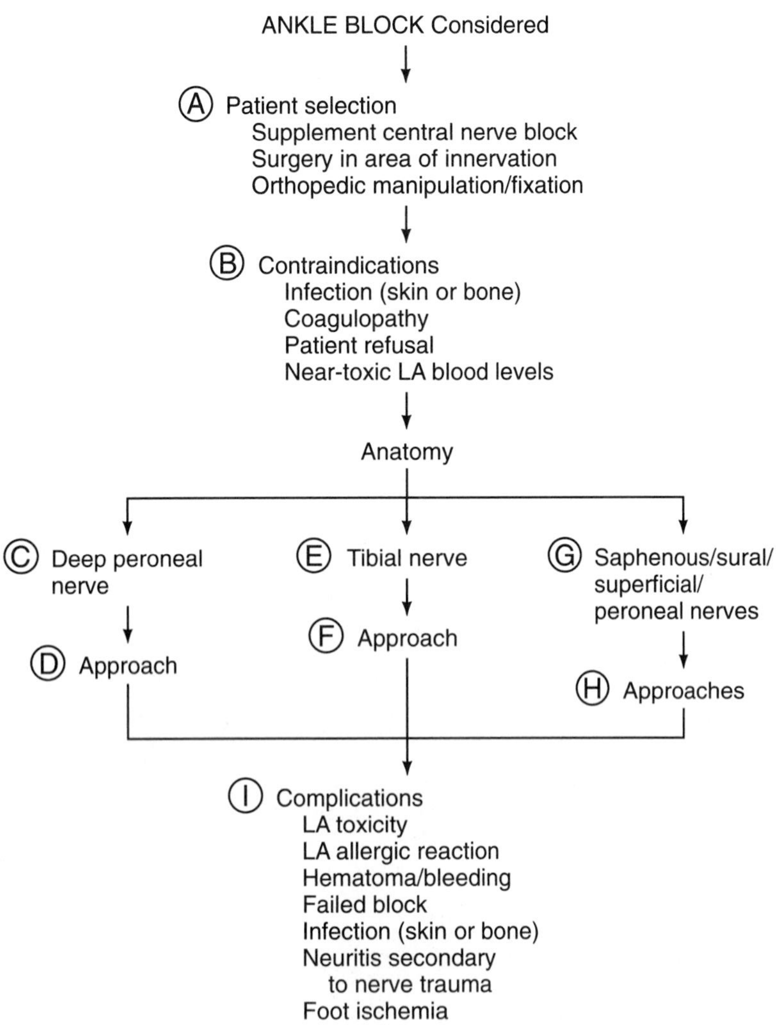

lateral malleolus, and innervates most of the skin on the dorsal surface of the foot and toes.

H. These nerves can be blocked with a subcutaneous infiltration in a ring fashion around the ankle at any level from the malleoli to 5 cm more proximal. Although individual nerves can be blocked using 5 ml of local anesthetic for subcutaneous infiltration in the distributions mentioned above, all three nerves can be safely and reliably blocked with a complete ring of LA anesthetic using 15 to 20 ml of solution. Failed blocks can occur with individual nerve blocks because of overlap in areas of innervation. A 25-gauge long needle is recommended. Epinephrine can safely prolong the block.

I. No major complications of ankle block have been reported. Systemic LA toxicity can result from unintended intravascular injection and additive systemic absorption from previously placed central neural blocks. Bleeding and hematoma formation are unlikely and usually of little consequence. Other complications include infection of the skin or bone, failure to block any of the intended nerves, an allergic reaction to the anesthetic, and neuritis after the injection. Use of a 25-gauge needle may reduce the incidence of neuritis. Ischemia of the foot due to vascular occlusion associated with a complete ring block around the ankle has not been reported and is highly unlikely. Separating the needle from the syringe by flexible tubing can help provide better needle control and better fixation if paresthesias occur.

References

Adriani J. Labat's regional anesthesia: Techniques and clinical applications. 4th ed. St Louis: Green, 1985:380.

Bridenbaugh P. Nerve blocks at the ankle. In: Cousins MJ, Bridenbaugh PO, eds. Neural blockade in clinical anesthesia and management of pain. 2nd ed. Philadelphia: JB Lippincott, 1988:434.

Hoerster W. Blocks in the area of the ankle (foot block). In: Hoerster W, ed. Regional anesthesia. 2nd ed. St. Louis: CV Mosby, 1990:133.

Scott DB. Nerve block at the ankle. In: Techniques of regional anesthesia. East Norwalk: Appleton & Lange, 1989:134.

APPENDICES

APPENDIX 1: DEFINITIONS OF COMMON PAIN TERMS

Allodynia Pain resulting from a stimulus that otherwise would not cause pain.

Analgesia Absence of pain despite stimulation that otherwise would be painful.

Dysesthesia An abnormal, unpleasant, either spontaneous or evoked sensation such as hyperalgesia or allodynia.

Hyperalgesia An increased response to a normally painful stimulus.

Hyperesthesia An increased sensitivity to stimulation. It can include touch or thermal sensation and may or may not include pain.

Hyperpathia An increased painful reaction to a stimulus, especially repetitive with increased threshold. Pain is often explosive in nature.

Hypoalgesia Diminished pain in response to a painful stimulus.

Hypoesthesia Decreased sensitivity to stimulation.

Paresthesia An abnormal spontaneous or evoked sensation, normally not unpleasant.

APPENDIX 2: OPIOIDS

	Route	*Equivalent Dose (mg)*	*Duration (hour)*	*T 1/2 (hour)*	*Usual Dose (mg)*	*Cancer Dose (mg)*
Weak Opioids						
Codeine	PO	30–200	3–4	3	30–40	32–128
Propoxyphene	PO	32–65	4–6	3.5	65	50–100
Potent Opioids						
Meperidine	IM	75–100	2–3	3.5	80	50–200
	PO	200–300			300	75–400+
Morphine	IM	10–15	3–5	2–3	10	5–35
	PO	30–60			30–60	10–200
Methadone	IM	8–10	4–8	15–30	10	5–35
	PO	10			20	10–200
Levorphanol	IM	2	5–8	12–16	2	1–6
	PO	4			4	2–12+
Oxymorphone	IM	1–1.5	3–5	2–3	1	
	PR				6	6–36+
Hydromorphone	IM	1–2	4–6	2–3	1–1.5	
	PO	2–4			2–4	6–12+
Oxycodone	PO	15	4–6	NK	30	30–120+
Mixed agonist/ antagonist						
Buprenorphine	IM	0.3–0.6	6–9	NK	0.3	0.2–1
	SL	0.4–0.8			0.4	0.2–1
Pentazocine	IM	40–60	3–4	2–3	60	40–300
	PO	50–200			180	120–400
Butorphanol	IM	2	4	3–4	1.5–2.5	1–6
Nalbuphine	IM	10–20	4–6	5	10	10–35

IM = Intramuscular; PO = oral; SL = sublingual; NK = not known; NA = not applicable.

APPENDIX 3: OPIOID SIDE EFFECTS AND TREATMENT

Nausea and vomiting	Phenothiazines, butyrophenones (chlorpromazine, 0.15–0.5 mg/kg PO q6h; perphenazine, 0.05–0.1 mg/kg IV or PO q6h; treat dystonic reactions with antihistamines)
Constipation	Stool softeners, cathartics
Pruritus	Antihistamines (diphenhydramine, 0.5–1 mg/kg IV or PO q6h)
Sleep disturbance (persisting despite adequate analgesia)	Low-dose tricyclics (imipramine, 0.2–0.4 mg/kg PO 1 hr before bedtime; may increase by 50% every 2–3 days up to 1–3 mg/kg)
Somnolence	Reduce opioid doses; consider regional techniques; psychostimulants (dextroamphetamine or methylphenidate, 0.1–0.2 mg/kg up to 0.3–0.5 mg/kg AM and noon; for children >age 6 yr, 5 mg at 8 AM and noon)
Respiratory depression: Mild	Apply oxygen; reduce opioid dose; stimulate; provide careful observation
Respiratory depression: Severe	Support ventilation; naloxone, 10 μg/kg—titrate slowly to effect

APPENDIX 4: ANTIDEPRESSANTS

(mg)		a	b	c	d	e	f	g	h	i	j	k	l	m
	Tricyclic													
25–100	Amitriptyline	+	++	++	+	+	+	++		−		4	3	4
50–100	Imipramine	++						+	+−		+	3	3	3
50–100	Trimipramine											3	3	4
25–100	Doxepin		+		++					+		3	3	4
25–50	Clomipramine	+							+			2	2	4
50–75	Desipramine											1	1	1
10–30	Protriptyline											1	1	3
25–100	Nortriptyline											2	1	3
1–200	Amoxapine											1	1	2
	Atypical													
50–200	Trazodone											0.5	2	3
20	Fluoxetine											1	1	0
1–200	Bupropion											1	1	0
50–100	Maprotiline											2	1	3
	MAOIs													
15–45	Phenelzine		+			+						1	3	0
10–40	Isocarboxazid											1	2	0
10–20	Tranylcypromine											1	2	0

+ = Study supporting use; − = study not supporting use; side effects graded scale: 0 = none to 4 = maximum.

a = arthritis
b = migraine headache
c = tension headache
d = psychogenic headache
e = facial pain
f = postherpetic pain
g = diabetic neuropathy
h = back pain
i = pain of mixed cause
j = neoplastic pain
k = anticholinergic side effects
l = orthostatic hypotension
m = sedation

APPENDIX 5: NONSTEROIDAL ANTI-INFLAMMATORY DRUGS

Kevin L. Kenworthy, M.D.

Class/Drug	*Usual Dose (mg PO)*	*Peak Effect (h)*	*Plasma T1/2 (h)*	*Analgesic Effect*	*Anti-Inflammatory Effect*	*Anti-Pyretic Effect*	*Anti-Platelet Effect*	*Comments*
Nonacidic NSAIDs								
Para-aminophenol								
Acetaminophen	325–1000 mg q4–8h	0.5–1h	1–4h	Yes +++	None 0	Yes +++	None 0	Minimal GI, renal side effects. Extensive hepatic metabolism. OD can cause hepatic damage with increased liver function tests.
Acidic NSAIDs								
Salicylates								
Acetylsalicylic acid (aspirin)	325–1000 mg q4–6h; "ceiling dose" 1300 mg/dose	2h	0.25h	Yes +++	Yes +++	Yes +++	Yes +++	Prodrug hydrolyzed by plasma esterase to salicylate, active for m. Irreversible platelet inhibition, must discontinue 7–14 days prior to surgery. Tinnitus, decreased hearing, dyspepsia, nausea/vomiting are signs of toxicity.
Choline magnesium trisalicylate (Trilisate)	870–1740 mg q3–4h	0.5–1h	9–17h	Yes +++	Yes +++	Yes +++	Min +/−	Advantage = minimal antiplatelet effect. Fewer side effects.
Salicylsalicylic acid (Salsalate) (Disalcid)	500–750 mg q12h			Yes +++	Yes +++	Yes +++	Yes +	Minimal GI & antiplatelet activity.
Diflunisal (Dolobid)	200–500 mg q12h	1–2h	8–20h	Yes +++	Yes ++	Yes +	Yes +	
Indoleacetic acids								
Indomethacin (Indocin)	25–75 mg q6h	2h	2–3h	Yes +++	Yes +++	Yes +++	Yes +++	Contraindicated in patients with psychiatric disorders, epilepsy, parkinsonism, and renal disease. Headache, confusion, dizziness, seizures, nausea/vomiting, syncope, signs of toxicity.
Sulindac (Clinoril)	150–200 mg q12h	1–2h	7–18h	Yes +++	Yes +++	Yes +++	Yes +++	Prodrug metabolized to active form by liver. Minimal renal side effects. Use for patient with renal disease.
Phenylacetic acid								
Diclofenac (Voltaren)	50–75 mg q12h	1.5–3h	2h	Yes +++	Yes +++	Yes ++	Yes ++	Risk of hepatotoxicity. Should check baseline and q8 weeks transaminases.
Pyrroleacetic acid								
Tolmetin	200–400 mg q6–8h	0.5–1h	1–3h	Yes ++	Yes +++	Yes ++	Yes ++	Frequent GI side effects. Increased risk of hepatotoxicity. Watch transaminase levels.

0 = no effect, +/− = minimal to none, + = minimal, ++ = moderate, +++ = severe, ++++ = maximal effects.

Continued.

Class/Drug	Usual Dose (mg PO)	Peak Effect (h)	Plasma T1/2 (h)	Analgesic Effect	Anti-Inflammatory Effect	Anti-Pyretic Effect	Anti-Platelet Effect	Comments
Pyrazole								
Phenylbutazone	100–200 mg q6h	2h	60–100h	Yes ++	Yes ++++	Yes ++	Yes +++	Very limited use in U.S. owing to toxicity, especially blood dyscrasias.
Fenamates								
Mefenamic acid (Ponstel)	500 mg q6–8h	2h	3–4h	Yes ++	Yes ++	Yes +	Yes ++	Not recommended for use beyond 1 week because of toxicity. Hemolytic anemia.
Propionic acid								
Ibuprofen (Motrin)	200–800 mg q6–8h	1–2h	2h	Yes +++	Yes +++	Yes ++	Yes +++	Monitor for hepatic toxicity with prolonged high dose. Over-the-counter so easy to obtain.
Naproxen (Naprosyn) (Anaprox)	250–500 mg q12h	2h	12–15h	Yes +++	Yes +++	Yes ++	Yes +++	GI side effects are common. Caution in patient with renal disease.
Fenoprofen (Nalfon)	300–600 mg q6–8h	2h	2–3h	Yes ++	Yes +++	Yes +	Yes +++	Monitor for renal toxicity (BUN, creatinine q month)
Ketoprofen (Orudis)	50–100 mg q6–8h	1–2h	1–35h	Yes ++	Yes +++	Yes +	Yes +++	High incidence of GI side effects.
Benzothazine (Oxicam)								
Piroxicam (Feldene)	20 mg q12–24h	2–4h	30–45h	Yes +++	Yes +++	Yes +	Yes +++	Longest T1/2. Good for noncompliant patient.

0 = no effect, +/− = minimal to none, + = minimal, ++ = moderate, +++ = severe, ++++ = maximal effects.

INDEX

C

D

E

F

G

H

I

J

K

L

O

P

Q

R

S

U

V

W